CHILD AND ADOLESCENT NEUROLOGY FOR PSYCHIATRISTS

CHILD AND ADOLESCENT NEUROLOGY FOR PSYCHIATRISTS

Edited by

DAVID MYLAND KAUFMAN, MD
Associate Professor of Neurology
Associate Professor of Psychiatry
Albert Einstein College of Medicine
Montefiore Medical Center
Bronx, New York

GAIL E. SOLOMON, MD
Associate Professor of Clinical Neurology in Pediatrics and Psychiatry
The New York Hospital-Cornell Medical Center
New York, New York

CYNTHIA R. PFEFFER, MD
Professor of Psychiatry
The New York Hospital-Cornell Medical Center
New York, New York

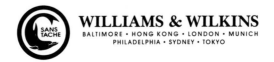

WILLIAMS & WILKINS
BALTIMORE · HONG KONG · LONDON · MUNICH
PHILADELPHIA · SYDNEY · TOKYO

Editor: Michael G. Fisher
Managing Editor: Carol Eckhart
Copy Editor: Dana Knighten
Designer: Karen Klinedinst
Illustration Planner: Ray Lowman
Production Coordinator: Barbara J. Felton
Cover Designer: Wilma E. Rosenberger

Printed in the United States of America

Library of Congress Cataloging-in-Publication Data

Child and adolescent neurology for psychiatrists / edited by David M.
   Kaufman, Gail E. Solomon, Cynthia R. Pfeffer.
       p.   cm.
   Includes bibliographical references and index.
   ISBN 0-683-04546-6
   1. Child psychiatry.   2. Pediatric neurology.   3. Developmental
neurology.   4. Nervous system—Diseases.   I. Kaufman, David Myland.
II. Solomon, Gail E., 1938–   . III. Pfeffer, Cynthia R.
   [DNLM: 1. Nervous System Diseases–diagnosis.   2. Nervous System
Diseases—in adolescence.   3. Nervous System Diseases–in infancy &
childhood.   4. Nervous System Diseases—physiopathology.   WS 340
C5354]
   RJ499.C48225   1992
618.92′8—dc20
DNLM/DLC
for Library of Congress   91-22858
                                                                    CIP

                                            92   93   94   95   96
                           2   3   4   5   6   7   8   9   10

FOREWORD

Unlike general psychiatry, which has strong historical links to clinical neurology, child psychiatry has never been clearly allied to the neurological sciences. Even Freud practiced neurology for a time, just as did many other "neuropsychiatrists" before World War I. In contrast, child psychiatry in America evolved largely from the Child Guidance movement, which itself was less interested in mental *illness* than it was in helping parents provide an optimal environment for the social and emotional development of their children. Today, however, child psychiatry appears to be moving in the direction of developing a better neurobiological understanding of mental illness in children and adolescents, while hopefully maintaining a strong affiliation with psychological, social, and humanitarian interests.

Has the time come, therefore, for a neurological textbook for the child psychiatrist? I believe it has.

Depending on one's type of practice, the need for neurological expertise may be more or less obvious. For child psychiatrists who work in consultation-liaison, such knowledge is especially important. I asked a colleague of mine who works in this field whether she could use such a text. She said, "I am asked to see cases with both neurological and psychiatric complications all the time. I get questions like, 'How much of this child's psychological problems are a result of the neurological complications of his radiation treatment?' or, 'Are his symptoms a result of his anticonvulsive medication?' " She added, "All too often I find that the children are in danger of falling between the disciplines. Ideally the neurologists should know enough psychiatry and the child psychiatrists enough neurology that they can have a reasonable dialogue with each other. Only in that way can you be sure that the child's illness will be comprehensively understood and effectively treated."

Of course, many child psychiatrists do not work extensively in the field of consultation-liaison, although more of us probably should. Nor do many child psychiatrists have practices that include autistic or mentally retarded children, two more groups for whom knowledge of clinical neurology is important. But child psychiatrists do see children with headaches or seizures, or who may need various brain imaging studies as part of their work-up. Each of these calls for an understanding of neurology by the child and adolescent psychiatrist.

But don't child psychiatrists learn neurology during their general residency? They do—to a point. After you have read this book, you may come to realize, as I did, that the symptoms of neurological disorders are different enough in children as compared with adults that child psychiatrists need a more specialized neurological database than one learns in the general residency. This applies even more so to child psychiatrists who are long beyond their initial training. After three years of training in general psychiatry, two years training in child and adolescent psychiatry, and additional years of practice, a little academic refreshment on the subject of neurology may not be a bad idea.

This is an excellent textbook. It is highly informative, concise, and readable. What's more, there is much in it that is immediately relevant to the practice of child and adolescent psychiatry.

My favorite chapters are those on epilepsy, neurological imaging, headaches, and neurology for psychiatrists who see patients in the emergency room. There are dozens of useful clinical suggestions or clinical facts in these and other chapters in the book. I learned that children with temporal lobe epilepsy may be better at drawing a picture of their aura than in describing it. Petit-mal attacks may be brought on by stress or exercise. Two percent of normal children may have spikes or sharp waves in their EEG without having epilepsy. T2-weighted MRI images are more sensitive in detecting psychopathology than are T1-weighted images. Migraine headaches can occur at any age, even early in childhood. Barbiturates and opiates lead to constriction of the pupils, while amphetamine, cocaine, and PCP cause pupillary dilation. These are, of course, examples of individual bits of knowledge. In-depth coverage of many major topics are presented, including chapters on sleep disorders, psychiatric symptoms in progressive neurological disorders, HIV in children, neuromuscular disorders in children, and Tourette's disorder.

I found the chapter on brain tumors in children to be both enlightening as well as cautionary. True, brain tumors are rare in children, but the sobering litany of missed diagnoses, fruitless therapies, and adverse outcomes illustrated in the case examples are more than enough to evoke "there but for the grace of God go I" anxiety in any child psychiatrist.

If the trend in the field of child and adolescent psychiatry continues, future child psychiatrists may function more and more as specialized consultants to other professionals. As such, the child and adolescent psychiatrist must be expert in evaluating, diagnosing, and treating a wide spectrum of behavioral disorders in children and adolescents. Having a good working knowledge of clinical neurology may be one of the attributes that defines such expertise. Training directors should welcome this text as a training resource, and practicing child psychiatrists should find it a first-rate reference text.

Peter E. Tanguay, MD
Professor of Child and Adolescent Psychiatry
UCLA Neuropsychiatric Institute
Los Angeles, California

PREFACE

The field of child and adolescent psychiatry has been advancing rapidly in the last two decades, especially in classification of psychiatric diagnoses, epidemiology of psychopathology, diagnostic assessment of psychiatric disorders, longitudinal course of symptoms and behavior, and treatment. The introduction of the DSM-III and the DSM-III-R defined standard diagnostic criteria specifically designated for children and adolescents, as well as the use of a multiaxial approach to indicate psychopathology related to primary psychiatric disorders on Axis I, developmental and/or personality disorders on Axis II, medical disorders that affect or interact with psychiatric disorders indicated on Axis III, degree of psychosocial stress indicated on Axis IV, and level of social functioning indicated on Axis V. This multiaxial system requires an appreciation of neurological factors affecting childhood and adolescent psychopathology.

Along with these advances in child and adolescent psychiatry, interest has been renewed in the neurological underpinnings of psychological and behavioral functioning. In fact, the decade of the 1990s has been termed "The Decade of the Brain" by the National Institute of Mental Health (NIMH) to highlight the intensive research and clinical efforts in the interface of neuroscience, neuropsychology, neurobiology, and psychiatry. Furthermore, a number of consensus conferences and reports sponsored by the Institute of Medicine, American Academy of Child and Adolescent Psychiatry and NIMH have strongly recommended research and effective clinical care for children and adolescents who exhibit or are vulnerable to psychopathology.

We offer this book, expressly written for psychiatrists, as an overview of important neurological disorders that occur in children and adolescents. Some of these disorders have traditionally been considered psychiatric problems, but new research has revealed their neurological aspects. Other disorders, primarily neurologically based, have demonstrated consequences for psychological adjustment. This book describes these pediatric disorders and provides information not only about their clinical presentations, course, and treatment but also about recognizing them and referring patients for a neurological evaluation. In the spirit of "The Decade of the Brain," we believe that clinical collaboration between psychiatrists and neurologists, as well as among other professionals who work with children and adolescents, is a key ingredient for promoting quality clinical care for children and adolescents and for preventing untoward sequelae of neurological and/or psychiatric disorders. We believe that the contents of this book will leave the reader prepared for the Decade.

We offer this book as a source for the psychiatrist who must identify some difficult clinical problems and manage them. With the knowledge gained from using this book, the psychiatrist can better communicate his/her findings and work with the neurologist in provding care for children and adolescents.

David M. Kaufman, MD
Gail E. Solomon, MD
Cynthia R. Pfeffer, MD

CONTRIBUTORS

JACQUELINE A. BELLO, MD
Associate Professor of Radiology
Director of Neuroradiology
Albert Einstein College of Medicine
Montefiore Medical Center
Bronx, New York

ANITA L. BELMAN, MD
Associate Professor
Department of Neurology
School of Medicine
State University of New York at Stony Brook
Stony Brook, New York

PIM BROUWERS, PhD
Senior Investigator, Pediatric Branch
National Cancer Institute
Bethesda, Maryland

ROBERT E. BURKE, MD
Associate Professor of Neurology
Department of Neurology
Columbia University
New York, New York

SANSNEE CHATKUPT, MD
Departments of Neuroscience and Pediatrics
University of Medicine and Dentistry of New
   Jersey
Children's Hospital of New Jersey
Newark, New Jersey

ABE M. CHUTORIAN, MD
Professor of Neurology and Pediatrics
The New York Hospital-Cornell Medical
   Center
New York, New York

MICHAEL E. COHEN, MD
Professor and Chairman of Neurology
State University of New York at Buffalo
School of Medicine and Biomedical Sciences
Buffalo, New York

RONALD E. DAHL, MD
Assistant Professor
Departments of Psychiatry and Pediatrics
University of Pittsburgh School of Medicine
Pittsburgh, Pennsylvania

PATRICIA K. DUFFNER, MD
Professor of Neurology
State University of New York at Buffalo
School of Medicine and Biomedical Sciences
Buffalo, New York

GERALD ERENBERG, MD
Child Neurologist
Cleveland Clinic Foundation
Cleveland, Ohio

ARNOLD P. GOLD, MD
Professor of Clinical Neurology
Professor of Clinical Pediatrics
College of Physicians and Surgeons
Columbia University
New York, New York

GERALD S. GOLDEN, MD
Director, Boling Center for Developmental
   Disabilities
Shainberg Professor of Pediatrics
Professor of Neurology
University of Tennessee, Memphis
Memphis, Tennessee

DAVID MYLAND KAUFMAN, MD
Associate Professor of Neurology
Associate Professor of Psychiatry
Albert Einstein College of Medicine
Montefiore Medical Center
Bronx, New York

DIANE KOCH, PhD
Departments of Pediatrics and Psychiatry
The New York Hospital-Cornell Medical
   Center
New York, New York

M. RICHARD KOENIGSBERGER, MD
Departments of Neuroscience and Pediatrics
University of Medicine and Dentistry of New
   Jersey
Children's Hospital of New Jersey
Newark, New Jersey

MARY ELIZABETH LELL, MD
Chief, Section of Pediatric Neurology
St. Vincent's Hospital
New York, New York
Clinical Assistant Professor of Pediatrics
New York Medical College
Valhalla, New York

WALTER J. MOLOFSKY, MD
Departments of Neuroscience and Pediatrics
University of Medicine and Dentistry of New
   Jersey
Children's Hospital of New Jersey
Newark, New Jersey

HOWARD MOSS, PhD
Research Psychologist
Medical Illness Counseling Center and
Pediatric Branch
National Cancer Institute
Chevy Chase, Maryand

EDWIN C. MYER, MD
Chairman, Division of Child Neurology
Professor of Neurology and Pediatrics
Medical College of Virginia
Virginia Commonwealth University
Richmond, Virginia

RUTH NASS, MD
Associate Professor of Neurology and
   Pediatrics
The New York Hospital-Cornell Medical
   Center
New York, New York

STEVEN G. PAVLAKIS, MD
Clinical Assistant Professor of Neurology and
   Pediatrics
The New York Hospital-Cornell Medical
   Center
New York, New York

JOHN M. PELLOCK, MD
Professor of Neurology and Pediatrics
Medical College of Virginia
Virginia Commonwealth University
Richmond, Virginia

HART PETERSON, MD
Clinical Professor of Neurology in Pediatrics
The New York Hospital-Cornell Medical
   Center
New York, New York

CYNTHIA R. PFEFFER, MD
Professor of Psychiatry
The New York Hospital-Cornell Medical
   Center
New York, New York

A. DAVID ROTHNER, MD
Chief, Child Neurology
The Cleveland Clinical Foundation
Cleveland, Ohio

SHLOMO SHINNAR, MD, PhD
Associate Professor of Neurology and
   Pediatrics
Director, Montefiore/Einstein Epilepsy
   Management Center
Montefiore Medical Center
Albert Einstein College of Medicine
Bronx, New York

GAIL E. SOLOMON, MD
Associate Professor of Clinical Neurology in
Pediatrics and Psychiatry
The New York Hospital-Cornell Medical
    Center
New York, New York

LISA M. TARTAGLINO, MD
Department of Radiology
Thomas Jefferson University Hospital
Philadelphia, Pennsylvania

CONTENTS

Chapter 1

EVALUATION AND DIAGNOSIS BY INSPECTION

Arnold P. Gold, MD

Pediatric neurologic disorders can be diagnosed by compiling a detailed history coupled with a careful evaluation of the child and performing appropriate supplementary studies. History, the cornerstone of psychiatric diagnosis, is of equal value in neurology. The history often suggests organicity and whether the condition is static or progressive. If at all possible, the history should be obtained from the child, even if young, prior to obtaining historical data from the parents. Not infrequently, this may generate information free of parental bias that often is invaluable in determining diagnosis as well as how the condition affects the child. Information supplied by the parents or other interested adults is essential, and a significant number of pediatric entities are diagnosed by history alone, with the child showing little or no evidence of neurologic dysfunction. The epilepsies, which affect 5% of the pediatric population, are rarely observed by the physician, and definition of the seizure type is in large part determined by the history. Absence epilepsy, or so-called petit mal seizures, often is precipitated by prolonged hyperventilation, and the diagnosis is confirmed by the classic findings on the electroencephalogram. The other generalized and focal seizure disorders are rarely observed, and the electroencephalogram (EEG) may show nonspecific findings or even be normal. The history should include the time at which developmental milestones were acquired, and this information often is invaluable in deter-

mining whether the neurologic condition is static or progressive.

Table 1.1 lists the major areas of inquiry essential in the neurologic history that are discussed with the parents, and this should be coupled with a history data questionnaire (Table 1.2) that was completed prior to the initial office visit. The general and neurologic examination includes the items listed in Table 1.3. More detailed techniques relative to the completion of the history and the evaluation of the child, whose nervous system is developing, are available in

Table 1.1.
Neurologic History—Outline

Chief complaint
Prenatal course
Neonatal course
Pattern of growth and development:
    Motor
    Speech
    Fine Motor
    Adaptive
Past medical history:
    Medicines
    Allergies
    Immunizations
    Hospitalizations
    Surgery
Behavioral history
School history
Family history
Review of systems; general
Review of systems; neurologic (historical examination)
Chronology of present illness

Table 1.2.
History Data Questionnaire

Answer the following to the best of your ability with regard to your child:

1. *PREGNANCY:*
   - _____ a) Duration of pregnancy
   - _____ b) Complications of pregnancy
   - _____ c) Medications during pregnancy
   - _____ d) Type of labor: Spontaneous   Induced
   - _____ e) Duration of labor
   - _____ f) Type of delivery and/or complications
   - _____ g) Birth weight
   - _____ h) Apgar score
   - _____ i) Complications or problems in the newborn period
     Suck
     Vomiting
     Infection
     Jaundice: level of bilirubin, if known
     RH factor; transfusion
     Incubator care; no. of days in nursery
     Convulsions
     Cry
     Respiratory distress
     Mucus accumulation
     Other

2. *DEVELOPMENTAL MILESTONES:* (answer when pertinent)
   (Write in age at which your child accomplished the following)
   MOTOR:
   - _____ a) Dominant handedness (state whether right, left, or both)
   - _____ b) Head control   _____ g) Walked unassisted
   - _____ c) Turned over   _____ h) Tricycle
   - _____ d) Sat alone   _____ i) Bicycle
   - _____ e) Crawled   _____ j) Special shoes or braces
   - _____ f) Stood alone unassisted   _____ k) Any physical or occupational therapy
   SPEECH:
   - _____ a) Difficulty with: drooling, chewing, swallowing
     Write in age at which your child accomplished the following:
   - _____ b) Spoke first words (other than "ma-ma" and "da-da")
   - _____ c) Spoke first phrase
   - _____ d) Spoke in complete sentences
   - _____ e) Is speech adequate for age? articulation; content:
   - _____ f) Speech therapy, if any

3. *COMPREHENSION OR UNDERSTANDING:*
   a) Do you consider your child to understand directions and situations as well as other children his or her age? If no, why?

4. *TOILET TRAINING:*
   - _____ a) At what age was the child toilet trained for day; for night?
   - _____ b) Problems

5. *COORDINATION:*
   Rate your child on the following skills:

	GOOD	*AVERAGE*	*POOR*
Walking			
Running			
Handwriting			
Catching			

Table 1.2.   (*Continued*)
History Data Questionnaire

	GOOD	*AVERAGE*	*POOR*

Throwing
Shoelace tying
Buttoning
Athletic abilities
At what age did your child accomplish the following:
_____ a) Buttons own clothes
_____ b) Ties own shoelaces

6. *SCHOOL:*
   Rate your child with regard to school experiences, learning adjustment in school:

	GOOD	*AVERAGE*	*POOR*

   a) Nursery school
   b) Kindergarten
   c) Current grade
   What is your child's current school grade placement?_____
   Describe any school problems.
   Note kinds of special therapy or remedial work the patient is currently receiving.

7. *PAST MEDICAL HISTORY:*
   If your child's history includes any of the following illnesses, please write in the age when the illness occurred and any other information regarding the illness:
   _____ a) Epilepsy or convulsions
   _____ b) Accidents, falls, trauma (type and age)
   _____ c) Hernia
   _____ d) Visual or eye problems
   _____ e) Childhood diseases (type and age)
   _____ f) Allergies (type and age)
   _____ g) Serious medical illnesses and operations (type and age)

8. *BEHAVIOR:*
   Please check any of the following that apply to your child's behavior:

Hyperactivity	Low frustration threshold
Poor attention span	Temper outbursts
Impulsiveness	Aggressiveness
Distractibility	Does not play well with peers
Cries easily	Sibling rivalry
Underactivity	Multiple fears
Behavioral problems: home/school	Other
HABITS:	
Movements	Thumbsucking
Nailbiting	Headbanging
Masturbation	Other

9. *FAMILY HISTORY—MOTHER:*
   _____ a) Age
   _____ b) Age of pregnancy with patient
   _____ c) Spontaneous abortions or miscarriages
   _____ d) Occupation
   _____ e) Highest grade completed in school
   _____ f) School problems:
        1) Learning
        2) Speech
        3) Behavior
   _____ g) Medical problems, neurologic disease
   _____ h) Note if any family members (not including siblings of the patient) are reported to have any of the following areas of difficulty:
        1) Learning problems

Table 1.2. (*Continued*)
History Data Questionnaire

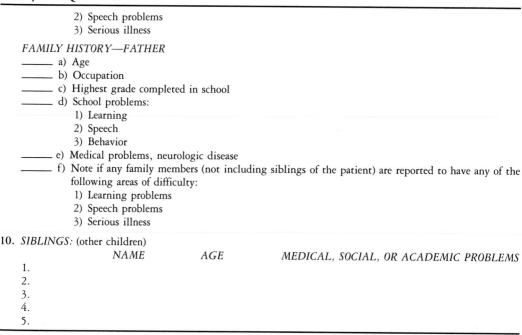

2) Speech problems
3) Serious illness

FAMILY HISTORY—FATHER

_____ a) Age
_____ b) Occupation
_____ c) Highest grade completed in school
_____ d) School problems:
    1) Learning
    2) Speech
    3) Behavior
_____ e) Medical problems, neurologic disease
_____ f) Note if any family members (not including siblings of the patient) are reported to have any of the following areas of difficulty:
    1) Learning problems
    2) Speech problems
    3) Serious illness

10. *SIBLINGS:* (other children)

	NAME	AGE	MEDICAL, SOCIAL, OR ACADEMIC PROBLEMS
1.			
2.			
3.			
4.			
5.			

the standard textbooks of child neurology and child psychiatry.

Observations may be more rewarding than examination, encouraging the clinician to acquire and use observational skills that may result in a diagnosis by inspection. This is obviously preferred to the performance of diagnostic studies that can be anxiety producing, painful, invasive, and expensive. Ultimately, selective neurodiagnostic studies may be necessary to confirm a diagnosis or follow the clinical course. Electrophysiologic studies include the EEG, which is important with the epilepsies; evoked potentials to determine the status of visual, auditory, and sensory function; and the electromyogram (EMG) and nerve conduction times with the myopathies and neuropathies. Neuroradiologic studies (CT and MRI scans) supply an invaluable window to the brain and spinal cord. Metabolic studies are essential with metabolic disorders, and the field of molecular biology includes chromosomal studies with genetic disorders.

Table 1.4 lists conditions in which the ability to observe and examine often produces a clinical diagnosis, and this resultant diagnosis by inspection enhances the relationship between clinician and family by providing a diagnosis and prognosis at the time of the initial evaluation. The head must be measured for size and configuration; the ear, for size and placement; the eyes, for pigmentation, pressure, and vasculature; the skin, for pigmentation and vascular changes; and the male genitalia, for the presence and size of the testes. Once an abnormality has been defined, it is mandatory that the parents be evaluated for a similar condition, since many of these disorders are of genetic etiology. This reinforces the diagnosis and often demonstrates the biologic variability of the condition, which may be mild in the parent and more severe in the child, or vice versa. On other occasions, a finding in both parent and child may suggest a genetic diagnosis in which there is no associated neurologic dysfunction. For example, a single pal-

Table 1.3.
Physical Examination

NAME: _____ DATE: _____
HEAD CIRCUMFERENCE   HEIGHT   WEIGHT   VITAL SIGNS
BRUITS
SKIN
HEENT
NECK
HEART
CHEST
ABDOMEN
PULSES
EXTREMITIES

NEUROLOGIC:
    I. DEVELOPMENTAL EVALUATION
        Developmental milestones
        R/L handed
        Speech: Comprehension
        Reading level
        Calculations
        General information
        Graphomotor skills
        Memory: Auditory/visual
        Perception: Auditory/visual
        Fund of knowledge
   II. MOTOR
        Gait patterns
        Bulk, tone, strength, abnormal postures, abnormal movements
  III. REFLEXES
        Deep tendon reflexes   Abdominal
        Babinski   Anal
        Cremasteric   Neonatal reflex
   IV. SENSORY
        Light touch, pain, position, vibrations, graphesthesia, stereognostic
    V. COORDINATION
        Finger-to-nose, heel-to-shin, rapid alternating movements, ataxia nystagmus
   VI. CRANIAL NERVES
        Smell   Corneal
        Visual acuity   Facial
        Visual fields   Hearing
        Fundus   Palate
        Pupils   Gag
        Extraocular movements   Sternocleidomastoid
        Lids   Tongue
        Nystagmus
 VII. OTHER

mar crease (simian line) when found in both typically is not associated with any impairment of neurologic function.

CRANIAL ABNORMALITIES

Head circumference measurements supply the most useful information relative to brain size and should be obtained in every pediatric neurologic evaluation. Measured around the forehead and occipital protuberance, serial measurements are invaluable in determining whether the increase in head circumference is physiologic, following a given percentile, or pathologic, crossing percentiles. Microcephaly and macrocephaly are

Table 1.4.
Diagnosis by Inspection

HEAD
  Measure size and shape
    Microcephaly
      Primary
      Secondary
    Macrocephaly
      Bone
        Achondroplasia
        Cleidocranial dysostosis
      Meninges—subdural
        Brain—neurodegenerative—Tay Sachs
    Cerebrospinal fluid—hydrocephalus
    Craniosynostosis

FACE
  Ears
    Fragile X syndrome
    Down's syndrome
  Eyes
    Shape—Down's and Prader-Willi syndromes
    Bulbar telangiectasia—ataxia telangiectasia
    Depigmented iris—tuberous sclerosis
    Glaucoma—trigeminal angiomatosis (Sturge-Weber syndrome)

SKIN
  Pigmentary changes
  Depigmented—tuberous sclerosis
  Pigmented
    Neurofibromatosis
    Incontinentia pigmenti
  Port wine nevus—trigeminal angiomatosis (Sturge-Weber syndrome)

GENITALIA
  Cryptorchidism
  Macroorchidism
  Prader-Willi syndrome
  Fragile-X syndrome

EXTREMITIES
  Down's and Prader-Willi syndromes
  Asymmetry—smaller hand and foot with congenital hemiparesis

---

measurements that are more than 2 standard deviations below or above the mean for age, sex, and race.

Microcephaly of early prenatal etiology is considered primary, while that of late prenatal, perinatal, or early postnatal is diagnostic of secondary microcephaly. *Primary microcephaly* can result from an intrauterine infection, notably cytomegalovirus, and from ionizing radiation, chemical exposure with drugs such as cortico-

steroids, aminopterin and nitrogen mustard, and genetic defects. Chromosomal and genetic disorders are often associated with microcephaly. Down's syndrome, or trisomy 21, typically has microcephaly; other conditions that should be considered include a genetically transmitted autosomal recessive microcephaly, migrational disorders (lissencephaly, macro- and microgyrus), and dysmorphic syndromes (Cornelia de Lange's, Seckel's, Rubinstein-Taybi's, and

Prader-Willi's). *Secondary microcephaly* results from anoxia, infections, and metabolic and nutritional problems. A developmental delay, primarily involving language, and a learning disability or retardation with or without seizures are the expected clinical manifestations of microcephaly.

Macrocephaly may be the result of a large brain (megalencephaly) with associated retardation, but cranial enlargement may be a dominantly inherited trait typically without neurologic deficit, a primary abnormality of the bony cranium (cleidocranial dysostosis, achondroplasia), or a condition secondary to chronic increased intracranial pressure (hydrocephalus, subdural collections) with the clinical presentation dependent upon the primary etiology. Hydrocephalus typically presents with progressive macrocrania with head circumference measurements that cross percentiles, and in the first 2 years of life this increase in intracranial pressure is almost never associated with papilledema.

Craniosynostosis, or premature closure of cranial sutures, most often results from a disorder of the bony mesenchymal matrix but rarely is secondary to a metabolic condition (hyperthyroidism, rickets) or hematologic disorder (sickle cell disease). In sharp contrast to the symmetric cranium of micro- or macrocephaly, craniosynostosis typically presents with an asymmetric cranium, and the skull shape is dependent upon the suture that is prematurely fused (see Table 1.5). Unless there is an associated anomaly of the brain, the child with craniosynostosis presents with no evidence of a neurologic deficit or with a developmental delay. The metopic suture is of interest, since the cranial asymmetry is self-corrected with age. Surgical correction is indicated in those rare cases of complicating increased intracranial pressure, but in the majority the decision for corrective strip craniectomy is based on cosmetic considerations.

CHROMOSOME DISORDERS

Recognition of facial dysmorphism often leads to a specific diagnosis, which can be verified by a chromosomal analysis.

Down's syndrome is the most common chromosomal abnormality to result in mental retardation. Trisomy, or an additional chromosome 21, is most commonly encountered; an identical clinical picture is encountered with a chromosome 21 translocation to another chromosome, usually 14 or 22. The incidence of Down's syndrome is related to maternal age for trisomy but not for translocation. In all newborns the incidence is 1 in 1000 live births, while with mothers aged 45 years or older the incidence approximates 1 in 50. Antenatal diagnosis by amniocentesis is indicated in mothers older than 35 years of age and in all mothers with a prior Down's syndrome pregnancy.

Down's syndrome pregnancy may be lethal, resulting in fetal death or stillbirth (approximately 25% of spontaneous abortions have Down's syndrome), while the remainder who are viable present with varied clinical manifestations that are dependent on the presence of associated

Table 1.5.
Craniosynostosis and Cranial Configuration

Suture Involved	Cranial Configuration
Sagittal	Scaphocephaly
Coronal	
Bilateral	Brachycephaly
Bilateral + face (basal skull)	Crouzon's syndrome
Bilateral + face + syndactyly	Apert's syndrome
Unilateral	Plagiocephaly
Metopic	Trigonocephaly
Lambdoidal—unilateral	Plagiocephaly

anomalies. The phenotype is complex and varied, with facies and extremities that are diagnostic. Microcephaly with large anterior fontanelle, depressed nasal bridge, bilateral epicanthic folds, mongoloid or upward-slanting palpebral fissures, Brushfield spots encircling the peripheral third of the iris, low-set and misshapen ears with a hypoplastic tragus and narrow external auditory meatus, and lingual protrusion with a small mouth are characteristic. Other observational diagnostic features include short stature, hands with a single transverse crease (simian line), brachyclinodactyly of the fifth finger with hypoplasia of the middle phalanx and resultant shortening and incurving, and feet with wide separation between the large and second toes. A dermatoglyphic pattern of the fingers and palms also shows diagnostic features.

Neuropathologically, there is a small brain with microcephaly and by age 30 premature senile changes such as those seen in Alzheimer's disease. Neurologically, there is a significant developmental delay and intellectual deficit. Generalized muscular hypotonia results in significant delay in the acquisition of motor milestones, and subsequently there is delayed development of language, both for articulation and content. In some, impaired hearing results from middle ear disease or a sensorineural hearing loss, and ultimately there is retardation or at least a learning disability. In less than 10% of children seizures can occur at any age and include infantile myoclonic spasms with hypsarhythmia. Quadriparesis can result at any time from a cervical subluxation of the atlantoaxial process. Life expectancy depends in part on associated malformations, including congenital heart disease with atrioventricular canals, ventricular septal defects, or a patent ductus arteriosus; and gastrointestinal anomalies with duodenal atresia and megacolon. Leukemia also occurs with increased frequency when compared with the normal population. Due to premature senility and changes involving both skin and brain, as well as increased susceptibility to infection, life expectancy is approximately 50 years.

Fragile X syndrome is another important genetic condition resulting in a learning disability or mental retardation, with an incidence of approximately 1 in 1000 male births. The diagnosis is established with documentation of a fragile site at the end of the long arm of chromosome X when cells are cultured in a reduced folic acid and thymidine medium. Prenatal diagnosis is possible only when the amniotic fluid cells are cultured in this special medium. The phenotype in boys is varied, but careful observation can result in a diagnosis by inspection. The infant presents with relative macrocrania and facial edema, while the older child and adult have a long face and a prominent chin. Large, floppy, seashell-shaped ears are characteristic at any age. Macroorchidism with normal-size penis is most frequently seen in the adolescent.

Neurologically, boys typically present with a significant language delay and behavioral problems, including an attention deficit disorder or behaviors with autistic-like features. Ultimately, there are academic difficulties and mental retardation.

Heterozygous girls with fragile X are usually phenotypically normal. Intellectually they may be normal or mildly retarded.

Prader-Willi syndrome is a recognizable condition that presents as a developmental delay or learning disability. Diagnosis is confirmed by documenting in most, but not all, a deletion or translocation of the long arm of chromosome 15.

Clinically, the child presents with the clinical tetrad of hypomentia, hypotonia, hypogonadism, and obesity. The infant and young child present with feeding problems and hypothermia and is floppy or hypotonic, resulting in a significant delay in the acquisition of motor milestones. The presence of a small penis, a hypoplastic scrotum, and cryptorchidism in a child with small hands and feet should suggest the diagnosis. At a later age, there is evidence of impaired expressive language, and the youngster, who often has a cheerful and outgoing personality, demonstrates pathologic polyphagia with resultant marked exogenous obesity and a significant learning disability and/or retardation. The individual is short in stature and the facies is also characteristically long, with a fishlike mouth and almond-shaped eyes.

Treatment includes specific remediation with physical, occupational, speech, language, and educational therapies. Management of the polyphagia includes behavioral modification and, when necessary, a residential program. Cryptorchidism should be corrected well in advance of puberty.

NEUROCUTANEOUS DISORDERS

Genetically and clinically distinct, these disorders are grouped together because each involves skin and nervous system. The distinctive features of each permit a clinical diagnosis.

Ataxia-telangiectasia is a highly characteristic disorder that is age dependent in its clinical presentation. The infant and young child present with a progressive truncal ataxia. At 3 to 5 years, increasing oculocutaneous telangiectasia involving the exposed areas of skin and bulbar conjunctiva suggests the diagnosis, and in later childhood there is complicating choreoathetosis, oculomotor apraxia, and nystagmus. By this time the child has a dull, expressionless facies and often has a learning disability or a mild intellectual deficit. Susceptibility to sinopulmonary infections, immunologic deficiencies, and a predilection for lymphoreticular and other neoplasias can occur at any age. In adolescence, many develop a form of insulin-resistant diabetes mellitus. The neurologic disability is progressive, and incapacitation and death from either infection or malignancy often occur in young adults.

Ataxia-telangiectasia is due in part to defective DNA repair mechanisms and is associated with chromosomal breaks involving chromosome 14. Other features include abnormalities of the immunologic globulins (low IgA, decreased to absent IgE, and low IgG^2 and IgG^4) and an elevated alpha-fetoprotein level.

Early recognition and treatment of infections and malignancies improve the quality of life in children affected with this progressive neurologic disorder.

Neurofibromatosis (NF) is highly varied in its clinical presentation but is readily diagnosed. Of dominant inheritance and apparently with 50% of cases resulting from mutations, there are two well-described genetic subtypes: NF-1, or generalized neurofibromatosis (von Recklinghausen's disease), assigned to chromosome 17; and NF-2, or neurofibromatosis, with bilateral acoustic neuroma that has been linked to chromosome 22. Other forms include segmental neurofibromatosis with café-au-lait spots and neurofibromas limited to a body segment, and cutaneous neurofibromatosis, which is limited to the pigmentary skin lesions without any other manifestations of the disorder.

Diagnostic criteria for NF-1 require two or more of the following:

1. Six or more café-au-lait spots larger than 5 mm in diameter in prepubertal children and larger than 15 mm in postpubertal children
2. Two or more neurofibromas or one plexiform neuroma
3. Freckling—axillary or inguinal
4. Optic nerve glioma
5. Bone lesion, such as defects in posterior superior orbital wall or long bone lesions with or without pseudoarthrosis
6. Two or more Lisch's nodules

Diagnostic criteria for NF-2 include either bilateral eighth nerve tumors or a first-degree relative with NF-2 and either a unilateral acoustic nerve tumor or two of the following: neurofibroma, meningioma, schwannoma, glioma, or juvenile posterior capsular cataract.

In addition to the genetic subtypes, NF characteristically has marked variability in its clinical presentation with involvement of skin, bone, and nervous system. Cutaneous lesions suggest the diagnosis, with the extreme variability of clinical presentation resulting from the variable expressivity of multisystem involvement. Diverse clinical manifestations such as learning disabilities, progressive visual loss, increased intracranial pressure, or scoliosis can all result from neurofibromatosis.

The café-au-lait macules, which increase in size and number and typically spare the face, are the pathognomonic lesion. Other cutaneous findings include freckling, which typically involves the axillary and other intertriginous areas, darkened hyperpigmented lesions often associated with an underlying plexiform neurofibroma, fibromas of varying sizes, hypopigmented macules, and angiomas. Pigmented iris hamartomas (Lisch's nodules), when present, are characteristic. Neurologic lesions, dysplasia, or neoplasia can involve either the central or peripheral nervous system. Static encephalopathies with resultant learning disability, attention deficit disorder, and macrocrania are often unrecognized, while the more dramatic and infrequent progressive encephalopathies due to neoplasm or vascular occlusive disease are frequently identified as a manifestation of neurofibromatosis. Neoplasia of the cranial nerves is age-related, with optic nerve glioma occurring before age 10 and bilateral acoustic neuroma after age 20. Tumors, most commonly an astrocytoma, may involve the brain, brainstem, and spinal cord, while less common are meningiomas, medulloblastomas, or ependymomas, with clinical manifestations determined by localization and tumor type. Precocious puberty and, less commonly, sexual infantilism result from a hypothalamic mass lesion or compression of the hypothalamus from an optic chiasm glioma. Neurofibromas arising from superficial or deep peripheral nerves or nerve roots are common and often have no symptoms other than pain, while plexiform neurofibromas are associated with overgrowth of tissues and, when extensive, elephantiasis. Typically, neurologic manifestations are slow and insidious in their development, but on rare occasions an acute onset with paralysis and seizures can result from occlusion of a major cerebral artery.

Other tumor types occur more frequently than in the general population, including leukemia, Wilms' tumor, sarcoma, neuroblastoma, ganglioglioma, medullary thyroid carcinoma, and pheochromocytoma. Hypertension can also result from intrinsic involvement of the renal artery.

Bone lesions characteristic of neurofibromatosis include progressive kyphoscoliosis, unilateral pulsatile exophthalmus due to a defect of the posterior superior wall of the orbit, pseudoarthrosis involving tibia and radius, enlargement of long bones, and "twisted ribbon" rib deformities.

There is no specific laboratory test or prenatal procedure that is diagnostic. It is anticipated that molecular biology will produce this invaluable data. Evaluation depends on clinical presentation and may require psychoeducational testing and/or neurodiagnostic studies, such as radiographs of skull, optic foramina, or spine; CT or MRI of brain or spine; EEG; visual studies for acuity and fields; and audiologic examinations.

Treatment depends on early diagnosis and prompt recognition of pathologic lesions. Evaluation at regular intervals with appropriate employment of diagnostic tools is essential in the formulation of a dynamic therapeutic regimen. There is no age that can be considered free of risk from a serious or even life-threatening complication. The child with the easily recognized café-au-lait macules may have cutaneous lesions with static or progressive multisystem involvement or may have a paucity of clinical manifestation, and both could die at age 40 to 50 from sarcomatous degeneration of a neurofibroma.

Tuberous sclerosis, a neurocutaneous disorder

with a highly varied presentation, should be readily diagnosed clinically. There is evidence of dominant inheritance involving chromosome 9 with variable penetrance, and approximately 50% of children are the result of a mutation. Prenatal testing is not yet available but is anticipated to be forthcoming.

The cardinal features of tuberous sclerosis include a triad consisting of age-related skin lesions, seizures, and mental retardation.

Depigmented macules that are present at birth, and persist throughout life may vary in size from a depigmented freckle to a macule of many centimeters in diameter. In an infant, its presence with infantile spasms should suggest the diagnosis. Facial adenoma sebaceum, the so-called pathognomonic cutaneous lesion, is never present at birth and becomes clinically evident after age 2 to 3 years. Involving the butterfly area of the face, the lesions are initially small in size with a telangiectatic component that is red in color; later the lesions enlarge and become fibrotic and tan. After the first decade, shagreen patches consisting of elevated plaques of yellowish-brown connective tissue develop and are most frequently localized to the lumbar area. At a similar or later age, periungual or subungual fibromas may develop.

Seizures are common and frequently are refractory to conventional anticonvulsant therapy. Infantile spasms, with or without hypsarhythmia, are the classic seizure type in the young infant, and in the presence of depigmented macules are diagnostic of tuberous sclerosis. Other seizure types, including generalized tonic-clonic or partial seizures, can occur at any age.

Developmental delay (above all for language), specific learning disabilities, and varying degrees of intellectual impairment are common, but normal intellect occurs in a significant number of affected children. Onset of seizures during the infancy period is often associated with mental retardation. Other neurologic manifestations include increased intracranial pressure resulting from obstruction of cerebrospinal fluid flow by intracranial tubers, most often at the foramen of Monro, or the development of an intraventricular glioma.

Ophthalmologically, retinal lesions, when present, can aid in diagnosis and include calcified multinodular hamartomas near or at the optic nerve, or relatively flat, smooth, whitish-pink hamartomas more peripherally placed. Depigmented lesions of the iris are comparable to the depigmented skin macule. Nonparalytic strabismus, cataracts, and optic atrophy are other nonspecific ophthalmologic findings.

Further variability in clinical presentation is due to visceral involvement. Tumors of the kidney include the common benign multiple angiomyolipomas and the rather rare renal carcinoma. Multicystic renal disease, when present, can significantly impair renal function. Cardiac rhabdomyomas may occur at any age, and their presence should suggest the diagnosis.

Clinical variability with multisystem involvement is characteristic of tuberous sclerosis. Despite this feature, the alert physician should be able to formulate a clinical diagnosis with confidence. In infants the depigmented skin macules and infantile spasms or in the older child the triad of facial adenoma sebaceum, seizures, and mental retardation should be diagnostic. Supplementary laboratory studies are essential in diagnosis and therapy. The computed tomographic (CT) scan is highly characteristic, with subependymal or periventricular calcified and frequently enhancing tubers that often encroach on the foramen of Monro. MRI scans may, in addition, demonstrate lesions that were isodense on CT. The electroencephalogram may be normal, nonspecifically abnormal with background slowing, or significantly abnormal with paroxysmal discharges, periodicity or hypsarhythmia. Renal ultrasound frequently demonstrates multiple and bilateral hamartomas (angiomyolypomas) and other renal pathology including renal cysts or tumors. Echocardiogram should be performed routinely to rule out a complicating rhabdomyoma.

Treatment should be individualized and depends on pathology and clinical manifestations. Complications must be anticipated, with clinical evaluation at regular intervals and the performance of supplementary studies as indicated.

Encephalotrigeminal angiomatosis (Sturge-Weber-Dimitri's syndrome) is a readily diagnosed condition with the port-wine facial nevus flammeus in the distribution of the ophthalmic branch of the trigeminal nerve. As with other neurocutaneous disorders, this is most often a diagnosis by inspection and is characterized by marked variability in clinical presentation. Genetic in origin, most cases are sporadic, and more than one affected sibling is rare. The gene has been linked to chromosome 3.

Typically, the facial nevus is associated neurologically with a triad of seizures, hemiplegia, and retardation, and ophthalmologically with glaucoma and homonymous hemianopsia. The port-wine facial nevus, present at birth, is often more extensive and may involve half of the face, neck, and even portions of the contralateral face. The neurologic syndrome is the result of a vascular anomaly of the brain, with unilateral leptomeningeal angiomatosis ipsilateral to the facial nevus and associated cerebral atrophy with classic curvilinear intracranial calcifications. Typically, the young infant presents with focal motor, partial complex, or generalized seizures that are not infrequently refractory to multiple and varied anticonvulsants. The contralateral hemiparesis, often progressive, is associated with hemiatrophy and homonymous hemianopsia. Developmental delay, specific learning disabilities, behavioral problems with an attention deficit disorder, and retardation are common. Intraorbital hypertension with buphthalmos and glaucoma is observed in approximately 30% of affected children.

Treatment is symptomatic. The facial nevus can be covered with cosmetics and at a later age treated with laser therapy. Recurrent seizures require anticonvulsants, and in selected children hemispherectomy is effective. Specific therapies, including physical, occupational, speech, and educational, are often required. The commonly observed behavioral problems require counseling and psychoactive compounds.

SUGGESTED READINGS

Alexander GL. Sturge-Weber syndrome. Handbook Neurol 1972;14:223–240.

Alexander GL, Normal FM. The Sturge-Weber syndrome. Baltimore: Williams & Wilkins, 1960.

Comez MR, ed. Tuberous sclerosis. New York: Raven Press, 1979.

Conference Statement, National Institutes of Health Consensus Development Conference: Neurofibromatosis. Arch Neurol 1988;45:575–578.

Donegani G, Gratarolla RF, Wildi E. Tuberous sclerosis. In: Vinken PH, Bruyn GW, eds. Handbook of Clinical Neurology, vol. 14. New York: Elsevier-North Holland, 1972:340–389.

Molofsky WJ, Gold AP. Pediatric neurological evaluation. In: Handbook of clinical assessment of children and adolescents. Kestenbaum CJ, Williams DT, eds. New York: New York University Press, 1988.

Paterson MC, Smith PJ. Ataxia-telangiectasia an inherited human disorder involving hypersensitivity to ionizing radiation and related DNA-damaging chemicals. Ann Rev Genet 1979;13:291.

Riccardi VM, Eichner JE. Neurofibromatosis. Baltimore: The Johns Hopkins University Press, 1986.

Rubenstein AE, Bunge RP, Housman DE, eds. Neurofibromatosis. Ann NY Acad Sci 1986;486:1–414.

Sedgwick RP, Boder E. Ataxia-telangiectasia. In: Vinken PJ, Bruyn G, eds. Handbook of clinical neurology, vol. 14. Amsterdam: North Holland Publishing, 1972.

Wisniewski KE, French JH, Fernando S, et al. Fragile-X syndrome: associated neurological abnormalities and developmental disabilities. Ann Neurol 1985;18:665.

Zellweger H. Down syndrome. In: Vinken PJ, Bruyn GW, eds. Congenital malformations of the brain and skull. Part II. Handbook of clinical neurology, vol. 31. Amsterdam: North Holland Publishing, 1977.

Zellweger H, Ionasescu V, Simpson J, Waziri M. Chromosomal aneuploidies excluding Down syndrome. In: Vinken PH, Bruyn GW, eds. Congenital malformations of the brain and skull. Part II. Handbook of clinical neurology, vol. 31. Amsterdam: North Holland Publishing, 1977.

Zellweger H, Patil SR. Down syndrome. In: Myriantho-poulous NC, ed. Handbook of clinical neurology, vol. 6: Malformations. New York: Elsevier Science Publishing, 1987.

Zellweger H, Schneider JH. Syndrome of hypotonia-hypomentia-hypogonadism-obesity (HHHO) or Prader-Willi syndrome. Am J Dis Child 1968;115:588.

Zellweger H, Soyer RT. The Prader-Willi syndrome. Med Hygiene 1979;37:3338.

Chapter 2

EXAMPLES OF PROBLEMS IN CHILD AND ADOLESCENT NEUROLOGY

David M. Kaufman, MD
Gail E. Solomon, MD
Cynthia R. Pfeffer, MD

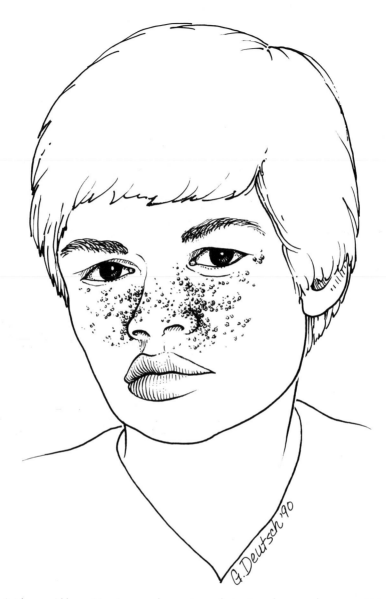

Figure 2.1. A 14-year-old boy with seizures and mental retardation has adenoma sebaceum, which is characteristic of tuberous sclerosis. The lesions consist of red papules over the nose and malar region that develop between the ages of 1 and 5 years (see Chapter 1).

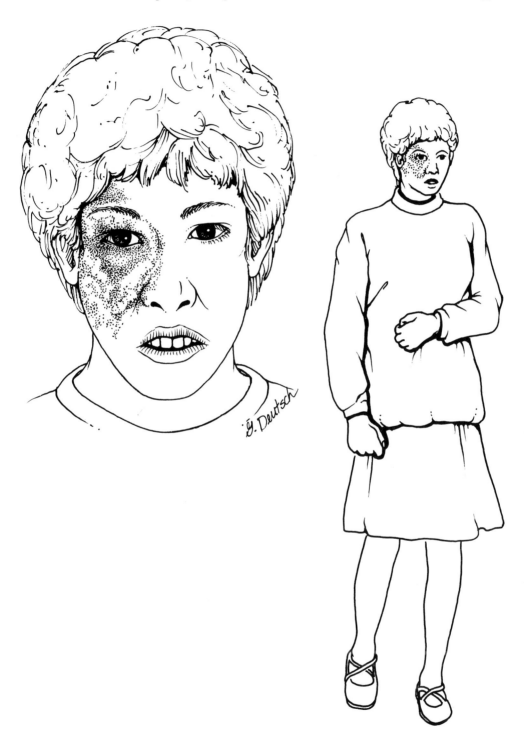

Figure 2.2.   This 13-year-old girl with Sturge-Weber syndrome has a "port-wine stain" hemangioma in the distribution of the right fifth cranial nerve and a left spastic hemiplegia. Note the flexed pronated, fisted left arm (Chapter 1).

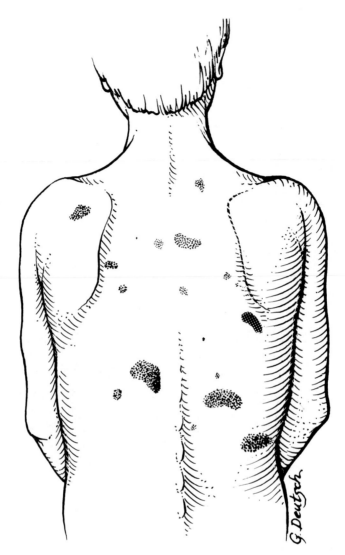

Figure 2.3.   This 8-year-old boy has café-au-lait spots that consist of 1.5 cm or larger flat, light brown, well-demarcated areas. In prepubertal children, neurofibromatosis is indicated in the presence of six or more café-au-lait spots with a diameter of at least 0.5 cm. In older children, the café-au-lait spots must be at least 1.5 cm (Chapter 1).

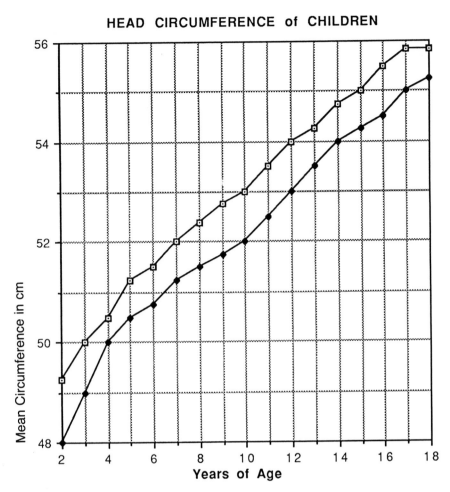

Figure 2.4.   The head circumference, greater in boys than in girls, increases in an almost linear fashion from ages 4 to 17 years. Ninety-eight percent of children fall within 2 standard deviations, which is approximately 2.5 cm, from the mean. Microcephaly usually has its onset in utero or in the early postnatal period. Macrocephaly is usually caused by hydrocephalus, but it may be caused by subdural effusions, storage diseases, neurofibromatosis, or benign familial factors (see Figure 2.5, **A** and **B**, and Chapters 1 and 13).

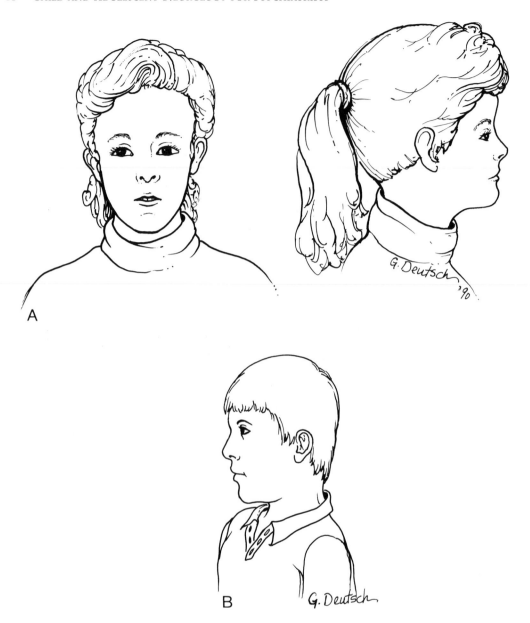

Figure 2.5.   A, This is an 11-year-old girl with macrocephaly, which is defined as a head circumference greater than 2 standard deviations above the mean for age, sex, race, and gestation. The cause of the macrocephaly in this child is hydrocephalus that has been treated with a shunt (Chapters 1 and 13). **B,** This boy, who is also 11 years old, has microcephaly, which is defined as head circumference 2 standard deviations below the average with the same provisos as for macrocephaly. Microcephaly is usually associated with mental retardation.

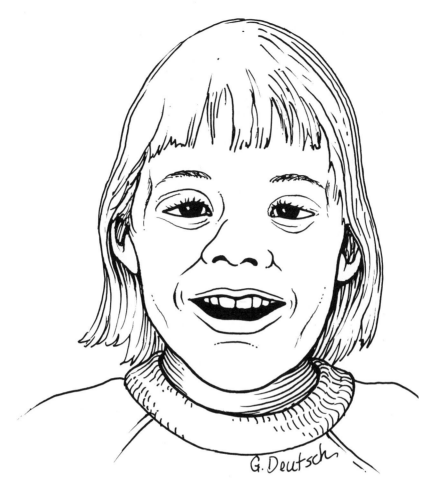

Figure 2.6.   This 9-year-old girl has Down's syndrome, which is most often caused by trisomy 21. This girl has the characteristic facial appearance that consists of palpebral fissures that are oblique and narrow, prominent epicanthal folds, and ears that are small, low-set, and with only a simple helix (Chapters 1 and 15).

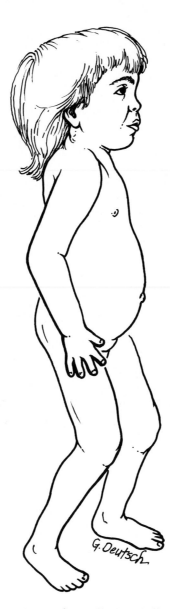

Figure 2.7. This 6-year-old girl has Hurler's syndrome. She is typically short with a large head and coarse facial features. Her eyes are widely spaced. The bridge of her nose is flat. Her jaw is slack. There is corneal clouding. She has dwarfism with kyphosis, a protuberant abdomen with a tendency toward umbilical hernia, and hepato-splenomegaly. Her hands are wide and the fingers are short and stubby (Chapter 14).

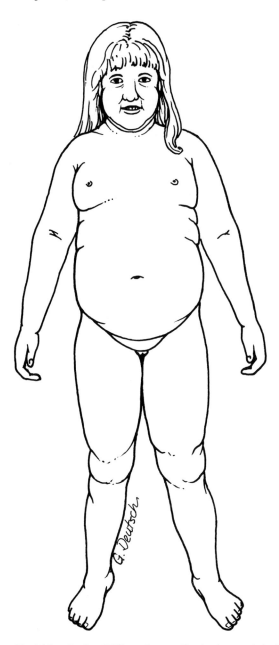

Figure 2.8. This 14-year-old girl has Prader-Willi syndrome. She is characteristically short, hypotonic, obese, and mentally retarded. She has a small stature with small hands. There is a tendency toward strabismus. Her forehead is narrow, and her eyes oval. Approximately 50% of children have abnormalities of chromosome 15 (Chapters 1 and 15).

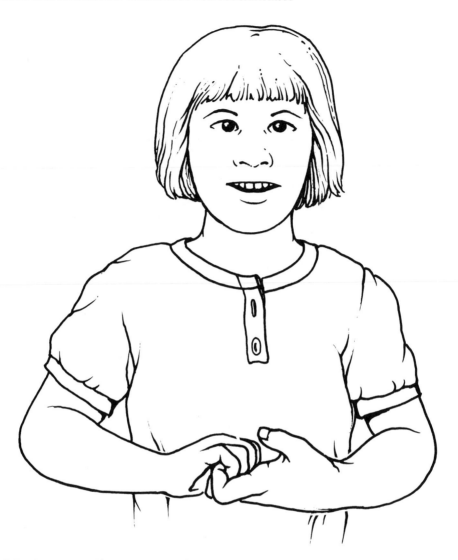

Figure 2.9.   This 5-year-old girl has Rett syndrome. She had developed normally until 10 months of age, when she began to have regression in her developmental milestones. She had the onset of autistic behavior, acquired microcephaly, hypotonia, ataxia, and the characteristic "hand-washing" or "hand-wringing" movements (Chapters 1, 5, and 15).

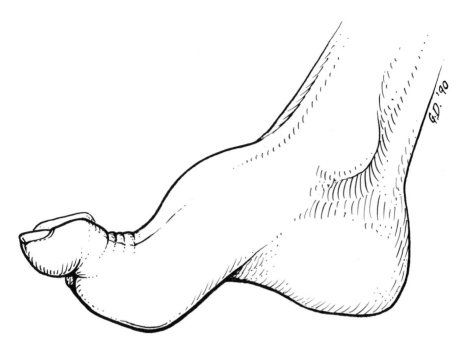

Figure 2.10.   The foot of this 15-year-old boy has a typical pes cavus deformity. This deformity is seen in spinocerebellar degenerations, which are not usually associated with mental impairment. It is characterized by a high arch, an elevated dorsum of the foot, and a retraction of the metatarsal joint (Chapter 3).

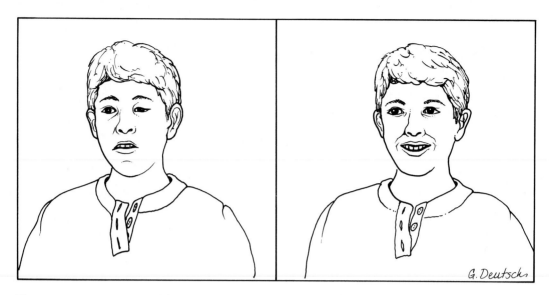

Figure 2.11.   This 13-year-old boy with myasthenia gravis is pictured before and after treatment with Tensilon (edrophonium). Before treatment, the boy has a flat, expressionless face with ptosis and strabismus that is more marked on the left. Also, he has loss of his nasolabial folds and a downward, depressed look of his mouth (Chapter 3).

After the injection of Tensilon, for several minutes, his face has a normal expression and his eyes have normal function. This dramatic response to the Tensilon test is diagnostic of myasthenia gravis.

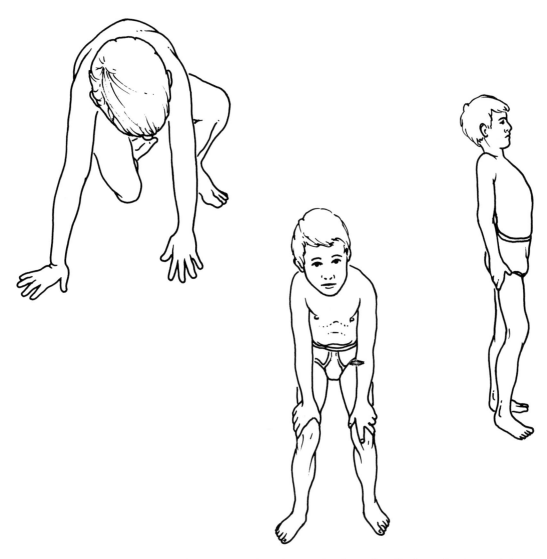

Figure 2.12.   This is an 8-year-old boy with Duchenne's muscular dystrophy. He shows the characteristic exaggerated pseudohypertrophy of his calves and marked lumbar lordosis. The illustration shows the Gowers' sign, which is an early indication of weakness of the pelvic muscles: When the child tries to get up from a sitting or kneeling position, he must rise from the floor by progressively "climbing up his thighs" (Chapter 3).

NEUROMUSCULAR DISEASES IN CHILDHOOD

M. Richard Koenigsberger, MD, Walter J. Molofsky, MD,
and Sansnee Chatkupt, MD

INTRODUCTION

Neuromuscular diseases in children are classified primarily by the location in the nervous system responsible for the motor impairment, and secondarily by the etiology. The clinician's initial goal is to localize the disease to a specific region of the brain, spinal cord, anterior horn cell, peripheral nerve, neuromuscular junction, or muscle.

Diseases associated with impairment in cognition and mental status affect the cerebral cortex; however, in certain circumstances, diseases at other locations may also be associated with impairment of cognitive function or mental status. Also, any illness may secondarily produce mental status changes.

The motor system consists of the upper motor neuron (UMN), which originates in the Betz cells in the cortex. It leads via myelinated tracts through the centrum semiovale, internal capsule, brainstem, and, in the spinal cord, corticospinal tracts to the anterior horn cells, which give rise to the lower motor neuron (LMN). The LMN consists of the peripheral nerve, neuromuscular junction, and muscle. In general, diseases of the UMN cause asymmetric weakness, increased muscle tone (spasticity), increased reflexes, and Babinski signs. Since UMN injury often results from cerebral injury, it is associated

with mental status changes, headaches, and convulsions.

Diseases of the LMN generally cause symmetrical weakness, decreased muscle tone (hypotonia), decreased or absent reflexes, and possibly fasciculations. There are also diseases of both the UMN and LMN where overlapping features are seen.

The physical characteristics of neuromuscular diseases in terms of their localization are summarized in Table 3.1. Examples of specific diseases for each of these locations are summarized in Table 3.2 and explained in detail in the latter part of this chapter.

HISTORY

A thorough history allows the physician to characterize the development of the problem and to search for physical disabilities that may not be readily apparent or demonstrable (Table 3.3). The goal is to characterize the onset of the problem as acute or chronic, localize the region of dysfunction, and decide whether the problem is static or progressive. Specific features then indicate a more definite etiology.

Chief Complaint. Evaluation begins with a statement regarding the chief complaint and a chronology of the present illness. In children older than 4 or 5 years, the physician should try

Table 3.1.
Regional Localization—Characteristic Findings

	Brain	Spinal Cord	Anterior Horn Cell	Peripheral Nerve	Nerve Muscle Junction	Muscle
Cognition	↓	N	N	N	N	±
Dysmorphic Features	+	+	—	—	—	±
Distribution	Q,H,PP	L	P	D	V,F	P
Reflexes	↑	Below lesion ↑	absent	↓ or absent	N	N, ↓
Fasciculations	—	—	+	—	—	—

Key:
Cognition: Refers to intellectual function or change in mental status. N = Normal
Dysmorphic Features: Refers to facial or systemic features seen in some chromosomal or metabolic diseases such as Down's, Hunter's, and Hurler's syndromes and to the presence of systemic abnormalities, such as increased liver, kidney, spleen size, or to orthopedic malformations.
Distribution of Weakness: Quadriparesis (Q), Hemiparesis (H), Paraparesis (PP), Level (L), Proximal (P), Distal (D), Variable (V), Facial (F)
Key:
↑, increased
↓, decreased
+, present
—, absent
±, variable

to obtain as much information as possible from the child. In most instances, however, it is provided by the parents.

Chronology of Present Illness. The intent here is to determine whether the onset of the illness is acute, subacute, or chronic. Acute onset—minutes, hours, or days—suggests trauma, infections, postinfectious processes, ingestion, overmedication, or conversion reactions. Subacute onset—of days to weeks—suggests postinfectious neuromuscular disorders, such as Guillain-Barré syndrome, myositis, or myasthenia gravis, or a systemic disease. A chronic disorder—of weeks, months, or years—may suggest a more chronic muscle or nerve problem, a congenital brain anomaly or meta-

Table 3.2.
Regional Localization—Examples of Specific Diseases

BRAIN	SPINAL CORD	ANTERIOR HORN CELL
Static encephalopathy	Meningomyelocele	Werdnig-Hoffmann disease
Down's syndrome	Tethered cord	Poliomyelitis
Hunter's syndrome	Spinal tumors	
Hurler's syndrome	Arteriovenous malformations	
Tay-Sachs disease		
Congenital anomalies		
Asphyxia		
Tumors		
PERIPHERAL NERVE	NERVE MUSCLE JUNCTION	MUSCLE
Polyneuritis	Myasthenia gravis	Duchenne dystrophy
Guillain-Barré syndrome	Botulism	Mitochondrial myopathy
Lyme disease		Fascioscapulohumeral dystrophy
Tick paralysis		Limb girdle dystrophy
AIDS		Steroid myopathy
Toxins		Nemaline rod myopathy
Hereditary sensory motor neuropathy		Myotonic dystrophy
		Polymyositis

Table 3.3.
History—Outline

Chief complaint
Chronology of present illness
Prenatal course
Neonatal course
Pattern of growth and development:
Motor
Speech
Fine motor
Adaptive
Past medical history:
Medicines
Allergies
Immunizations
Hospitalizations
Surgery
Behavioral history
School history
Family history
Review of systems—general
Review of systems—neurologic
(historical examination)

Table 3.4.
Developmental Milestones

BEHAVIOR	
1–2 months	Smiles
4 months	Expresses displeasure
6 months	Recognizes parents
8 months	Responds to "no"
10 months	"Patty-cake" and "Bye-Bye"
12 months	Understands names of objects
15 months	Imitates and requests by pointing
18 months	Follows simple commands
2 years	Organized play and body parts
LANGUAGE	
Birth	Cries
4 months	Sounds of pleasure
5 months	Primitive sounds "ah"
8 months	Syllables "baba, dada, mama"
12 months	2–3 words
2–3 years	Sentences
GROSS MOTOR	
Birth–1 month	Lifts head prone
3 months	Head control supine
5 months	Turns over
8 months	Sits without support
10 months	Crawls and stands
15 months	Walks alone
3½ years	Tricycle
6 years	Bicycle
HAND SKILLS	
Birth	Fists
3 months	Opens hands
4 months	Midline play
6 months	Reaches
7 months	Transfers
12 months	Pincer grasp
5 years	Rigid tripod pencil grip
8 years	Dynamic tripod pencil grip

bolic disease. Although the physician should also try to establish whether the process is a static or progressive one, the distinction can sometimes be difficult because a static brain lesion may produce what appears to be increasing impairment as a child gets older.

Neonatal Course. Lack of fetal movement in the last trimester suggests intrauterine weakness. Such weakness, which may be found at birth, can result from chronic anterior horn cell disease or congenital myopathy. Premature birth, as well as asphyxia in the full-term neonate, can result in a hypotonic (floppy) infant. Hypotonicity without weakness generally suggests a central rather than peripheral basis. Breech delivery is more frequent in infants with an early onset or intrauterine lower motor neuron disorder.

Growth and Development. An infant who is slow in the major developmental milestones (Table 3.4) is likely to have a cerebral injury. In contrast, one who is slow only in motor development is more likely to have a lower motor neuron disorder.

Past Medical History. Substance abuse, especially in adolescents, usually leads to central nervous system or systemic symptoms. Cocaine, amphetamine, and barbiturate abuse may lead to certain neuromuscular disorders. Heroin abuse gives rise to radiculopathy and myopathy. Glue sniffing may lead to neuropathy. Unintentional or occupational exposures to acromid and heavy metal may produce neuropathy. Infections, such as mononucleosis or Lyme disase, may explain peripheral as well as central disease. Similarly, AIDS in children can lead to nervous system disease that is more likely to be central than peripheral.

Family History.   Myotonic dystrophy, facio-scapulohumeral dystrophy, and certain types of Charcot-Marie-Tooth (CMT) disease are examples of autosomal dominant disorders in which successive generations are afflicted. Autosomal recessive disorders, such as Werdnig-Hoffmann disease, may also present with involvement of other family members. A few disorders, such as Duchenne muscular dystrophy, are X-linked recessive and may be present in other male family members. There are also other metabolic disorders, such as the MELAS syndrome (discussed below), that are inherited in a non-Mendelian manner through the variably affected mother's mitochondria and affect both boys and girls.

Review of the System.   This section provides information on both general and neurologic function. It is particularly important in children when specific information cannot be found easily during the actual examination. It characterizes the child's level of function and focuses the physical examination on certain areas.

PHYSICAL EXAMINATION

The physical examination documents abnormalities suggested in the history and determines specific localization (Table 3.5). The following comments refer to specific sections of the physical examination.

Table 3.5.
Physical Examination

NAME:		DATE:	
Head circumference Height		Weight	Vital Signs

Bruits
Skin
HEENT
Neck
Heart
Chest
Abdomen
Pulses
Extremities

NEUROLOGIC

   I. Developmental evaluation
  II. Motor
       Gait patterns
       Bulk, tone, strength, abnormal postures, abnormal movements
 III. Reflexes
       Deep tendon reflexes
       Babinski
 IV. Sensory
       Light touch, pain, position, vibration, graphesthesia, stereognosis
  V. Coordination
       Finger-to-nose, heel-to-shin, rapid alternating movements, ataxia, nystagmus
 VI. Cranial Nerves

Smell	Nystagmus
Visual acuity	Corneal
Visual fields	Facial
Fundus	Hearing
Pupils	Palate
Extraocular movements	Gag
Lids	Sternocleidomastoid
	Tongue

General Examination

Vital Signs.   Elevated temperature or pulse suggests systemic disease, including infection, collagen vascular disease, or drug fever. Cardiac involvement and cardiomyopathy may be seen in some chronic neuromuscular disorders. Difficulty breathing or hyperpnea may suggest bulbar palsy or weakness of the respiratory muscles from myasthenia gravis, Guillain-Barré syndrome, or advanced chronic myopathic disease.

Skin.   Drug rashes are usually red, macular, papillar, and often confluent, and they may involve the palms and soles. Linear itchy lesions located where clothes meet skin suggests tick bites, which can lead to tick paralysis or Lyme disease. Telangiectatic lesions on the extensor surfaces of joints are pathognomic of dermatomyositis. A malar butterfly rash suggests systemic lupus erythematosus (SLE). Joint pain and swelling are seen in Lyme disease and collagen vascular disease. Palpably enlarged nerves, such as the ulnar at the elbow and the peroneal at the knee, suggest a chronic peripheral neuropathy such as CMT.

HEENT Examination.   Abnormal facial features may be diagnostic. Congenital facial abnormalities are characteristic of certain syndromes, chromosomal anomalies, and neuromuscular diseases. Failure of the face to move in a normal fashion suggests bilateral facial weakness indicative of chronic myopathies and some acute neuropathies. A long, expressionless face suggests a myopathic process. A lack of facial movement may be mistaken for a sign of depression.

Extremities.   A chronic orthopedic deformity, such as contractures or short limbs, suggests an old poliomyelitis, which is rare today in young people, or a chronic neuromuscular process. Scoliosis, which is often idiopathic in adolescent girls, should prompt an investigation for vertebral anomalies or neuromuscular diseases. Foot deformities should be noted. For example, equinovarus deformities acquired at birth may be seen in congenital myopathies and early-onset myotonic dystrophy. Also, pes cavus, an imbalance of the intrinsic foot musculature, is observed in chronic neuropathies, such as CMT, and some spinocerebellar degenerative diseases, such as Friedreich's ataxia.

Abdomen.   Hepatosplenomegaly may be indicative of systemic diseases, such as mononucleosis; chronic diseases, such as AIDS; or some storage diseases with neurologic aspects, such as mucopolysaccharidosis.

Neurologic Examination

Developmental Examination.   Abnormalities in the developmental examination often indicate cortical as well as peripheral neuromuscular dysfunction.

Motor Examination.   Much of the motor examination is best completed by observation of infants and young children. Initially, the physician should observe the child's walk, because gait patterns are a guide to normal development and abnormalities may suggest certain neurologic conditions.

A normal toddler by 13 to 18 months should be walking steadily on a slightly wide-based gait with only occasional stumbling or falling. He should be running by 18 to 24 months; climbing stairs with support by 2 years; and climbing independently, with alternation of feet, by 3. He should be able to stand from a sitting position without needing to be pulled up or climbing up himself (Gowers' signs) by 18 months—unless she is very obese or has proximal weakness.

Abnormal gaits that should arouse suspicion are a waddle, a slapping gait (heard as well as seen), toe walking, and an ataxic gait. Abnormal postures include increased lumbar lordosis and genu recurvatum (hyperextension of the knee, giving the leg a backward curve at the knee)—they imply muscle weakness from myopathy or anterior horn cell disease.

Lower Extremities.   Detecting mild weakness in older children may be difficult. Even a weakened child's legs may be more powerful than the examiner's arms. It is important to discern whether the weakness is predominantly proximal or distal. Proximal (hip) muscles are tested by asking the patient to move against the resistance of the examiner's hands. The testing can also be done by asking the patient to rise from a knee-squat position or by eliciting a Gowers' sign. Distal (ankle and knee) muscles are similarly tested against resistance by asking the patient to heel- or toe-walk.

Upper Extremities. Strength of the shoulder girdle is tested by looking for muscle wasting and scapular winging. The muscles are then tested against gravity by asking the child to extend the arms. The muscles are then tested against resistance. The muscles of the elbow and and wrist joints are tested against extension and flexion. The fingers are hard to test, but poor grip and wasting in the palmar, thenar, and hypothenar areas suggest intrinsic hand muscle weakness.

The importance of distinguishing between proximal and distal weakness is that most myopathic and anterior horn cell weakness is proximal and, in contrast, peripheral nerve disorder weakness is distal. The few exceptions to the rule are the ones to learn. Myotonic dystrophy is the only common myopathy with predominantly distal weakness. Of the neuropathies, Guillain-Barré syndrome is sometimes proximal. Diphtheria, rare in this country, starts in the oral and facial muscles, and spreads centripetally—proximally to distally.

Sensory Findings. Anterior horn cell diseases, myoneural processes, and muscle diseases should be devoid of sensory findings, except for muscle tenderness is acute polymyositis or dermatomyositis. However, sensory abnormalities can be found in neuropathies, where they usually have a "stocking-glove" distribution, with loss of sensation of temperature, light touch, position, and vibration. Since a good, reproducible sensory examination may be difficult to obtain in children, inconsistent results should be almost disregarded.

Cranial Nerves. Persistent bilateral ptosis often indicates a myopathic disease. Variable ptosis after the child looks up and down a few times points to myasthenia. Failure of tight closure of the lids with good effort points to neurogenic or muscular facial weakness. A squint that changes is not paralytic and is probably visual. On the other hand, a squint that is fixed or paralytic indicates myasthenia, myopathy, or a brainstem disorder. Optic fundus changes do not usually reflect neuromuscular disease, but retinitis pigmentosa may suggest a metabolic myopathy. Papilledema and optic atrophy usually suggest central pathology; however, optic atrophy may be seen in hereditary leukodystrophy with neuropathy. Bulbar weakness, with changes of voice, swallowing, and drooling may be central or peripheral. Pseudobulbar palsy with a normal-appearing tongue and brisk gag reflex may be due to cerebral or high brainstem involvement; whereas bulbar palsy, with a wasted tongue and depressed or absent gag reflex, suggests anterior horn cell disease, myopathy, or myasthenia. Tongue fasciculations, wormlike spontaneous fine movements, definitely point to disorders of the anterior horn cells of the lower brainstem.

Psychogenic Findings. When the examination does not show a consistent anatomic pattern that suggests one or more common neuromuscular diseases, the physician should consider that the findings may be psychogenic. For example, of the many bizarre gaits that cannot be explained by either motor or cerebellar findings, the best known psychogenic gait disturbance is astasia-abasia. In this disturbance a child staggers from pillar to post but never falls, does not suffer serious injury, and exhibits neither ataxia nor weakness of individual muscles. Some patients with psychogenic weakness appear to be totally paralyzed. All of these conditions can confound the most experienced examiner.

Laboratory

The basic laboratory investigations include an assessment of muscle enzymes, electrophysiologic studies, and muscle biopsy. Specific diagnostic testing may be confirmatory. Genetic molecular biologic techniques, which are now available, are described.

Serum transaminase (SGOT), lactic acid dehydrogenase (LDH), aldolase, and creatinephosphokinase (CPK) are elevated in any disease that causes destruction of striated muscle. CPK is the most sensitive indicator of muscle damage. Marked CPK elevations occur in the muscular dystrophies, particular the Duchenne and Becker varieties, myositis, and severe muscle injury. Although elevations of CPK are important, normal CPK levels do not exclude neuromuscular disease.

Electrodiagnostic testing, which is extremely useful in neuromuscular disease, includes the measurement of nerve conduction velocities (NCV), needle electromyography (EMG) studies, and other special techniques. NCV is normal in diseases of the anterior horn cell, neuromuscular junction, and muscle. Abnormal NCV is seen in neuropathies (Aminoff, 1986). The interpretation of results should be compared with standard values for a particular age group (Koenigsberger, 1981): NCV is normally slower in children than adults.

EMG needle studies often separate a neurogenic from a myopathic process. Neurogenic findings include fibrillations, sharp waves, and fasciculations. In myopathic processes, motor units are abnormally small and polyphasic but normal in numbers. Myopathic features in EMGs are seen in inflammatory myopathy and muscular dystrophy; however, congenital myopathy frequently demonstrates normal EMGs. In acute inflammatory myopathy (i.e., polymyositis), fibrillations and positive sharp waves resembling neurogenic findings may be seen. Myotonia on insertion of the needle into a muscle, with resulting decrescendo positive waves on the monitor, accompanied by a dive-bomber sound, is characteristic of myotonic dystrophy, but it may be seen in storage disease and periodic paralysis (Aminoff, 1986).

Repetitive stimulation techniques are useful in diagnosing myoneural junction disorders. In myasthenia gravis, repetitive stimulation at low frequencies shows a decremental response (fatigue) of the evoked muscle. In botulism, the contrary may happen: repetitive stimulation at high rates provokes an incremental response from an increased release of acetylcholine (Aminoff, 1986).

The edrophonium (Tensilon) test is a pharmacologic means to diagnosis myasthenia gravis. In this illness, weakness temporarily improves within a minute after intravenous injection of edrophonium. Atropine should be available at the time of testing to counteract any unpleasant muscarinic effects of the edrophonium.

Muscle biopsy is essential to confirm a diagnosis of muscle disease. A myopathic, neuropathic, and sometimes a normal, biopsy may be obtained. In addition, in some patients with peripheral nerve disease, nerve biopsy may be indicated to obtain a specific diagnosis.

SPECIFIC DISEASES
Anterior Horn Cell Disease

HRONIC

The prototype of anterior horn cell disease in children is spinal muscular atrophy. This illness, often known by its eponym, Werdnig-Hoffmann disease, is inherited in an autosomal recessive manner that characteristically presents with the floppy infant syndrome (Dubowitz, 1978). Spinal muscular atrophy causes symptoms and signs 2 to 3 months or earlier after birth. Weakness is generalized, symmetric, and slightly more proximal than distal. Swallowing and respiratory difficulties are evident early. Tongue fasciulations, which are practically pathognomonic when present, are evident in about one-half of cases. The diagnosis is confirmed by an EMG showing neuropathic changes with normal motor conduction velocities and a muscle biopsy showing neurogenic atrophy.

Children with early-onset spinal muscular atrophy are unlikely to survive beyond 2 years. They usually die of pneumonia from bulbar or respiratory muscle weakness. However, milder forms of spinal muscular atrophy can become evident after 1 year of age, and even in the first and second decade. When the disease develops after the child is walking, it has a very slow progression and is known as Kugelberg-Welander syndrome (Dubowitz, 1978; Kugelberg et al., 1956). Described originally by its Swedish authors as a form of anterior horn cell disease resembling muscular dystrophy, this illness presents with a slow onset of proximal weakness. The main symptoms are difficulty in running, climbing stairs, and lifting heavy objects. The physical findings are proximal weakness, hypo- or areflexia, and fasciculations of tongue and axial musculature. These children frequently are alert and have normal intellectual function. The disease resembles limb-girdle dystrophy, but serum CPK is, at most, only mildly elevated. EMG studies, as with Werdnig-Hoffmann disease, sometimes show fasciculations. These studies and a neurogenic muscle biopsy make the distinction from dystrophy. Recently, in the more chronic forms of anterior horn cell disease, the locus for the disease has been found on the long arm of chromosome 5 (Brzustowicz, et al., 1990). The course is variably progressive over many years, but it eventually leads to a wheelchair. Longevity depends on the degree of respiratory muscle involvement.

ACUTE

Acute anterior horn cell disease, which was rampant before poliomyelitis immunization, is now rare. Most current cases are vaccine-related (Sutter et al., 1989). Fever with upper respiratory symptoms is followed in 2 to 5 days by meningeal signs. During this preparalytic stage, children may have headache, confusion, irritability, and emotional instability. They quickly progress to a paralytic stage. The clinical picture of asymmetric paralysis with depressed or absent reflexes and normal mental status is indicative of poliomyelitis (Price et al., 1978), although some echoviruses and other summer viruses (Chonmaitree et al., 1981) can present in this manner. The diagnosis is made by finding cells (mainly mononuclear) in the cerebrospinal fluid and culture or serologic evidence of the virus in throat, stool, or blood. Prognosis ranges from minimal deficit in most cases to severe and permanent paralysis in some. A very small number of children die when the anterior horn cells of the medulla become infected (i.e., bulbar poliomyelitis).

Peripheral Nerve Disease

Acquired peripheral nerve diseases usually present in an acute or subacute manner. Hereditary peripheral nerve diseases usually have an insidious presentation and a chronic course.

ACUTE AND SUBACUTE NEUROPATHIES

Acute postinfectious polyneuritis, commonly called Guillain-Barré syndrome (Fenichel, 1988), is the most common acute neuropathy encountered in this country. It can evolve over a few days to a few weeks. All physcians should be aware of its manifestations, since proper recognition and supportive care can prevent death. The disease has its onset 7 to 14 days following an acute, but often mild, upper viral respiratory or gastrointestinal syndrome. Many viruses and bacteria have been implicated. Weakness usually begins in the feet and ascends at a variable rate to involve the hands and arms. The facial muscles are involved in 50% of cases. In 10 to 15% of cases there is involvement of the bulbar and respiratory muscles, which can cause morbidity and death. Examination reveals distal weakness, areflexia, leg and back tenderness, and, probably from radiculitis, pain on straight leg raising. There is no alteration in consciousness. With severe leg weakness, incontinence, and a sensory level, the diagnosis of acute transverse myelitis should be considered.

The disease plateaus in 2 to 3 weeks, remains static for a time, and finally slowly starts to improve. Early in the disease the cerebrospinal fluid (CSF) may be normal, but then it develops a cytoalbuminologic dissociation (normal cell count with protein elevation in the 100 to 300 mg/dl range). In most cases, bed rest with careful observation is the only therapy needed. Until the illness plateaus, the patient should be observed in an intensive care unit so that supportive measures, such as tracheostomy and ventilation, can be administered. If the disease is diagnosed within 7 to 10 days from its onset, plasmapheresis may prevent progression of the disease and shorten ventilatory dependence and hospitalization (Guillain-Barré Study Group, 1985). More recently, intravenous gamma globulin has been helpful in some cases.

Other infections can cause an acute neuropathy. Diphtheria-induced polyneuritis (Dyck et al., 1984), now rare in this country, can be distinguished from Guillain-Barré syndrome by a history of incomplete immunization, a longer interval—up to 6 weeks—following a respiratory infection, and paresis of ocular accommodation. These patients often develop carditis.

Epstein-Barr virus infection can cause an acute polyneuritic syndrome with pharyngitis, adenopathy, hepatosplenomegaly, and peripheral neuropathy that is indistinguishable from any other postinfectious neuropathy. Alternatively, it can cause a chronic fatigue syndrome. The diagnosis can be confirmed by serology against Epstein-Barr virus.

Lyme disease (Steere, 1989), an infection with a spirochete, Borrelia burgdorferi, transmitted to man by Ixodes ticks, causes polyneuritis, VIIth nerve palsies (Bell's palsy), and meningitis. It can also cause a pure sensory neuropathy with dysesthesias of the hands and feet. Exposure to ticks, migrating rashes, and joint involvement suggest Lyme disease. Serologic testing for Lyme antibody titres (both IgG and IgM) can confirm the diagnosis. In early stages of the illness, oral tetracycline, amoxicillin, or erythromycin are ef-

fective, but with neurologic involvement, intravenous cetriaxone or penicillin is recommended. Interestingly, a larger tick, Dermacentor variabilis, causes an acute ascending neuropathy only while it is attached to the child's body, usually in the hair. This "tick paralysis" remits rapidly once the tick is removed (Brooke, 1986; Swift et al., 1975).

Neuropathy is a well-recognized complication of adults with human immunodeficiency virus type I (HIV-I) infection (Bailey et al., 1988), but so far it has not been clearly documented in children (Belman, 1990).

Among the hereditary neuropathies that can present acutely, porphyria-induced polyneuropathy is of particular interest to psychiatrists (Becker et al., 1977). This disorder, usually dominantly inherited, is usually not observed before the teenage years. Psychiatric disturbance, especially psychotic behavior, and abdominal pain usually accompany a Guillain-Barré like neuropathy, Crisis and exacerbations of the porphyria-induced constellation may be set off by barbiturates and other drugs. The diagnosis is confirmed by elevated urine porphobilinogen and delta-aminolevulinic acid levels. Treatment with intravenous glucose and hematin has been reported to relieve the symptoms.

The heavy metals, ingested or inhaled accidentally, may lead to acute, subacute, and even chronic neuropathy. Common examples are arsenic in rat poisons; lead in paint chips from old buildings, lead smelters, and old batteries; mercury in skin medications, tooth powders, and fish from contaminated waters; and thallium, also in rat poisons (Heyman et al., 1956; Miyakawa et al., 1970, Bank et al., 1972). Before neuropathy is evident, these heavy metals give rise to rashes, alopecia, gastrointestinal disorders, and systemic illness. Lead usually causes encephalopathy in young children, but it may produce a neuropathy characterized by wrist drop in the older child and adolescent (Fenichel, 1988; Dyck et al., 1984).

Toxic substances taken by adolescents for

"highs," as well as prescribed medications, also cause acute or subacute neuropathy. N-hexane and toluene (glue-sniffing) and methyl N-butyl ketone are among several industrial solvents inhaled for pleasure by adolescents that cause a subacute neuropathy with distal weakness (Towfigli et al., 1976; Editorial, 1979). Opium derivatives, particularly heroin (Richter et al., 1973), have reportedly led to painful radiculitis as well as acute peripheral neuropathy.

Chronic abuse of high doses of vitamin B_6 can cause a sensory neuropathy. On the other hand, adolescents treated for tuberculosis with isoniazid may develop polyneuropathy from lack of B_6 (Rowland, 1989). Nitrofurantoin, in patients with chronic renal disease, causes neuropathy. Lastly, certain drugs used for chemotherapy of childhood malignancies and leukemia, particularly vincristine and cisplatin, almost always lead to areflexia and sometimes to distal weakness (Kaplan, 1982).

Chronic Neuropathies

The most common disorders of the hereditary chronic peripheral neuropathies (Dyck et al., 1984), now designated as hereditary sensory and motor neuropathies (HSMN Types I–V or more), are Charcot-Marie-Tooth disease (CMT) and peroneal muscular atrophy (particularly Type I [HSMNs Type I and II]) (Hagberg et al., 1981). These disorders present in the first decade well into advanced adulthood. In children and adolescents, the main difficulty is in awkward gait, toe walking, frequent falling, and an inability to stand still. The main findings may be orthopedic or neurologic. The most common skeletal finding is a very arched foot, "pes cavus," or curling of the toes, "hammer toes," resulting from weakness and imbalance in the intrinsic foot musculature. The feet may be in an "equinus" position, in which patients are unable to get off their toes because weak peroneal muscles are overcome by the more intact gastrocnemius muscles. The foot deformities result in

the patient's inability to stand still, and the wasting of the lower leg muscles may result in a "stork" or "inverted champagne bottle" appearance of the lower legs. These deformities may lead to a "steeping gait," in which the patient may have to lift the legs high with each step to avoid tripping. If the deformities are not too fixed or severe, a slapping gait, heard as well as seen, ensues. As the disease progresses very slowly, weakness and wasting of the hand and later the paraspinal muscles results in a progressive scoliosis. Deep tendon reflexes, particularly those at the ankles, are frequently absent. There may be a stocking-glove sensory impairment. Enlarged peroneal nerves may be palpable.

Both Types I and II of HSMN are usually dominantly inherited; however, rare sporadic, autosomal recessive, and X-linked recessive cases are also observed. The diagnosis of Type I is confirmed by finding severely reduced motor and sensory conduction velocities (suggesting demyelination), neuropathic EMG findings (fibrillations, positive waves, and a reduced interference pattern), and elevated spinal fluid protein. In Type II, nerve conduction is usually normal or slightly decreased; however, neurogenic findings are apparent in EMGs. If the diagnosis is in doubt, a nerve biopsy can confirm and differentiate the two entities (Harding and Thomas, 1980).

The differential diagnosis includes Friedreich's ataxia, in which areflexia is combined with Babinski signs and prominent ataxia. This disease is rapidly progressive during the second decade, and it may induce mental change, depression, and psychosis. Other forms of HSMN are usually obviously different. Type III, Déjérine-Sottas disease (Ouvrier et al., 1987), is rapidly progressive in the first decade and causes a very high CSF protein. Type IV, Refsum's disease, is extremely rare and causes ichthyosis of skin, deafness, and retinitis pigmentosa (Dyck et al., 1984). Type V, sensorimotor neuropathy with progressive spastic paraplegia (Dyck et al., 1984), has spasticity and increased tendon reflexes, although it may superficially resemble the two types of CMT on first inspection.

Chronic relapsing polyneuritis, important although rare, is often amenable to treatment (Dyck et al., 1984; Dalakas and Engel, 1981). It most likely presents like an ordinary Guillain-Barré syndrome, but then either fails to improve or runs a relapsing course. When steroids or other immunosuppressants are administered, the process usually improves, but the patient may remain medication-dependent. Recently, a number of these cases have been successfully treated with intravenous gamma globulin (van Doorn et al., 1990). Clues to the diagnosis are a persistent elevation of CSF protein concentration and NCV that is much slower than in Guillain-Barré syndrome.

Neuromuscular Junction Disease

JUVENILE MYASTHENIA GRAVIS

Myasthenia gravis, perhaps not quite the threat to life its name implies, may have its onset by age 10 in 4% of patients and before the age of 20 in 24% of patients (Fenichel, 1988; Engel, 1984; Rodriguez et al., 1983). A number of familial syndromes have been described, most of which present at birth or in infancy (Engel, 1984). Juvenile myasthenia, an acquired disease, is a treatable entity that may mimic psychogenic disease. It is now thought to be an autoimmune disease caused by the production of autoantibodies directed toward the acetylcholine receptors (AChRs) at the neuromuscular junctions. The altered junctions produce weakness, particularly following strenuous or repetitive muscle use. As the disease progresses, usually slowly but sometimes very rapidly, the muscles become severely paretic after very little effort. The thymus is thought to be the source of the abnormal antibodies, consequently its removal may be curative. Although increased anti-AChR circulating antibodies confirm the diagnosis in 85% of cases, no clear relationship between the antibody titre and the severity of the disease has been established.

Although the eye muscles are frequently involved early in the disease, the signs and symptoms of myasthenia are variable. When the eye muscles are not involved or are only intermittently involved, the patient may be thought to have a "chronic fatigue syndrome," systemic disease, or psychogenic illness. To paraphrase Dubowitz (1978), a careful history usually reveals typical effects of muscle fatigability related to exertion, such as diplopia or ptosis brought on by prolonged visual activity, thickening or slurring of speech after prolonged use of any particular muscle group. Since symptoms typically have their onset after stress or psychogenic trauma and the examination may be normal during an initial evaluation, it is easy to understand why psychogenic disease may be suspected.

The neurologic examination usually reveals a variable degree of ptosis or extraocular muscle paralysis that may become more dramatic by making the patient look up and down or side to side. There may be weakness of the muscles of the jaw, neck, shoulder, and hip. The weakness, which is more proximal than distal, may be brought out by exercising a particular set of muscles. Reflexes are generally normal. If the weakness is not readily apparent, the diagnosis can be confirmed in the office by the injection of a choline esterase inhibitor such as edrophonium (Tensilon). More subtle weakness can be documented by the use of repetitive EMG stimulation, which shows a decrement of the evoked muscle action potential, and single fiber EMG (Aminoff, 1986). Increased levels of serum AChR receptor antibodies confirm the diagnosis. However, early in the disease, all laboratory tests may be negative.

Myasthenia gravis is ultimately a clinical diagnosis. The diffential diagnosis, which is short, includes psychogenic disease, metabolic myopathy, and remotely, brainstem neoplasms and multiple sclerosis. The Lambert-Eaton syndrome, due to remote effects of a neoplasm, resembles myasthenia in adults but has not been reported in children. Botulism is seen in infants

3 to 4 months of age after ingesting botulinum spores or organisms and in adults from eating toxin-contaminated foods (Fenichel, 1988; Guillain-Barré Study Group, 1985; Dyck et al., 1984; Sumaya, 1987; Steere, 1989; Brooke, 1986). It immediately results in neuromuscular blockade that follows gastrointestinal symptoms of constipation and results in total paralysis within hours. Botulism differs from myasthenia in the acuteness of the onset, involvement of pupillary muscles, and an EMG pattern that increases in amplitude, rather than decreases, as stimulation rates increase.

Some children may have ocular myasthenia that never progresses to generalized myasthenia and may or may not require therapy before its resolution. Once the disease becomes generalized, although anticholine esterase agents, such as neostigmine and pyridostigmine, may alleviate symptoms temporarily, modern therapy now suggests a more aggressive treatment. After a relatively short period using high-dose steroids or plasmapheresis to bring the patient to optimal status, patients undergo a surgical thymectomy. After the thymectomy, juvenile myasthenia recovers partly or fully over a few months to 5 years. Although anticholine esterase agents may be needed after thymectomy, the disease should no longer cause significant mortality.

Myopathies

Diseases that affect the muscle directly, the myopathies, may be inherited or acquired. The inherited myopathies may be divided into three broad groups: the congenital myopathies, metabolic myopathies, and dystrophies. Myositis is acquired.

CONGENITAL MYOPATHIES

The congenital myopathies (Dubowitz, 1978; Brooke, 1986) are a group of generally nonprogressive entities that frequently present at birth with the floppy infant syndrome. Neonates have difficulty feeding and breathing and have a weak cry. They have a myopathic facies, with little facial expression, sometimes with ptosis, extraocular muscle paresis, and generalized hypotonia, and suppressed or absent deep tendon reflexes. These children, who ordinarily have normal intelligence, go on to achieve most of their motor milestones at a delayed age, but they may show residual weakness and secondary orthopedic deformities.

The EMG may be myopathic or normal. CPK levels are usually within the normal range; however, the muscle biopsy often shows specific morphologic abnormalities. Among these abnormalities are fibers with a central defect (central core disease); central nuclei (myotubular myopathy); or inclusion rods (nemaline myopathy).

One other illness in which the biopsy may be normal or nonspecifically abnormal is the Prader-Willi syndrome. It presents with severe hypotonia at birth and at the age of 3 years with the "HHHO" constellation (hypomentia, hypogonadism, hypotonia, and obesity). Many of these children are mentally deficient. They can be diagnosed by the HHHO constellation, an almond-like facies, and small hands and feet. Many have a deletion in the long arm of chromosome 15 (Butler and Palmer, 1983).

METABOLIC MYOPATHIES

McArdle's syndrome (Dubowitz, 1978; Brooke, 1986), a glycogen storage disease type V, may present in adolescence with chronic fatigue, cramps, and myoglobinuria. Although their examination may be normal, muscle biopsies of affected children contain excess glycogen. The accumulation of glycogen is due to an absence of muscle phosphorylase which leads to an inability to metabolize glucose and release lactate during muscle activity. A form of lipid myopathy due to carnitine palmotyl transferase deficiency can present with the same features as McArdle's syndrome (Brooke, 1986). The muscle biopsy shows excess lipid droplets.

A host of mitochondrial myopathies with abnormal or deficient mitochondria have recently been elucidated (DiMauro et al., 1985). In these conditions, a lack of electron transport, which is required to sustain energy, leads to improper metabolism. In the entity with the acronym MELAS (mitochondrial myopathy, encephalopathy, lactic acidosis, and stroke-like episodes) (Pavlakis et al., 1984), symptoms may be either muscular weakness with extraocular involvement, or central with migraine headaches and stroke-like syndromes. Serum lactic and pyruvic acids are elevated, and muscle biopsy shows specific collections of clumped mitochondria known as ragged red fibers. Biochemical analysis of a muscle biopsy may reveal the precise enzymatic error in the deficient mitochondria (Ichiki et al., 1988). Some mitochondrial myopathies may be treated with coenzyme Q (Ogasahara et al., 1986).

MUSCULAR DYSTROPHIES

The muscular dystrophies are a heterogeneous group of muscle diseases that are usually inherited but occasionally occur sporadically. Duchenne muscular dystrophy (DMD) and myotonic dystrophy are the two most common dystrophies with which the child psychiatrist should be familiar, because the illnesses are common, present in childhood, and may have mental symptoms (Dubowitz, 1978; Brooke, 1986).

DMD is an X-linked recessive disease that is inherited by boys through their carrier mother. It has been in the limelight because advances in molecular genetics have localized the Duchenne genetic defect to the short arm of the X chromosome at Xp21 (Hyser and Mendell, 1988). The absence of the normal gene product dystrophin, a muscle protein, appears to be responsible for the disease, although the exact mechanism has not been elucidated (Hyser and Mendell, 1988; Hoffman et al., 1989).

Boys with DMD may be normal or slightly slow in their milestones in the first 2 years. Then they have trouble running, climbing stairs, and getting off the floor without using their arms. Examination usually reveals normal facial musculature, perhaps some proxial arm muscle weakness, and definite proximal leg weakness best exemplified by a waddling gait and having to climb up their legs to stand from a sitting position (Gowers' sign). The boys may have distal leg weakness with toe walking and abnormally large, firm calves (pseudohypertrophy). Reflexes in the first few years may be normal. Approximately 30 to 50% of these children have subnormal intelligence (Dubowitz, 1978; Brooke, 1986; Hyser and Mendell, 1988).

The diagnosis is made by finding very elevated CPK levels in the serum. Aside from DMD, only dermatomyositis (below) and acute rhabdomyolysis can give such levels. The EMG is myopathic, and muscle biopsy reveals classic dystrophic changes with degeneration of muscle fibers and a lrage amount of replacement by fat and fibrosis. With the new genetic technology, two-thirds of cases will be shown to have the gene deletion or duplication. Unless the patient represents a spontaneous mutation, the carrier mother will also show the deletion.

Such testing is most useful in providing genetic counseling. In further pregnancies, the deletion may be detected in amniotic fluid cells. Linkage analysis of the family members also provides useful information (Hyser and Mendell, 1988). A deletion similar to that in DMD is found in Becker's dystrophy, an entity much like Duchenne dystrophy, whose onset is later in the first decade and whose course is more protracted (Dubowitz, 1978; Brooke, 1986; Hyser and Mendell, 1988; Hoffman et al., 1989). Dystrophin analysis in the muscles can distinguish these two entities.

Children with DMD usually lose ambulation near the end of the first decade. They become wheelchair dependent for the next 10 to 20 years, after which they succumb to pulmonary complications of progressive scoliosis and muscle weakness. Children with Becker's dystrophy may survive considerably longer.

Myotonic Dystrophy

Myotonic dystrophy is a multisystem disease transmitted as an autosomal dominant trait. The onset of symptoms is toward the end of the first decade, adolescence, or later. It is probably the most common of the dystrophies because many patients live long enough to reproduce.

A neonatal form is peculiar in that it occurs only in offspring of myotonic mothers (Harper, 1975). These children present as floppy infants with myotonic facies, ptosis, and ophthalmoparesis. They often have talipes equinovarus. If they survive the neonatal period, when respiratory complications may supervene, they have slow acquisition of milestones, physical handicaps, and, often, mental impairments.

When myotonic dystrophy is recognized at the end of the first decade, parents complain that the child is awkward, weak, or having learning problems. A syndrome complex of myotonic dystrophy which is rarely seen before the age of 30, includes weakness (due to dystrophy), a disturbance in muscle relaxation after forceful muscle contraction (myotonia), frontal baldness, cataracts, gonadal atrophy, multiple endocrinopathies, and variable mental retardations (Dubowitz, 1978; Brooke, 1986).

Children with myotonic dystrophy exhibit a long, myopathic facies with hollowed cheek regions and a degree of ptosis. Their face is characteristic and gives the impression of sadness. Frontal baldness may develop late in the second decade in both sexes. The muscular weakness is more distal than proximal, an exceptional finding in myopathies. Thus, an awkward slapping gait may be observed. In addition, myotonia may be exhibited by the child having difficulty letting go shaking hands. Myotonia can also be demonstrated by prolonged dimpling of the thenar muscles on percussion. The thumb can remain abducted for several seconds after the thenar muscles are struck. Likewise, excessive tongue dimpling can be demonstrated. If the patient does not demonstrate myotonia, then almost surely one of the parents will.

The diagnosis is made on EMG insertion when motor units wax and wane in decrescendo fashion and sound like dive-bombers. The EMG is critical because the muscle biopsy may be equivocal. Biopsies may not always show central nuclei, type I fiber atrophy (Brooke, 1986), or ringbinden (muscle fibrils oriented in the wrong plane). The genetic marker for myotonic dystrophy has recently been located on chromosome 19 (Pericak-Vance et al., 1986).

Treatment of myotonia can be accomplished with membrane stabilizing drugs, such as quinine, procainamide, phenytoin, and carbamazepine (Brooke, 1986). However, there is no treatment for the slowly progressive weakness except bracing and eventual respiratory support.

Other Dystrophies

Three other forms of dystrophy deserve brief mention. Facioscapulohumeral dystrophy (FSH), which has autosomal dominant inheritance (Brooke, 1986), usually has an onset in the second decade; however, with an affected parent, it can be recognized earlier. Weakness may start in the shoulder girdle or in the face. Patients may develop a change in facial expression, an inability to purse the lips to whistle, and subsequently, possible difficulty with speech. Leg weakness usually appears late in the disease in either the peroneal or quadriceps muscles. FSH is diagnosed by a myopathic EMG and muscle biopsy. The course of this syndrome is usually benign, with ambulation being preserved and normal longevity.

Limb-girdle dystrophy (Brooke, 1986), which may be dominant, recessive, or, most frequently, sporadic, may resemble late-onset Becker's dystrophy but without a male preponderance. There is a late first decade or teenage onset of proximal shoulder and leg muscle weakness and atrophy. CPK levels are moderately elevated, but not as high as in Duchenne's or Becker's dystrophy. Limb-girdle dystrophy should be differentiated from late-onset spinal muscular atrophy, metabolic and endocrine myopathies, and chronic polymyositis. The entity is slowly progressive and not as devastating as Duchenne's and Becker's dystrophies.

Finally, among the dystrophies, an X-linked recessive entity known as Emery-Dreifuss muscular dystrophy has an onset between 5 and 15 years of age (Merlini et al., 1986). It may be misclassified as a dystrophy because of atypical EMG and biopsy changes (Fenichel, 1988). Progressive contractures and a cardiomyopathy that may be treated with a pacemaker occur. CPK is moderately elevated. Recently, the genetic locus for this entity has been mapped on the long arm of the X chromosome at Xq26–q28 (Human Gene Mapping 10, 1989).

INFLAMMATORY ACQUIRED MYOPATHIES

With polymyositis being rare until the teenage years, dermatomyositis is the principal myositis observed in children (Brooke, 1986). Dermatomyositis was thought to be viral in origin because viral particles were sometimes observed in biopsies, but many authorities recently have thought the illness is more likely to be an autoimmune disorder (Whitaker, 1982). The illness presents after the first year of life with fever, lassitude, rash, muscle pain, and tenderness, and weakness that is proximal. The rash may be very particular, with heliotrope discoloration of the eyelids, sometimes with swelling in the periorbital area, and a scaly, telangiectatic rash over the extensor surfaces of joints, the knuckles, elbows, and knees. Serum erythrocyte sedimentation rate (ESR) is often elevated, and serum CPK is as dramatically high as in severe dystrophy. The illness is acute or subacute in presentation and, before the rash is evident, may be confused with rheumatic fever, systemic illness, collagen vascular disease, or leukemia. It is occasionally thought to be psychogenic.

The EMG is myopathic, and the biopsy shows perifascicular atrophy, inflammatory cell infiltration, and capillary necrosis. If treated early

with daily corticosteroids, which are subsequently given on alternate days to avoid long-term complications (even myopathy; see below), most patients respond in a few weeks. Some authorities believe that alternate day steroid therapy should be maintained for a least a year to avoid relapse. Untreated dermatomyositis can go on to severe wasting, contractures, and muscle calcification (Bowyer et al., 1982). Unlike the situation in adults, neoplasms or other collagen-vascular diseases seldom, if ever, underlie the disease. Polymyositis, with the same muscle involvement as dermatomyositis, is quite rare in children.

A painful myositis confined to the calves, which lasts less than a week, can occur in epidemic form in children. It is due often to an influenza virus (Fenichel, 1988). The CPK is markedly elevated. A painless myositis due to AIDS has been reported in children (L. Sharer, personal communication). In areas where raw pork is consumed, cysticercosis and trichinosis can produce a painful myositis with eosinophilia (Brooke, 1986).

Steroid Myopathy

Steroids are frequently used for treatment of many childhood diseases. Exogenous administration or excessive endogenous production of glucocorticoids can produce myopathy (Kaminski and Ruff, 1989). Approximately 2 to 21% of patients who receive steroids for more than 4 weeks develop muscle weakness sufficient to limit ambulation. The weakness involves the legs more than the arms. Also, it is generally more proximal than distal, and more severe in disused muscles. Cranial nerves are spared. Myalgia may be associated with weakness. Reflexes are normal or reduced. Muscle enzymes are frequently normal. EMG findings are variable. Muscle biopsy often shows type II fiber atrophy, aggregation of mitochondria, and vacuolization.

Steroids may produce changes in mental status, usually euphoria; however, depression and psychosis can also occur. Diffuse cognitive impairment is demonstrated in formal psychological testing (Kaminski and Ruff, 1989).

REFERENCES

Aminoff MJ, ed. Electrodiagnosis in clinical neurology, 2nd ed. New York: Churchill Livingstone, 1986.

Bailey RO, Baltch AL, Venkatesh R, et al. Sensory motor neuropathy associated with AIDS. Neurology 1988; 38:886–891.

Bank WJ, Pleasure DE, Suzuki D, et al. Thallium poisoning. Arch Neurol 1972;26:456–464.

Becker DM, Kramer S. The neurological manifestations of porphyria: a review. Medicine 1977;56:411–423.

Belman AL. AIDS and Pediatric Neurology. Neurol Clin 1990;8:571–603.

Bowyer SL, Blane CE, Sullivan DB, et al. Childhood dermatomyositis: factors predicting functional outcome and development of dystrophic calcification. J Pediatr 1982;103:882–888.

Brooke MH. A clinician's view of neuromuscular diseases, 2nd ed. Baltimore: Williams & Wilkins, 1986.

Brzustowicz LM, Lehner T, Castilla LH, et al. Genetic mapping of chronic childhood-onset spinal muscular atrophy to chromosome 5q11.2–13.3. Nature 1990;344:540–541.

Butler MG, Palmer CG. Parental origin of chromosome 15 deletion in Prader-Willi syndrome. Lancet 1983;1:1285.

Chonmaitree T, Menegus MA, Schheruish-Swierkosz EM, Schwalenstocker E. Enterovirus 71 infection: report of an outbreak with two cases of paralysis and a reivew of the literature. Pediatrics 1981;67:489–493.

Dalakas MC, Engel WK. Chronic relapsing (dysimmune) polyneuropathy: pathogenesis and treatment. Ann Neurol 1981;9:134–145.

DiMauro S, Bonilla E, Zeviani M, Nakagawa M, DeVivo DC. Mitochondrial myopathies. Ann Neurol 1985; 17:521–538.

Dubowitz V. Muscle disorders in childhood. In: Schaffer AJ, ed. Major problems in clinical pediatrics. 1st ed. London: WB Saunders, 1978, p. 16.

Dyck PJ, Thomas PK, Lambert EH, Bunge R, eds. Peripheral neuropathy. Philadelphia: WB Saunders, 1984.

Editorial. Hexacarbon neuropathy. Lancet 1979;2:942–943.

Engel AG. Myasthenia gravis and myasthenic syndromes. Ann Neurol 1984;16:519–534.

Fenichel GM. Clinical pediatric neurology. A signs and symptoms approach. Philadelphia: WB Saunders, 1988.

The Guillain-Barré Study Group: Plasmapheresis and acute Guillain-Barré syndrome. Neurology 1985;35:1096–1104.

Hagberg B, Lyon NG. Pooled European series of hereditary peripheral neuropathies in infancy and childhood. Neuropediatrics 1981;12:9–17.

Harding AE, Thomas PK. The clinical features of hereditary motor and sensory neuropathy types I and II. Brain 1980;103:259–280.

Harper PS. Congenital myotonic dystrophy in Britain. Arch Dis Child 1975;50:514–521.

Heyman A, Pfeiffer JB Jr, Willet RW, Taylor HM: Peripheral neuropathy caused by arsenical intoxication. N Engl J Med 1956;254:401–409.

Hoffman EP, Kunkel LM, Angelini C, Clarke A, Johnson M, Harris JB. Improved diagnosis of Becker muscular dystrophy by dystrophin testing. Neurology 1989; 39:1011–1017.

Human Gene Mapping 10. New Haven Conference (1989). Cytogenet Cell Genet 1989;51:419.

Hyser CL, Mendell JR. Recent Advances in Duchenne and Becker muscular dystrophy. Neurol Clin 1988;6:429–453.

Ichiki T, Tanaka M, Nishikimi M, et al. Deficiency of subunits of complex I and mitochondrial enceophalomyopathy. Ann Neurol 1988;23:287–294.

Kaminski HJ, Ruff RL. Neurologic complications of endocrine diseases. Neurol Clin 1989;7:489–508.

Kaplan RS, Wiernik PH. Neurotoxicity of antineoplastic drugs. Semin Oncol 1982;9:103–123.

Koenigsberger MR. Electrodiagnostic studies in infants and children. In: Kelly VC, ed. Practice of Pediatrics. Philadelphia: Harper & Row, 1981.

Kugelberg E, Welander L. Heredofamilial juvenile muscular atrophy simulating muscular dystrophy. Arch Neurol Psychiatry 1956;75:500–509.

Merlini L, Granata C, Dominici P, et al. Emery-Dreifuss muscular dystrophy: report of five cases in a family and review of the literature. Muscle Nerve 1986;9:481–485.

Miyakawa T, Deshimaru M, Sumiyoshi S, et al. Experimental organic mercury poisoning—pathological changes in peripheral nerves. Acta Neuropathol (Berl) 1970; 15:45–55.

Ogasahara S, Nishikaa Y, Yorifuji, et al. Treatment of Kearns-Sayre syndrome with coenzyme Q10. Neurology 1986;36:45–53.

Ouvrier RA, McLeod JG, Concin TE. The hypertrophic forms of hereditary motor and sensory neuropathy. A study of hypertrophic Charcot-Marie-Tooth disease (HMSN type I) and Dejerine-Sottas (HMSN type III) in childhood. Brain 1987;110:121–148.

Pavlakis S, Phillips PC, DiMauro S, DeVivo DC, Rowland LP. Mitochondrial myopathy, encephalopathy, lactic acidosis, and stroke like episodes. Ann Neurol 1984;16:481–488.

Pericak-Vance MA, Yamaoka LH, Assinder RIF, et al. Tight linkage of apolipoprotein C2 to myotonic dystrophy on chromosome 19. Neurology 1986;36:1418–1423.

Price RW, Plum F. Poliomyelitis. In: Vinken PJ, Bruyn GW, Klawans HL, eds. Handbook of clinical neurology. New York: Elsevier-North Holland, 1978;34:93–132.

Richter RW, Pearson J, Bruun B, et al. Neurological complications of heroin addiction. Bull NY Acad Med 1973;49:3–21.

Rodriguez M, Gomez MR, Howard FM, et al. Myasthenia gravis in children: Long term follow-up. Ann Neurol 1983;13:504–510.

Rowland LP, ed. Merritt's textbook of neurology. 8th ed. Philadelphia: Lea & Febiger, 1989.

Steere AC. Lyme disease. N Engl J Med 1989;321:586–596.

Sumaya CV. Epstein-Barr virus infections in children. Curr Probl Pediatr 1987;17:681–722.

Sutter RW, Brink EW, Cochi SL, et al. A new epidemiologic and laboratory classification system for paralytic polio-myelitis cases. Am J Public Health 1989;79:495–498.

Swift TR, Ignacio OJ. Tick paralysis: electrophysiologic studies. Neurology 1975;25:1130–1133.

Towfigli J, Gonatas N, Pleasure D, Cooper H, McCree L. Glue sniffer's neuropathy. Neurology 1976;26:238–243.

van Doorn PA, Brand A, Strengers PFW, Meulstee J, Vermeulen M. High-dose intravenous immunoglobulin treatment in chronic inflammatory demyelinating polyneuropoathy. Neurology 1990;40:209–212.

Whitaker JN. Inflammatory myopathy: a review of etiologic and pathogenetic factors. Muscle Nerve 1982;5:573–592.

Chapter 4

ATTENTION DEFICIT HYPERACTIVITY DISORDER

Gerald S. Golden, MD

Children with attention deficit hyperactivity disorder (ADHD) present with the cardinal features of inattention and impulsivity that are inappropriate for the child's developmental level. These symptoms frequently are associated with motor hyperactivity, especially in preschool and young school-age children. The behavior is often disruptive and is seen in all social settings, including at home, with peers, and in school.

Although there is general consensus that a biologic substrate for inattention is present in many children with this condition, there is no agreement as to its exact nature. The ability to attend to a stimulus first requires that the child be fully alert. If alertness is impaired, the desired stimulus may not be noted, and so it would not be perceived. The second requirement for maintaining effective attention is the ability to filter out irrelevant sensory stimuli. If competing stimuli are perceived and acted upon, there will be a loss of selective attention. Alertness gives the system sensitivity; the ability to ignore competing stimuli provides selectivity.

The underlying neurobiologic basis for alertness and attention is not fully understood. The reticular activating system appears to be important in maintaining attention. This system, involving the upper brainstem and hypothalmus, is central to integrating stimuli from the periphery and special sense organs and activating the cerebral cortex. Although this activation is essential for alert wakefulness, attention must be focused. This is aided by the inhibitory action of norepinephrine, derived largely from the locus ceruleus, which is also in the brainstem.

A previously popular but no longer used construct, "minimal brain dysfunction," implies that relatively minor degrees of brain damage can produce abnormalities in all areas of brain function that are unassociated with classic signs of neurologic disease. These abnormalities include ADHD, learning disabilities, soft signs on the neurologic examination, and an abnormal electroencephalogram (EEG). It is clear now that these clinical findings are not reliably interrelated and that very few of these children actually have had cerebral injuries from perinatal events or insults in later life.

Since first-degree relatives appear to be affected more than the general population, there may be a genetic component underlying the condition. Families of affected children also have an increased incidence of other psychiatric disorders.

PREVALENCE

In general, the prevalence is difficult to determine in any condition that depends entirely on a clinical diagnosis and for which there is no biologic marker. In some geographic areas, the diagnosis of ADHD is made in as many as 10% of all school-age boys. A recent study showed that 6% of all public school elementary students were receiving drug treatment for hyperactivity and inattentiveness (Safer and Krager, 1988). Stimulant drugs were prescribed in 99% of this group, and methylphenidate was the drug used in 93% of cases. The ratio of treated boys to girls was 5:1. The authors estimated that in 1987 at least 750,000 children were receiving drugs for ADHD.

In contrast, perhaps reflecting cultural differences in the frequency with which the diagnosis of ADHD is made, in Great Britain only 1.5% of school-age boys are given this diagnosis (Sandberg et al., 1978). The difference between the reported prevalence in the United States and that in the United Kingdom appears to be a bias toward the use of the diagnosis of ADHD in the United States and that of conduct disorders in Great Britain.

CLASSIFICATION

The DSM-III divided symptoms into three groups and provided descriptors for the types of behaviors: inattention, impulsivity, and hyperactivity. The diagnosis of attention deficit disorder required the presence of inattentiveness and impulsivity and could be made with or without associated hyperactivity. The DSM-III-R does not differentiate between symptoms in each of these three categories but lists 14 clinical features by the power with which they proved important in a national field trial (Table 4.1). At least eight of these features must be present and must have persisted for at least 6 months. The disorder always begins before 7 years of age. It is essential to remember that all of the behavioral symptoms should be compared with age-specific norms. Quantitative norms are not available, so clinical experience and judgment are required. The ability to sustain attention to a task and the ability to inhibit impulsive behaviors increase with age in all children. It is obvious that a

Table 4.1.
Features of ADHD[a]

Onset before age 7 years
Does not meet criteria for pervasive developmental
  disorder
Duration at least 6 months
At least eight of the following:
  1. Fidgets or squirms
  2. Has difficulty remaining seated
  3. Is easily distracted by extraneous stimuli
  4. Has difficulty awaiting turns
  5. Blurts out answers to questions
  6. Has difficulty following through on
     instructions
  7. Has difficulty sustaining attention
  8. Shifts from one activity to another
  9. Has difficulty playing quietly
  10. Talks excessively
  11. Interrupts or intrudes on others
  12. Does not seem to listen
  13. Loses things
  14. Engages in physically dangerous activities

[a] Adapted from American Psychiatric Association: Diagnostic and Statistical Manual of Mental Disorders, 3rd ed., revised, 1987.

normal 4-year-old child should not be expected to have the attention span of an 8-year-old. Differences in average activity levels between boys and girls should also be taken into account, as should the normal range of temperament and personality styles seen in children.

An aid to diagnosis is the use of scales that help to structure and quantitate the observations of parents, teachers, and other professionals. The Conners scales are the most commonly used (Conners, 1969; Wilson and Kiessling, 1988). These scales consist of a list of behaviors (e.g., disturbs other children), each of which is rated "not at all", "just a little", "pretty much", or "very much" (Table 4.2). Numeric values are given and a total score calculated; this is compared with a set of norms. There are a number of versions of varying length and complexity. In addition to providing assistance in the diagnostic process, these scales are useful for monitoring the response of individual children to treatment with drugs.

DIAGNOSIS

History

The behavioral history must focus on two central issues: what is the disruptive behavior, and when does it occur? These are not fully independent variables, but it is important to be certain that the problem behavior is not context-specific, which would imply that the symptoms are a response to environmental stress. The major complaint in the preschool child is typically that of excessive motor activity and, unless the child is in a structured preschool program, this complaint is voiced by the parents. The symptoms often are said to have started early in life, with the comment that the child never walked but went from crawling to running. Parents state that the child will never sit still or focus on any activity, even television, for more than a minute or two. Other complaints are that the child will not follow instructions, tends to break things, is accident prone, and does not respond to the usual disciplinary methods.

If the child is in a preschool program, there are often complaints of disruptive behavior, interference with the work of others as a result of intrusive or aggressive behavior, and failure to attend and to complete assignments. The child is frequently disciplined for moving about the room rather than staying at his or her desk. It should be noted that at this age, as is the case with older children, there is some overlap in the symptoms of ADHD and those of conduct disorder.

If these same symptoms continue into the school years, they interfere with academic progress and frequently lead to disciplinary action on the part of the school authorities. Inattentiveness, impulsivity, and motor hyperactivity are all viewed as negative characteristics in the classroom setting. Many children with ADHD have learning disabilities, and these may go unrecognized, with the failure to learn being blamed on the ADHD.

The core symptoms also continue into adolescence in many children. Impulsiveness is a major problem and frequently causes the child to have trouble with school or legal authorities. There is evidence now that these personality traits may continue into adulthood in some individuals.

If the abnormal behavior occurs only in one setting, either in school or at home, it suggests that ADHD is not present; rather similar symptoms are occurring as a result of inappropriate relationships and interactions in the affected setting. This can also occur if either the parent or teacher is not a good observer or has a serious misconception concerning the normal levels of attentiveness, impulsivity, and motor activity in a given age group. A useful approach to aid in sorting out the possibilities is to have both the teacher and the parent complete a structured scale and also provide a narrative statement of the child's general level of function and the disruptive behaviors.

Risk Factors

The issue of biologic risk factors underlying the production of ADHD is not clearly settled. As noted, there are significant questions about the validity of the construct of minimal brain dysfunction and the role of adverse perinatal events in the production of problems of behavior and learning. A number of specific neurologic conditions, such as fetal alcohol syndrome, seem to have an association with symptoms similar to ADHD. However, the issue is often clouded by subnormal intelligence and its effect on learning and behavior, as well as the need to examine the attention span as a function of mental, rather than chronologic, age. Although there have been attempts to correlate many biologic risk factors with ADHD, most of the relationships are weak or nonspecific (Rapoport and Ferguson, 1981).

There is current interest concerning possible long-term effects of low-level lead exposure on cognition and behavior of children. A relation-

Table 4.2.
Abbreviated Parent-Teacher Questionnaire[a]

Patient Name _____   Patient Number _____

Study Number _____

Parent's Observations

Information obtained _____   by _____
Month   Day   Year

Observation	Degree of Activity			
	Not at all	Just a little	Pretty much	Very much
1. Restless or overactive				
2. Excitable, impulsive				
3. Disturbs other children				
4. Fails to finish things he starts—short attention span				
5. Constantly fidgeting				
6. Inattentive, easily distracted				
7. Demands must be met immediately—easily frustrated				
8. Cries often and easily				
9. Mood changes quickly and drastically				
10. Temper outbursts, explosive and unpredictable behavior				

Teacher's Observations

Information obtained _____   by _____
Month   Day   Year

Observation	Degree of Activity			
	Not at all	Just a little	Pretty much	Very much
1. Restless or overactive				
2. Excitable, impulsive				
3. Disturbs other children				
4. Fails to finish things he starts—short attention span				
5. Constantly fidgeting				
6. Inattentive, easily distracted				
7. Demands must be met immediately—easily frustrated				
8. Cries often and easily				
9. Mood changes quickly and drastically				
10. Temper outbursts, explosive and unpredictable behavior				

Table 4.2.   (*Continued*)
Abbreviated Parent-Teacher Questionnaire[a]

Other Observations of Parent or Teacher (Use reverse side if more space is required)

_____

_____

_____

_____

_____

[a] From Conners CK: Rating scales for use in drug studies with children. *Psychopharmacol Bull* 9 (Special Issue): 24–84, 1973, with permission.

ship between elevated lead levels and hyperactivity was suggested by David et al. (1976). More recent research has confirmed that permanent deficits in school performance and a number of neuropsychologic measures do occur (Needleman et al., 1990). Deficits in memory and concentration, but not attention, have also been defined (Faust and Brown, 1987). It would seem, therefore, that low lead levels can impair performance and behavior in school but do not produce a typical picture of ADHD.

Sociocultural risk factors are somewhat clearer, since the child under significant stress for any reason will manifest symptoms of ADHD. These problems should be explored as part of the initial history and include intrafamilial stresses, family disorganization, physical or sexual abuse, peer group influences, and a mismatch between the child's personality and the expectations of the school or home setting.

Physical Examination

After the behavioral history has been obtained, it is important to perform a general medical history and physical examination. Unrecognized impairment of vision or hearing can be associated with symptoms similar to those found in ADHD and can cause poor scholastic performance. Screening evaluation of these functions should always be carried out. Children with any type of chronic illness, such as renal insufficiency, asthma, or congenital heart disease may also have difficulty in maintaining concentration. Reasons for this difficulty include factors such as chronic fatigue, decreased exercise tolerance, and dyspnea. Certain chronic illnesses, especially renal and hepatic disease, may also be associated with some degree of metabolic encephalopathy. These disorders should be recognized and treated or the child referred for appropriate treatment. If the child is taking medication for any reason, side effects of the drug could produce behavioral symptoms. Sedative drugs, psychotropic agents, and anticonvulsants, especially barbiturates, can all have adverse effects on behavior and learning.

Occasionally, the history will suggest the presence of a seizure disorder, or evidence of seizures will be found during the examination. These are most typically absence or partial complex seizures and, if frequent, may present as an abnormality in behavior or cognition.

A standard neurologic examination should be performed next. Although this rarely defines an underlying problem as the cause of ADHD, it may reveal the presence of a previously unrecognized neurologic disorder such as cerebral palsy. In rare instances, evidence of a neurodegenerative disorder, with progressive change in cognitive and behavioral function, is found.

Soft signs can best be defined as abnormalities in motor function that are abnormal only as a function of the child's age. The most commonly tested functions are coordination, rapid repetitive movements, ability to maintain fixed postures, and balance. Structured examinations have been developed that set performance criteria and allow for semiquantitative assessment of performance (Shaywitz et al., 1984). However, many clinicians rely on qualitative descriptors, with norms based on their clinical experience. It is essential to remember that motor skills, like cognitive abilities, improve with age. As a general guideline, motor performance in the areas tested begins to mature by age 7 years; by age 10 years, the child should perform nearly as well as an adult.

A second group of soft signs, which can be differentiated from the developmental soft signs, is defined by the presence of neurologic abnormalities found on examination but unassociated with functional impairment. An example is the presence of a unilateral Babinski sign or reflex asymmetry with no other evidence of a hemiparesis.

Severe impairment of motor skills occurs in children with developmental dyspraxia. This is defined as difficulty in planning or carrying out skilled purposeful movements in the absence of weakness, spasticity, ataxia, or a sensory deficit. Dyspraxic children are extremely clumsy and do not improve rapidly, even with optimal physical and occupational therapy.

Children with ADHD and learning disabilities may or may not show soft signs, and so these findings have no specific diagnostic utility (Shaywitz et al., 1984). However, these signs are important as markers for abnormal motor skills that may have an adverse impact on tasks that require an intact motor system (Landman et al., 1986). In school, the child may have difficulty with writing and, occasionally, spelling. Inadequate athletic abilities are a source of difficulties with peers and may further impair self-esteem in a child who already has a poor self-image.

Rapid assessment of cognitive function should be carried out if these data are not available through school reports or previous psychological tests. It is important to determine whether the child's general cognitive level is normal or close to normal, since the behavior expected of the child with mental retardation is different from that seen in the normal child. Instruments useful for the preschool child are the Denver Developmental Screening Test and the Peabody Picture Vocabulary Test. The Denver Developmental Screening Test uses historical and examination data to assess the child's performance in the gross motor, fine motor/adaptive, personal-social, and language areas. This is a screening test and if a failure occurs, the child should be referred for a more complete evaluation. The Peabody Picture Vocabulary Test relies on a series of pictures to evaluate the child's vocabulary and receptive language skills. Although the results of this test often give a good approximation of the child's verbal IQ, the data should be viewed with caution.

Children who are in school can be given a test of school achievement such as the Wide Range Achievement Test, and cognitive tests such as the Peabody Picture Vocabulary Test and Raven's Progressive Matrices. This latter examination tests increasingly complex cognitive skills ranging from visual matching to thinking by analogy. These examinations do not replace a full test battery administered and interpreted by a trained psychologist, but they can be used as part of the initial examination.

Laboratory Evaluation

Laboratory examinations do not provide primary diagnostic information concerning ADHD but can be used to help clarify the differential diagnosis and detect underlying neurologic or medical disorders. Routine tests such as complete blood count and urinalysis are not required unless the medical history suggests a specific problem.

Neuroimaging studies such as computed tomography (CT) scans or magnetic resonance imaging (MRI) of the head are unnecessary unless a specific indication is found on the history or neurologic examination. No diagnostic changes have been found in studies of children with ADHD (Caparulo et al., 1981). Although there may be abnormalities in some children with learning disabilities, the findings currently have interest for research but no clinical utility.

Electroencephalography also has no place as a routine diagnostic procedure. There is an increase in minor nonspecific abnormalities in children with ADHD, but these are of no importance for either diagnosis or treatment. If there is reason to suspect that the child has a seizure disorder, an electroencephalogram (EEG) should be obtained. It is important to remember that the diagnosis of a seizure disorder is made on analysis of the clinical features of the history, and up to 15% of individuals with seizures will have a normal EEG, even on repeated studies. It is less common to have an active seizure focus in a child without seizures, although this may occur also.

Brain mapping is still primarily a research tool. The technique, based on computer analysis of EEG activity (Duffy et al., 1980), is displayed in any one of a number of modes and compared with data obtained from an age-specific reference group. Results obtained by the use of this technique are of interest, but it is still too early to determine whether or not they will be useful for improving diagnostic precision or defining appropriate treatment.

DIFFERENTIAL DIAGNOSIS

The differential diagnosis must explore both psychosocial and neurologic factors that can produce similar complaints and findings (Cantwell and Baker, 1987). The child from a disrupted, stress-filled family may have difficulty concentrating and often develops an impulsive, aggressive approach to those around him.

Children with mood disorders also have an impaired attention span and can show other features suggestive of ADHD. Children with mania almost always have a significant family history of affective disorder. The Personality Inventory for Children correctly classifies patients with mania but incorrectly classifies as many as 20% of children with ADHD as being manic-depressive (Nieman and DeLong, 1987). This issue must be considered carefully during the diagnostic evaluation. A detailed family history is most important.

Similar symptoms are seen as part of a pervasive developmental disorder; DSM-III-R does not permit the diagnosis of ADHD to be made if a pervasive developmental disorder is present.

The child with mental retardation can also be diagnosed as having ADHD. Before this can be done, however, there must be certainty that the child's attention span and level of impulsivity are clearly abnormal for his or her mental age and adaptive level.

There is a strong association between Tourette's syndrome and ADHD (Erenberg et al., 1986). Approximately one-third of children with Tourette's syndrome also have evidence of attention deficit and impulsivity. This group of children also has a high incidence of learning disabilities. Treatment, to be discussed later, is problematic, as some children with Tourette's syndrome have an exacerbation of their tics when treated with psychostimulant drugs.

Other neurologic disorders may affect behavior and cognitive function in such a way as to raise the diagnostic possibility of ADHD. Unrecognized absence or partial complex seizures, if occurring frequently during the day, may impair attention and disrupt the learning process. The drugs used to treat these conditions, especially barbiturates and benzodiazepines, may also interfere with attention and learning, and so the situation requires close analysis and a skilled approach to treatment.

An unrecognized language disorder, a visual or hearing handicap, a learning disability, mild mental retardation, or borderline intelligence often present with symptoms suggestive of

ADHD. A diagnostic clue in these children is that the complaint of an attention disorder is typically made first after the child enters school and is exposed to the stress of learning in an academic setting. If no behavioral abnormalities were present in the preschool years, one of these conditions should be suspected.

On rare occasions a serious neurologic or medical disorder, such as a brain tumor, neurodegenerative disease, subacute sclerosing panencephalitis (SSPE), Sydenham's chorea, or endocrine disorders such as hypothyroidism or hyperthyroidism will first come to clinical attention because of behavioral abnormalities. Here again, the most important diagnostic clue is the change in behavior of a child who previously functioned well.

INDICATIONS FOR NEUROLOGIC CONSULTATION

Based on this differential diagnosis, a number of indications for neurologic consultation are apparent. The first is the suspicion of underlying neurologic disease, which may present with symptoms similar to those of ADHD. This may be a static disorder, such as mental retardation or cerebral palsy, which can either mimic or coexist with ADHD. Diagnosis is important in order to help frame expectations for the child's behavior and to ensure that both conditions are being treated appropriately.

Consultation is critical if the presence of a metabolic or degenerative disease is suspected, so that treatment, if available, can be instituted and an accurate prognosis developed. The clinical clues suggesting a degenerative disorder are loss of preexisting developmental achievements or a decrease in the rate of development. These changes often are associated with new or changing abnormalities on the neurologic examination.

Once the child is past infancy, metabolic disorders typically present only as static deficits in cognition. They should be suspected if there is no other definable cause for the mental retardation or a family history of a similar disorder is found. Screening tests are available for the most common disorders.

The suspicion of a seizure disorder is also an indication for neurologic consultation. Although the diagnosis of seizures, ultimately, is clinical and not made on the basis of the EEG, the differentiation between daydreaming, absence seizures, and complex partial seizures may require the use of this procedure. This is important for defining the most effective treatment and determining the prognosis.

Another reason for referral for neurologic consultation is the coexistence of ADHD and another neurologic disease, such as Tourette's syndrome, that may be closely related. Treatment of one condition may exacerbate the other or may produce unacceptable drug interactions. Related to this is the onset of new neurologic symptoms when treatment for ADHD is initiated. Psychostimulant drugs can produce tics, headaches, and adverse behavioral changes.

Finally, neurologic consultation should be considered any time that the child's behavior is atypical of ADHD and does not adequately fit any other psychiatric diagnostic category. The yield of specific diagnoses is not high, but if one can be made it has the greatest importance for the patient and his or her family.

TREATMENT

The role and efficacy of behavioral strategies in the treatment of ADHD is a matter of some controversy. The child with mild symptoms may benefit from cognitive behavioral self-control therapy, although this is less likely to be effective with severely involved children (Brown et al., 1986). Some workers have recommended a multimodal treatment plan in which medication is combined with one or more psychological treatment approaches (Satterfield et al., 1981). Although short-term benefits can be documented, it is less easy to demonstrate a sustained effect after treatment is discontinued.

There are indications for the use of psychotherapy beyond the treatment of the ADHD itself. These children often suffer from a poor self-image, impaired peer and family relationships, anxiety, and depression. Anything that can be done to relieve these symptoms will be reflected in a better level of general function and may have a positive impact on the ADHD.

The use of medication should be considered for treating the child who has ADHD that produces serious impairment of function at home, in school, or with peers, and in whom behavioral strategies provide inadequate benefit (American Academy of Pediatrics, 1987; Golden, 1989). The diagnosis should be firmly established before embarking on drug therapy, and associated neurologic conditions should be under control to the greatest extent possible.

Psychostimulants are the primary pharmacologic agents used for the treatment of ADHD (Table 4.3). Methylphenidate is the drug most frequently prescribed. Pemoline is used somewhat less frequently, and dextroamphetamine is used rarely at this time. The specific therapeutic mode of action of these agents is not known, although they appear to increase the activity of central dopaminergic and norepinephrinergic systems. When these drugs were first introduced, it was thought that they had an idiosyncratic effect, producing calming and sedation in the hyperactive child while acting as stimulants in unaffected individuals. It now appears that most children, with or without ADHD, show a decrease in motor activity, increased attention span, and improved performance on short-term learning tasks when given psychostimulants (Rapoport et al., 1978). The child with ADHD

obviously starts from a different baseline and may show greater changes, but the drug effects are not specific to this group of children.

Other classes of drugs, such as anxiolytics and neuroleptics, do not have a specific effect on ADHD and, if they provide any benefit at all, it is through sedation and the reduction of anxiety. Since these drugs may have an adverse effect on cognition and learning, they cannot be recommended.

There is evidence that antidepressants may provide therapeutic benefits for some patients with ADHD. Despiramine, with a maximum daily dose of 4 to 5 mg/kg, has been shown to be clinically and statistically more effective than placebo (Biederman et al., 1989A). The drug appeared to be useful in previously untreated patients as well as those who failed to respond to methylphenidate. Although high doses of desipramine were used in this study, the authors did find changes in cardiac rate and conduction with doses higher than 3.5 mg/kg and blood levels above 150 ng/ml (Biederman et al., 1989B). These changes were generally asymptomatic and consisted of sinus tachycardia, prolongation of the QRS interval, and a slight increase in diastolic blood pressure. They recommended monitoring of serum drug levels and the electrocardiogram at higher doses. Sudden death in three children being treated with desipramine has been reported to the manufacturer (Medical Letter, 1990). In each case plasma levels were in the therapeutic range or lower.

Methylphenidate is started at a dose of 5 mg daily to determine whether or not the patient has an idiosyncratic sensitivity to the drug. The

Table 4.3.
Drugs for Treatment of ADHD

	Initial Dose	Maximum Dose
Methylphenidate	5 mg b.i.d	60 mg daily
Dextroamphetamine sulfate	5 mg/day	40 mg daily
Pemoline	37.5 mg/day	112.5 mg daily
Imipramine hydrochloride	25 mg/day	2.5 mg/kg/day
Clonidine	0.05 mg/day	0.3–0.4 mg/day

dose can then be increased in 5-mg increments every 3 to 4 days until the desired therapeutic effect is obtained or the maximum recommended dose is reached. In general, an optimal dose is between 0.3 mg/kg/day and 0.6 mg/kg/day, given in two divided doses. A dose of 1.0 mg/kg/day or higher rarely provides any additional benefit, and there is evidence that these doses are associated with a decline in certain cognitive abilities (Brown and Sleator, 1979). Some clinicians used a placebo-controlled trial when starting the drug for the first time in a new patient. Although this may be useful under certain circumstances, it is not necessary to do this with most children.

One problem with methylphenidate is a short duration of action. Some children demonstrate large swings in behavioral control associated with the pharmacokinetic characteristics of the drug. If this is a major problem, it can often be managed by giving three divided doses daily. If the last dose is taken late in the day, however, insomnia may occur. A sustained release preparation is available, but many children do not have an adequate response to this form of the drug.

Pemoline is preferred by some clinicians because it has a longer duration of action than methylphenidate, can be given in a single daily dose, and is useful for those children who do not have a sustained effect with methylphenidate. However, a problem with pemoline is that the therapeutic effect may not be seen until the drug has been administered for 3 to 4 weeks. The usual starting dose is 37.5 mg daily. This is increased in increments of 18.75 mg at 1 week intervals until a therapeutic response is achieved or a maximum dose of 112.5 mg daily is reached. The average therapeutic dose is 56.25 to 75 mg daily.

There is controversy concerning the use of drug holidays for the child taking psychostimulant drugs. Most children who clearly need medication should take it continuously, including weekends. Parents should be discouraged from giving the medication on an irregular basis only "when it is necessary for the child to be good." This presents the message that the child is unable to take any responsibility for his or her own behavior, but that the situation can be fixed with a drug. It is reasonable to try to discontinue the medication during prolonged school holidays, to assess whether or not the need for treatment continues. Before attempting a drug holiday or discontinuation of the medication, the family should be warned that a rebound may occur and that there will be a period of time during which the symptoms of ADHD appear to increase markedly. Failure to recognize this rebound often results in reinstitution of therapy and treatment beyond the point at which the drug could be permanently discontinued.

However, some workers in the field believe that drug holidays are inappropriate and that the need for medication may continue into adulthood. An increase in attention span and the ability to control impulsive behavior typically occurs in many children with ADHD in the preteen and adolescent years. Whether or not significant symptoms can continue into adulthood, and the need for treating this group, is under study.

Psychostimulants generally are free of serious medical side effects. Young children, especially those less than 5 years of age, often have adverse behavioral effects. Their parents describe them as subdued and without spontaneity. Anorexia may be associated with weight loss and decreased linear growth, but height and weight are regained during drug holidays. Other common complaints are sedation, abdominal pain, and insomnia. There have been reports of methylphenidate and pemoline lowering the seizure threshold in patients with epilepsy, but this does not appear to be a problem in most children (Feldman et al., 1989).

The precipitation or exacerbation of tics, including Tourette's syndrome, has been reported following the use of psychostimulant drugs (Lowe et al., 1982). The situation is complex, in that at least one-third of children with Tourette's syndrome also have symptoms of ADHD. It may be this group in which the tic disorder begins following initiation of therapy. If this should occur, the drug should be discontinued and the situation thoroughly evaluated. Attempts at nonpharmacologic treatment should be tried. If other treatment modalities are not successful and drug treatment of ADHD is essential, it may be necessary to accept the increase in tics. If they become severe, haloperidol can be added to the treatment regimen, but this may have adverse effects on behavior and learning. Clonidine and tricyclic antidepressants have also been recommended (Table 4.3) in this clinical situation, but experience with this approach is limited.

UNORTHODOX THERAPIES

Unorthodox treatment approaches for ADHD appear at least monthly, often promulgated through publication of a book and enhanced by an author's appearance on a television interview show. Families are eager to grasp new approaches that do not require the use of drugs and are based only on dietary modification or the use of "natural" substances such as vitamins. These therapies have a number of characteristics in common. They are usually based on an idiosyncratic theory, and the proponents claim that they are effective for a wide range of problems and free of serious side effects. The therapies are rarely introduced in the peer-reviewed scientific literature, and when controlled studies fail to confirm their efficacy, the originator of the theory claims that there is a conspiracy on the part of the medical establishment not to accept its usefulness.

The best known of these approaches is the additive-free diet, based on the elimination of food colorings and other additives. Controlled studies have provided no conclusive evidence that this approach is effective (Wender, 1986). Although there are no medical contraindications to such a diet, it is complicated, time consum-

ing, and expensive. The child, who is already stigmatized, can become further alienated from peers as a result of the rigid dietary requirements and his or her inability to participate in social functions where food plays an important role.

Megavitamins and megadose mineral therapy have been put forward as treatment for a large range of psychiatric and neurologic conditions, including ADHD. There are no properly constructed clinical trials that support the hypothesis, and a number of studies fail to confirm it. All of the vitamins used can have serious toxic side effects when given in large doses. One study not only demonstrated that megavitamins were ineffective but also found an increase in disruptive behavior when vitamins were being taken as well as an elevation in serum levels of hepatic enzymes, probably representing niacin toxicity (Haslam et al., 1984).

The lay public and many practitioners appear to believe that dietary sugar, especially sucrose, increases the activity level of sensitive children. As with the other therapies discussed, this cannot be documented in double-blind placebo-controlled studies. Reduction of refined sugar in the diet certainly helps prevent dental caries but appears to have no effect on ADHD. Other techniques that have been recommended but are unproved include vestibular stimulation, motion sickness drugs, anticonvulsants, and biofeedback. New treatment modalities should be approached with caution and should not be accepted unless the studies meet the standards of rigorous scientific design.

PROGNOSIS

Studies of the long-term prognosis of children with ADHD are difficult to interpret for several reasons. The conceptual framework in which the disorder is viewed and diagnostic criteria have changed over time. Even under the best of circumstances, the diagnosis is made on the basis of nonquantitative criteria, and these are often employed in retrospective studies. Finally, there is a good deal of overlap between the symptoms of ADHD and those of other disruptive behavior disorders.

The results of a 15-year follow-up study at Montreal Children's Hospital is of interest because of the long study period and the use of a matched control group (Weiss and Hechtman, 1985). A total of 63 hyperactive adults and 41 matched controls were evaluated. At least one symptom of ADHD was present in 66% of the subjects and 10% of controls. The WAIS IQ was significantly lower for the subject group, although the groups were matched at the initiation of the study. The only consistent psychiatric diagnosis that was made was antisocial personality disorder, and the subject group had more court appearances and committed more antisocial acts. There were no differences in the rate of alcoholism, but there was a higher incidence of suicide attempts.

Another study reviewed the status of 101 hyperactive children diagnosed 6 to 11 years previously (Gittleman-Klein et al., 1985). The diagnosis of ADHD was still present in 31% of the subject group and 3% of controls. The subject group showed an increase in conduct and antisocial disorders and in substance abuse.

This second study raised the important issues of the relationship between the persistence of the symptoms of ADHD and antisocial behavior. It was demonstrated that those subjects who maintained symptoms of ADHD made up the bulk of the group with antisocial or substance abuse disorders. The subjects who no longer had symptoms of ADHD did not differ from control subjects in the frequency of substance abuse and antisocial behavior.

Although these studies suggest a poor prognosis for many individuals with ADHD, especially the group with continuing symptoms, there is a built-in bias in that the subjects were those who were referred to psychiatric clinics. In addition, there was no attempt to determine whether there was a differential outcome when comparing children presenting with "pure" ADHD and those with ADHD and conduct disorder or antisocial behavior.

REFERENCES

American Academy of Pediatrics. Committee on Children with Disabilities, Committee on Drugs: medication for children with an attention deficit disorder. Pediatrics 1987;80:758.

American Psychiatric Association: Diagnostic and Statistical Manual of Mental Disorders, 3rd ed., rev. Washington, DC: American Psychiatric Association, 1987.

Biederman J, Baldessarini RJ, Wright V, et al. A double-blind placebo controlled study of desipramine in the treatment of ADD: I. Efficacy. J Am Acad Child Adolesc Psychiatry 1989A;28:577–584.

Biederman J, Baldessarini RJ, Wright V, et al: A double-blind placebo controlled study of desipramine in the treatment of ADD: II. Serum drug levels and cardiovascular findings. J Am Acad Child Adolesc Psychiatry 1989B;28:903–911.

Brown RT, Sleator EK. Methylphenidate in hyperkinetic children: differences in dose effect on impulsive behavior. Pediatrics 1979;64:408–411.

Brown RT, Wynne ME, Borden KA, Clingerman SR, Geniesse R, Spunt AL: Methylphenidate and cognitive therapy in children with attention deficit disorder: a double-blind trial. J Devel Behav Pediatr 1986;7:163.

Cantwell DP, Baker LB. Differential diagnosis of hyperactivity. J Devel Behav Pediatr 1987;8:159–165.

Caparulo B, Cohen D, Rothman S, et al. Computed tomographic brain scanning in children with developmental neuropsychiatric disorders. J Am Acad Child Adol Psychiatr 1981;20:339.

Conners CK: A teacher rating scale for use in drug studies which children. Am J Psychiatr 1969;126:884–888.

Conners CK. Rating scales for use in drug studies with children. Psychopharmacol Bull 1973;9(special issue):24–84.

David OJ, Hoffman SP, Sverd J, et al: The role of lead in hyperactivity. Psychopharmacol Bull 1976;12:11–13.

Duffy FH, Denckla MB, Bartels PH, et al. Dyslexia: automated diagnosis by computerized classification of brain electrical activity. Ann Neurol 1980;7:421–428.

Erenberg G, Cruse RP, Rothner AD: Tourette syndrome: an analysis of 200 pediatric and adolescent cases. Cleve Clin Q 1986;53:127–131.

Faust D, Brown J: Moderately elevated blood lead levels: effects on neuropsychologic functioning in children. Pediatrics 1987;80:623–629.

Feldman H, Crumrine P, Handen BL, et al. Methylphenidate in children with seizures and attention-deficit disorder. Am J Dis Child 1989;143:1081–1086.

Gittleman-Klein R, Manuzze SD, Skenker R, et al. Hyperactive boys almost grown up. Arch Gen Psychiatr 1985;42:937–947.

Golden GS. Pharmacologic intervention in attention deficit disorder. In: French JH, Harel S, Casaer P, eds. Child neurology and developmental disabilities. Baltimore: Paul H. Brooks Publishing, 1989, p. 245.

Haslam RHA, Dalby JT, Rademaker AW. Effects of megavitamin therapy on children with attention deficit disorder. Pediatrics 1984;74:103–111.

Landman GB, Levine MD, Fenton T, Solomon B. Minor neurological indicators and developmental function in preschool children. Devel Behav Pediatr 1986;7:97–101.

Lowe TL, Cohen DJ, Detlor J, et al. Stimulant medications precipitate Tourette's syndrome. JAMA 1982;247:1729–1731.

McBride MC. An individual double-blind cross-over trial for assessing methylphenidate response in children with attention deficit disorder. J Pediatr 1988;113:137.

Medical Letter. Sudden death in children treated with a tricyclic antidepressant. Medical Letter 1990;32:53.

Needleman HL, Schell A, Bellinger, et al. The long-term effects of exposure to low doses of lead in childhood: an 11-year follow-up report. N Engl J Med 1990;322:83–88.

Nieman GW, DeLong R. Use of the Personality Inventory for Children as an aid in differentiating children with mania from children with attention deficit disorder with hyperactivity. J Am Acad Child Adolesc Psychiatr 1987;26:381–388.

Rapoport JL, Buchsbaum MS, Zahn TP, et al. Dextroamphetamine: cognitive and behavioral effects in normal prepubertal boys. Science 1978;199:560–563.

Rapoport JL, Ferguson HB. Biological validation of the hyperkinetic syndrome. Devel Med Child Neurol 1981;23:667–682.

Safer DJ, Krager JM. A survey of medication treatment for hyperactive/inattentive students. JAMA 1988;260:2256.

Sandberg S, Rutter M, Taylor E. Hyperkinetic disorder in psychiatric clinic attenders. Devel Med Child Neurol 1978;20:279–299.

Satterfield JM, Satterfield BT, Cantwell DP. Three-year multimodality treatment study of 100 hyperactive boys. J Pediatr 1981;98:650.

Shaywitz SE, Shaywitz BA, McGraw K, et al. Current status of neuromaturational examination as an index of learning disability. J Pediatr 1984;104:819–825.

Weiss G, Hechtman L. The psychiatric status of hyperactives: a controlled prospective 15-year follow-up of 63 hyperactive children. J Am Acad Child Adol Psychiatr 1985;24:211–221.

Wender EH. The food additive-free diet in the treatment of behavior disorders: a review. J Devel Behav Pediatr 1986;7:35–42.

Wilson JM, Kiessling LS: What is measured by the Conners' Teacher Behavior Rating Scale? Replication of factor analysis. J Devel Behav Pediatr 1988;9:271.

Chapter 5

PERVASIVE DEVELOPMENTAL DISORDERS

Ruth Nass, MD, and Diane Koch, PhD

INTRODUCTION

Almost one-half century ago Kanner (1943) reported on 11 patients with impaired social skills, deficits in both verbal and nonverbal communication, poor development of imaginative play skills, and stereotyped and repetitive behaviors. Kanner's description remains a classic and his patient population is prototypic of autistic disorder (AD), the most severe subclass of pervasive developmental disorders (PDD) (defined by consensus in the Diagnostic and Statistical Manual III-Revised (DSM III-R) and presented in adapted form in Table 5.1). Cases that meet the general description of PDD but not autistic disorder are called "PDD not otherwise specified."

Early-onset impairments of sociability, verbal, and nonverbal communication and restricted activities and interests are required for the diagnosis of autistic disorder. Autistic disorder varies markedly in severity. Its incidence is estimated at 2 to 4.5/10,000, and as with other developmental disorders of childhood, there is a male preponderance, with a male:female ratio of 3:1. The high concordance in monozygotic twins and the presence of multiple siblings affected within the same family suggest a genetic component (Golden, 1987).

CLASSIFICATION

Subtyping systems have concentrated on the three potentially defining aspects of autistic dis-

orders: deficits of cognitive function, sociability, and language.

Cognitive Function

Children with AD may function in the inferior, average, or superior range of intellectual ability. The majority (70 to 85%), however, are mentally retarded. Fein and colleagues (1985) have defined four main cognitive skill profiles based on the different patterns of verbal, perceptual, quantitative, and memory strengths and weaknesses (Table 5.2). There were no age, IQ, or sex differences among the four subgroups, suggesting that the subgroups did not merely reflect the level of intellectual functioning or extent of maturation. By contrast, behavioral and attentional deficit patterns were not related to cognitive subgroups, suggesting that behavioral/psychiatric features may occur independently of cognitive deficit patterns and may be separately localized in the brain.

Sociability

Fein and colleagues (1986) have argued that the sociability deficit is primary to autism. Several different types of sociability deficits have been described. Based on a social interaction scale (Table 5.3) that rates sociability on a continuum from aloof and indifferent to normal and a checklist that assesses for the presence of specific play, social, and language skills, Wing (Wing and

Table 5.1.
Main Diagnostic Criteria for Autistic Disorder[a]

A. Impairment in reciprocal social interaction
    1. Unawareness of others' feelings or existence
    2. Failure to seek comfort in distress
    3. Impaired imitation
    4. Abnormal social play
    5. Inability to make peer friendships

B. Impairment in verbal and nonverbal
    communication
    1. No mode of communication
    2. Abnormal nonverbal communication such
       as eye-to-eye gaze
    3. Absent imaginative play
    4. Abnormal speech prosody
    5. Abnormal speech content
    6. Inability to maintain a conversation

C. Restricted activities and interests
    1. Stereotyped body movements
    2. Preoccupation with object parts or
       attachment to unusual objects
    3. Distress over trivial changes
    4. Excess insistence on routines
    5. Restricted range of interests

D. Onset during infancy or childhood

[a] Modified from Diagnostic and Statistical Manual-Revised (DSM III-R). Washington, DC: American Psychiatric Association, 1987.

Gould, 1979; Wing and Attwood, 1987) distinguished three social deficit patterns: aloof, passive, and interactive but odd.

The *aloof* group is most similar to the popular notion of autism. Signs of abnormal attachment are apparent in the first years. These children do not follow their parents around, do not run to greet them, and do not seek comfort when in pain. This subgroup tends to be low functioning in verbal skills and nonverbal communication and also exhibits very little symbolic play.

Table 5.2.
Cognitive Profiles in Autism[a]

I.   Visuospatial strength and variable receptive
     language skills
II. Verbal strength
III. Quantitative and verbal strength
IV. Flat profile

[a] Modified from Fein D, Waterhouse L, Lucci D, Snyder D. Cognitive subtypes in developmentally disabled children: a pilot study. J Autism Devel Disord 1985;15:77–95.

Table 5.3.
Wing's Social Interaction Scale

0	Does not interact—aloof and indifferent
1	Interacts to obtain needs, otherwise indifferent
2	Responds to (and may initiate) *physical* contact only, including rough and tumble games, chasing, cuddling, etc.
3	Generally does not initiate, but responds to *social* (not just physical) contact, if others, including peers, make approaches. Joins in passively (e.g., as baby in game of mother and father). Tries to copy, but with little understanding. Shows some pleasure in passive role (unlike Groups 0, 1, 2, who move away once physical needs are satisfied).
4	Makes social approaches actively, but these are usually inappropriate, naive, peculiar, or bizarre—"one-sided". The behavior is not modified according to (approached) situation/interpersonal feedback.
5	Shy, but social contacts appropriate for mental age with well-known people, including peers. Also use for children who refuse to talk to adults but interact with other children.
6	Social contacts appropriate for *mental* age with children and adults. Looks up with interest and smiles when approached. Responds to the ideas and interests of people of similar mental age and contributes to the interactions. Nonmobile people without speech can show social interest by means of eye contact and pointing.

The *passive* group is somewhat higher functioning. The children do not make social approaches, but they accept such approaches when made by others. They join in games, but they take a passive role, (e.g., the baby in the game of mothers and fathers).

The children in the *interactive but odd* group make spontaneous social approaches to others, but they do so in a peculiar, naive and one-sided fashion. They tend to talk *at* other people, and their approach may be so persistent as to become unwelcome. Their language lacks pragmatic constraints. For example, questions are used as conversational openers without preceding social graces. These children are capable of pretend symbolic play, but it is extremely repetitive.

Allen (1988) provided an alternative subtyping system that defines autism as a spectrum disorder with four types of sociability deficits as the universal variable and different language and play deficits as additional subtyping factors. The *socially unavailable* pattern includes the most severely impaired children, who are unavailable for interpersonal contact. The *socially remote* category includes children who engage in solitary activity. The child may be interested in the activities of another person, but not in the person. If someone attempts to intrude, these children ignore, move away, or vocally protest. The *inappropriately interactive* category includes children who are easier to engage but who have difficulty initiating or maintaining social interactions. The *pseudosocial* category includes the most verbal children, who are engagable, although their attempts at social interaction are immature, inadequate, or bizarre.

Language

Abnormal language is a major symptom of autism. When autistic children have language it is generally parrot-like; repetitive, stereotyped phrases are uttered with no conversational give-and-take. Comprehension of language is literal. Questions are repeated rather than answered (echolalia). Similarly, the repetition of personal pronouns results in reversals; the child speaks of himself as "you" and of the person addressed as "I". Young autistic children typically ignore verbal instruction, often leading to the erroneous suspicion of deafness.

Several developmental language disorders (Rapin and Allen, 1983) are discernible in preschool autistic children. In *verbal auditory agnosia,* meaningful language cannot be understood despite intact hearing. Expressive speech, when present, is poorly articulated and dysprosodic. (Prosody is the intonation of speech that allows us to do things like ask questions or express surprise). This language deficit pattern has been reported on a congenital (Rapin et al., 1977) and an acquired epileptic basis (Landau and Kleffner, 1957) in children with developmental language disorders. Paroxysmal EEG findings with and without seizures have been reported in autistic children with this language syndrome, some of whom show good behavioral response to anticonvulsants (Nass and Pietrucha, 1990; Payton and Minshew, 1987).

Children with the *semantic pragmatic syndrome* are fluent, even verbose. Phonologic (letter sounds) and syntactic (grammar) skills are intact. These children fall short in the basic semantic (vocabulary) skills required for meaningful conversation. Comprehension is impaired. They do not learn the basic rules that govern the use of language in context—pragmatics. Turn-taking, topic maintenance, and style changes when talking to people of different ages are limited. Their speech often has a sing-song quality and they cannot convey the additional pragmatic intentions that prosody affords (Rapin and Allen, 1983).

The *phonologic-syntactic syndrome* consists of omissions, substitutions, and distortions of consonants in all word positions. The sounds produced are unpredictable and unrecognizable. The syntactic deficit is generally evidenced by lack of small grammatical words (e.g., "and", "but") and the absence of appropriately inflected endings (e.g., "-ed", "-ing"). Sentences are aberrant, not just immature—"the baby is cry". In general, although not wholly spared, comprehension exceeds expressive skills. Neuromotor dysfunction is commonly seen in these children (Rapin and Allen, 1983).

In the *lexical syntactic syndrome,* speech is generally dysfluent with many hesitancies and false starts, because of word-finding difficulties and poor grammatical (syntactic) skills. Paraphasias (use of the wrong word) are notable. Phonology is spared and repetition skills exceed spontaneous speech. Comprehension is relatively spared, although complex questions taxing syntactic capabilities may be affected. When this language disorder subtype is seen in the setting of autism, pragmatics are generally affected, too.

The prominence of the language deficits in autism is suggestive of left hemisphere dysfunction as autism's underlying neurologic cause. Consistent with this, a number of neuropsychologic and electrophysiologic studies have documented a higher than normal incidence of right hemisphere specialization for language processing (Dawson et al., 1982; Prior and Bradshaw, 1979; Dawson et al., 1986). Left-handers and ambidexters are found in increased numbers among autistics (Golden, 1987; Soper et al., 1986). Fein and colleagues (1984) argue against a left hemisphere dysfunction interpretation because language behaviors like prosody and pragmatics, which are considered right-hemisphere (Nass and Gazzaniga, 1987) dominated, are also abnormal in autism. In addition, the types of language disorders found among children with autism are not specific but are seen among non-autistic children as well (Rapin and Allen, 1983).

CLINICAL HISTORY

The child with autism generally presents during the preschool years with developmental motor delay, developmental language delay, or impaired social skills, depending on the severity of the disorder. Motor milestones are generally achieved on time in the nonretarded child. Items in the clinical history suggestive of autism are shown in Table 5.4 (Rapin, 1988). Some studies suggest that the obstetric history may be suboptimal; second trimester bleeding, in particular, is found in excess (Tsai, 1987). The "suboptimality" may reflect a fetal abnormality resulting in preperinatal problems, rather than the perinatal problems causing autistic disorder. Congenital infections such as toxoplasmosis, rubella, syphilis, and cytomegalovirus occasionally result in autism. Problems in the perinatal period, particularly hypoglycemia, hyperbilirubinemia, and respiratory distress associated with prematurity, have been associated with autistic outcome (Table 5.5).

Table 5.4.
Items in the History Suggesting an Autistic Spectrum Disorder[a]

1. Is aloof or indiscriminately affectionate. While affectionate to family members, is unduly afraid of strangers.
2. Is a loner, does not know how to interact with other children, prefers adults to children, tolerates solitude.
3. While he or she may seek to interact with others, does so ineptly, especially in unstructured social situations.
4. Has a labile affect, unexplained mood swing. and terrors.
5. Is aggressive when unprovoked.
6. Is negativistic, wants everything on own terms.
7. Language was delayed, comprehension is impaired.
8. Has difficulty communicating wants, pointing was absent or appeared late.
9. Has gaze avoidance, turns back to others.
10. Talks to talk rather than because he or she has something to say.
11. Verbose, may prefer to talk rather than play, but conversation is limited to narrow range of favorite topics.
12. Is echolalic, uses verbal scripts, talks to self.
13. Speech is sing-song, or monotonous and robotic.
14. Prefers puzzles and mechanical objects to symbolic toys.
15. Has little or no interactive, social, or pretend play.
16. Has overspecialized interests (e.g., letters and numbers, maps, timetables, lists, etc.).
17. Is rigid in choice of activities, insists on sameness.
18. Perseverates, has stereotypic compulsive movements (e.g., finger flicking, flapping, twirling hair).
19. Walks on toes, is clumsy.
20. Has a history of head-banging, rocking, self-mutilation.
21. Licks, smells, taps at lights, appears deaf yet is intolerant of loud sound.
22. Has sleep problems.
23. Has an attention deficit or overfocused attention.
24. Has a phenomenal memory for places and routes.
25. Has a phenomenal verbal memory, repeats verbatim.
26. Is gifted in some areas (e.g., puzzle solving) despite severe deficiency in others.
27. Can read but will not listen to a story or look at pictures.

[a] From Rapin I. Disorders of higher cerebral function in preschool children. Am J Dis Child 1988;142:1178–1182.

Table 5.5.
Medical Problems Associated with Autism[a]

Prenatal	Metabolic
Midtrimester bleeding	Phenylketonuria
Toxemia	Histidinemia
Rubella	Lipidosis
Toxoplasmosis	Addison's disease
Lues	Hyperuricosuria
Cytomegalovirus	Hurler's syndrome
Perinatal	Hyperthyroidism
Hypoglycemia	Celiac disease
Trauma	Adrenoleukodystrophy
Hyperbilirubinemia	Lead ingestion
Respiratory distress syndrome	Chromosomal
Congenital	Trisomy 21
Cornelia de Lange syndrome	XYY syndrome
Microcephaly	XXX syndrome
Möbius' syndrome	Fragile X syndrome
Tuberous sclerosis	Acquired
Hydrocephalus	Infantile spasms
Dandy-Walker syndrome	Vascular occlusion
Oculocutaneous albinism	Encephalitis
	Meningitis

[a] Modified from Golden GS. Neurological functioning. In: Cohen DJ, Donnellan AM, Paul R, eds. Handbook of autism and pervasive developmental disorders. New York: Wiley and Sons, 1987.

Physical Examination

The mental status exam of the child with autism should include assessments in areas of relatedness, play, affect, and language skills. Children with autism often evidence motor stereotypies like flapping, twirling, or rocking. Toe-walking is relatively common. Abnormalities of response to sensory stimuli (either increased or decreased) may be found. Aberrant attention is seen, including distractibility, overfocus, and tolerance for or even insistence on sameness. A number of medical problems have been associated with autism (Table 5.5). Minor physical anomalies such as abnormal ears and widely spaced eyes are reported (Steg and Rapoport, 1975). Children with definite chromosomal abnormalities like Down's syndrome evidence the typical epicanthal folds and antimongolian slant to the eyes. The long facies with large heads and prominent ears of fragile X patients should suggest the diagnosis (Figure 5.1). A careful examination for signs of a neurocutaneous disorder—café au laits and hypopigmented patches—should be undertaken.

Patients with tuberous sclerosis in particular may be autistic.

The neurologic examination is generally not abnormal, unless the child has a specific neurologic disorder manifesting as an autistic phenotype (Table 5.5) (Golden, 1987). Gubbay et al. (1970) do, however, report tremor, hypotonia, spasticity, hyperactive tendon reflexes, asymmetric tendon reflexes, and extensor plantars among a cohort of 24 children, many with presumed idiopathic autism. Particular care in the assessment of gait, which may be slow, festinating, and stooped, is indicated because such Parkinsonian features led Damasio and colleagues (Damasio and Maurer, 1978; Vilensky et al., 1981) to speculate that autism represents a disorder of the mesolimbic dopaminergic system.

Evaluation

Evaluation for the etiology of autism should include a basic metabolic screening including complete blood count, chemical profile, and lactate

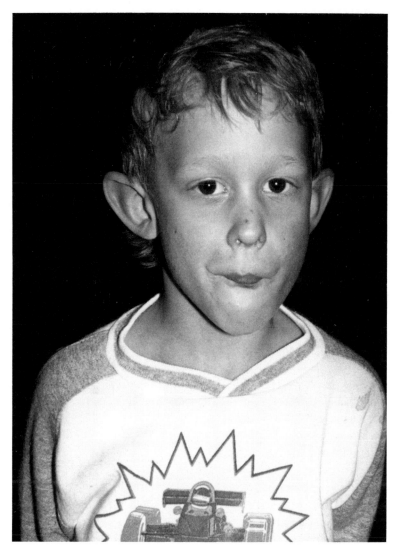

Figure 5.1. Note the large head, prominent ears, and characteristic facies of this boy with fragile X syndrome. Macroorchidism is not necessarily present prior to puberty. (Courtesy of Randi Hagerman, MD, The Children's Hospital, Denver, Colorado.)

and amino acids (see Table 5.5). An evaluation of endocrine function, particularly thyroid and adrenal, may be appropriate. In view of the frequency of the fragile X chromosome disorder in autism (approximately 8% of autistic males are fragile X positive and approximately 12% of fragile X positive males manifest autistic symptoms; Opitz, 1986), its genetic implications, and its potential for prenatal diagnosis, all patients with autism should be screened for this disorder. Macroorchidism may not be present until after puberty. An evaluation of hearing is essential. Depending on the child's age and level of function, this may be done by behavioral audiometry or by brainstem auditory evoked responses. Speech and language evaluation may be useful, particularly for determining school placement. An assessment of level of intellectual functioning is crucial both for immediate planning and for prognosis.

The frequency of seizures ranges from 11 to 42% (Jacobson and Janick, 1983; Schain and Yannet, 1960). The first year of life (usually infantile spasms-myoclonic seizures with hypsarhythmia EEG) and adolescence are the most common times of onset, and the cumulative risk of developing epilepsy by age 19 years is 23% (Deykin et al., 1979). All seizure types have been reported. Recent reports suggest a beneficial effect of seizure treatment on the autistic disorder (Payton and Minshew, 1987; Nass and Pietrucha, 1988). Electroencephalograms ought to be obtained at the slightest hint of seizures and certainly if there is an active seizure disorder.

Neuroimaging studies have provided some information about the basis of autism. Although the majority of patients who have been imaged by CT and MRI have normal studies, ventricular enlargement is found in up to 25% of patients (Campbell et al., 1982; Gillberg and Svendsen, 1983). Evaluating 10 relatively high-functioning autistics using MRI, Minshew et al. (1986) found ventricular dilation and atrophy only in the autistics functioning in the 70 to 85 IQ range and not in those functioning above 85. Cerebral asymmetries have also been assessed in the autistic patient. Hier et al. (1979) found a reversed parietal occipital asymmetry pattern in 57% of 116 autistic patients (in contrast to the approximately 20% with this pattern that would be anticipated among normal right-handers). However, this study can be criticized for not controlling for sex and handedness. Others have not confirmed the high frequency of reversed asymmetry (Tsai and Stewart, 1983; Prior et al., 1984; Damasio et al., 1980; Rosenbloom et al., 1984; Creasey et al., 1986).

Although previous studies found no relevant gross abnormalities at biopsy or postmortem of 10 patients with autism (Golden, 1987), Bauman and Kemper (1985) recently reported important cytoarchitectonic (cell morphology) abnormalities: reduced neuronal size and increased cell packing density in hippocampal complex and amygdala. Bilateral and symmetric loss of Purkinje and granular neurons were seen in the neocerebellum and confirmed by Ritvo and colleagues (1986) in four more autistics. Both CT and MRI studies showing a proportionately smaller cerebellum with a relatively large fourth ventricle corroborate these pathologic findings (Bauman et al., 1985; Gaffney et al., 1987; Courchesne et al., 1988, per contra Ritvo and Garber, 1988).

Metabolic studies using the xenon inhalation technique (labeled gas is inhaled and its distribution mapped) revealed overall depressed regional cerebral blood flow (similar to that found in dementia) and an abnormal resting landscape with the usual hyperfrontal flow apparent only on the left (Sherman et al., 1984). Positron emission tomography resting state studies of 10 high-functioning autistics using 2-deoxyglucose revealed hypermetabolism 13 to 21% greater than that in controls throughout the brain (Duara et al., 1984). Horwitz et al. (1988) recently demonstrated atypical interhemispheric metabolic asymmetries.

DIFFERENTIAL DIAGNOSIS

Developmental Language Disorder and Nonautistic Mental Deficiency

The Child Neurology Society Nosology Task Force on Higher Cortical Function separates autistic spectrum disorder from developmental language disorders and nonautistic mental deficiency based on performance on an IQ test, a language test, and a sociability rating scale. Although children with developmental language disorders may exhibit linguistic phenomenology similar to that of those with autistic disorder, the two groups are clearly separable by their social skills. While retarded children may evidence an occasional autistic feature, in particular, motor stereotypies like rocking or twirling, they can be distinguished from low-functioning autistic children based on their social skills. Congenital or acquired brain damage does not militate against the diagnosis of autistic disorder.

Asperger's Syndrome

This syndrome is appropriately placed within the autistic disorders; however, since high functioning is the rule, the aberrant behaviors may not become apparent before 30 months, thereby excluding the DSM III-R diagnosis of autism. The criteria elaborated by Wing (1981) to define this syndrome include: (*a*) pedantic aprosodic bizarre speech; (*b*) clumsy and uncoordinated nonverbal communication; (*c*) withdrawn or clumsy interpersonal relatedness; (*d*) defect in empathy for others; (*e*) repetitive activity; (*f*) resistance to change in the environment; (*g*) stereotyped bodily movements; (*h*) adequate to excellent rote memory; (*i*) circumscribed interest patterns.

Rett's Syndrome

Rett's syndrome is distinguished from autism by its exclusive occurrence in girls and its progressive nature. It is X-linked dominant, with lethality in males and reproductive lethality in the female (Hass, Rapin, and Moser, 1988). Girls with this disorder have a normal pre- and perinatal history and their development is generally normal until 6 to 18 months. Deceleration of initially normal head growth with ultimate acquired microcephaly occurs between 6 and 48 months. Between the ages of 6 and 30 months (usually 18 to 24) there is a loss of previously acquired skilled hand movements and the appearance of pathognomonic hand stereotypies of twisting or wringing. Truncal ataxia, gait apraxia (wide-based, unsteady, stiff-legged), and toe-walking supervene in the child who has previously walked normally. Simultaneously with the motor deterioration there is a deterioration in language, communication, intellectual, and social skills. Although these children may have developed a several-word vocabulary, receptive and expressive language skills deteriorate to the point of mutism. Severe to profound mental retardation is the eventual cognitive outcome. Social interactions become impaired. Marked irritability with screaming fits tends to occur at this time. The aloofness and gaze avoidance in the Rett's syndrome child are often more pronounced than in the typical autistic child. Social interactions and eye contact actually tend to improve at approximately 4 to 5 years, coincident with a plateauing in neurologic deterioration. During the second decade, patients develop scoliosis, muscle wasting with peculiar trophic changes of feet more than hands, rigidity, and growth retardation.

Supportive criteria for the diagnosis include breathing dysfunction, which takes the form of periodic apnea during waking, intermittent hyperventilation, breath-holding spells, and forced expulsion of air or saliva. Seizures, intractable in one-third of cases, occur in the majority of patients prior to adolescence. Peripheral vasomotor disturbances such as mottling are common.

Distinguishing Rett syndrome with autism should be difficult only until age 3 to 5 years. Indeed, 78% of children ultimately diagnosed with Rett syndrome previously carried the diagnosis of autism (Witt-Engerstrom and Gillberg, 1987). The development of the distinctive hand stereotypies and progressive neurologic deterioration should assure the diagnosis.

Schizoid Disorder of Childhood

The essential feature of schizoid disorder of childhood (DSM III-R) is an inability to form social relationships. Schizoid children, like autistics (Dahl et al., 1986), may show little desire for social involvement, are uncomfortable or awkward in social situations, and can often appear aloof or withdrawn. This disorder can be diagnosed as early as 5 years. It can be differentiated from autism by its lack of association with deficits in multiple areas of functioning. The sociability deficit of the autistic is by definition in the context of pervasive deficits in other areas, such as communicative language.

Childhood Schizophrenia

The diagnosis of schizophrenia is extremely rare in childhood and requires not only disturbances in communication and affect similar to autistic disorder, but also the presence of prominent delusions or hallucinations (DSM III-R). This essential feature of psychosis needs to be distinguished from the stereotyped, repetitive acting out of the role of an object, animal, or person that may be seen in autistic disorder.

TREATMENT

Behavioral response to pharmacologic manipulation of dopaminergic and serotonergic neurotransmitter systems has been used as an argument for the possible neurochemical basis of autism. Lithium, tricyclic antidepressants, lysergic acid, L-dopa, and amphetamines have all been tried with little success (Campbell et al., 1987). A poor response to amphetamine, which may lead to worsened psychosis and stereotypies, is of clinical import, since on occasion in short-term assessment the high-functioning autistic child can appear hyperactive. Stimulants would not usually be the treatment. In some children with autism, low-dose stimulant medication may be helpful as part of the treatment plans (Birmaher et al., 1988; Strayhorn et al., 1988).

By contrast, dopamine blockers, particularly Haldol and Prolixin, appear to decrease behavioral symptoms and increase learning. These studies thus suggest that decreasing dopaminergic activity improves function in autism (a finding in direct contrast to the hypodopaminergic hypothesis put forward by Damasio and Maurer (1978)). Overall, the combination of behavioral modification in conjunction with medical therapy produces the best results (Campbell et al., 1987).

In 1982, Geller et al., using a 2-week placebo-drug-placebo design, reported that fenfluramine, an agent that depletes serotonin, improved the social responsiveness and IQ of three autistic males. Coincident with and continuing for several weeks after the drug was withdrawn was a decrease in blood serotonin level. Fenfluramine trials have now been reported in more than 100 autistic patients, with mixed success. With a sample size of 81 and using the placebo-drug-placebo design, Ritvo et al. (1986) report that in approximately 25% of patients unequivocal improvement occurred and in approximately 50% equivocal improvement occurred with decreased hyperactivity and stereotypies and improved social awareness and communication. The autistic patients with higher initial IQ and lower baseline serotonin levels showed the most improvement. Using a dose of 1.5/mg per kilogram per day, blood serotonin levels fell approximately 50%, regardless of initial level. By contrast, Campbell et al. (1987) report best success with lower IQ subjects. August et al. (1984) report no relationship between response and baseline serotonin level. Most recently, fenfluramine in 28 autistic children failed to show superiority over placebo (Campbell et al., 1988). Thus, the fenfluramine story shows some promise, but one must be cautious about overestimating its efficacy (Ho et al., 1986).

OUTCOME OF AUTISM

Long-term follow-up studies suggest a normal outcome in adulthood in 1 to 2% of the cases, an overall good outcome (employed) in 5 to 20%, a fair outcome (unemployed, but some independence) in 15 to 27%, and a poor outcome (dependent, institutionalized) in 60 to 75% (Paul, 1987). Follow-up studies suggest that initial language, initial social skills, and initial IQ are each predictive of outcome. Useful speech before age 5 years is generally an important positive prognostic sign for overall outcome. Forty percent of children with at least some speech at age 5 years developed conversational speech, contrasted with 30% with echolalia and 10% with muteness at intake. Sixty percent of the children presenting with speech sufficient to express immediate needs developed conversational speech (DeMyer et al., 1974). Ultimately, about one-third had no speech and one-half had communicatively useful speech. Six percent of 126 children had normal speech.

Social skills and IQ at presentation are also predictive of outcome. Whereas 75% of the higher IQ functioning (over 80) autistics were initially rated as withdrawn, only 25% were similarly rated at follow-up. In the middle- and low-functioning intellectual groups, 100% were withdrawn at intake and 80% remained withdrawn at follow-up (DeMyer et al., 1974). In Lockyer and Rutter's (1970) follow-up study the social features of autism became less marked over time in half the patients; in fact 14% were no longer termed autistic at follow-up. Most recently, a neuropsychologic study (Rumsey and Hamburger, 1988) of 10 adult males with normal intelligence and a history of childhood autism revealed no significant differences compared with controls on measures of visuoperceptual, memory, sensory perceptual, or motor skills. However, subtle differences were found in language skills and dramatic differences on tasks that measure frontal lobe functioning. These findings highlight the need for adequate outcome markers in follow-up studies.

REFERENCES

Allen D. Autistic spectrum disorder. J Child Neurol 1988; 3:548–556.

August GJ, Raz N, Papanicolaou AC, et al. Fenfluramine treatment in infantile autism. J Nerv Ment Dis 1984;172:604–612.

Bauman M, Kemper TL. Histoanatomic observations of the brain in early infantile autism. Neurology 1985;35:866–874.

Bauman, ML, LeMay M, Bauman RA. Computerized tomographic (CT) observations of the posterior fossa in early infantile autism. Neurology 1985;35(suppl I):247.

Birmaher B, Quintana H, Greenhill LL. Methylphenidate treatment of hyperactive autistic children. J Am Acad Child Adolesc Psychiatry 1988;27:248–251.

Campbell, M, Anderson LT, Greene WH, et al. Psychopharmacology. In: Cohen DA, Donnallan AM, Paul R, eds. Handbook of autism and pervasive developmental disorders. Wiley and Sons, New York, 1987.

Campbell M, Rosenbloom S, Perry R, et al. Computerized axial tomography in young autistic children. Am J Psychiatry 1982;139:510–512.

Campbell M, et al. Fenfluramine fails to show superiority over placebo in 28 autistic children. J Am Acad Child Adolesc Psychiatr 1988;27:434–439.

Courchesne E, Yeung-Courchesne R, Press GA, et al. Hypoplasia of cerebellar vermal lobules VI & VII in autism. New Engl J Med 1988;318:1349–1354.

Creasey H, Rumsey J, Schwartz M, et al. Brain morphology in autistic men as measured by volumetric computed tomography. Arch Neurol 1986;43:669–672.

Dahl EK, Cohen DJ, Provence S. Clinical and multivariate approaches to the nosology of pervasive developmental disorders. J Am Acad Child Psychiatry 1986;25:170–180.

Damasio AR, Maurer RG. A neurological model for childhood autism. Arch Neurol 1978;35:777–786.

Damasio H, Maurer RG, Damasio AR, Chui HC. Computerized tomographic scan findings in patients with autistic behavior. Arch Neurol 1980;37:504–510.

Dawson G, Finlay C, Phillips S, Galpert L. Hemispheric specialization and the language abilities of autistic children. Child Devel 1986;57:1440–1453.

Dawson G, Warrenburg S, Fuller P. Cerebral lateralization in individuals diagnosed as autistic in early childhood. Brain Lang 1982;15:353–368.

DeMyer MK, Barton S, Alpern GD, et al. The measured intelligence of autistic children: a follow-up study. J Autism Child Schizophr 1974;4:42–60.

Deykin EY, McMahon PH, McMahon B. The incidence of seizures among children with autistic symptoms. Am J Psychiatry 1979;136:1310–1312.

Diagnostic and Statistical Manual—Revised (DSM III-R). Washington, DC: American Psychiatric Association, 1987.

Duara R, Rumsey J, Grady C, et al. Cerebral glucose metabolism in adult autism. Neurology 1984;34:117.

Fein D, Humes M, Kaplan E, et al. The question of left hemisphere dysfunction in autism. Psychol Bull 1984;95:258–281.

Fein D, Pennington B, Markowitz P, et al. Toward a neuropsychological model of infantile autism: are the social deficits primary? J Am Acad Child Psychiatry 1986;25:198–212.

Fein D, Waterhouse L, Lucci D, Snyder D. Cognitive subtypes in developmentally disabled children: a pilot study. J Autism Devel Disord 1985;15:77–95.

Gaffney GR, Tsai LY, Kuperman S, Minchin S. Cerebellar structure in autism. Am J Dis Child 1987;141:1330–1332.

Geller E, Ritvo ER, Freeman BJ, Yuwiler A. Preliminary observations on the effects of fenfluramine on blood serotonin and symptoms in three autistic boys. N Engl J Med 1982;307:165–169.

Gillberg C, Svendsen P. Childhood psychosis and computed tomographic brain scan findings. J Autism Devel Disord 1983;13:19–32.

Golden GS. Neurological functioning. In: Cohen DJ, Donnellan AM, Paul R, eds. Handbook of autism and pervasive developmental disorders. New York: Wiley and Sons, 1987.

Gubbay S, Lobascher M, Kingarlee P. A neurologic appraisal of autistic children: results of Western Australia survey. Dev Med Child Neurol 1970;13:19–32.

Hass R, Rapin I, Moser H. Rett syndrome and autism. J Child Neurol 1988;3:52–593.

Hier DB, LeMay M, Rosenberger PB. Autism and unfavorable left-right asymmetries of the brain. J Autism Devel Disord 1979;9:153–159.

Horwitz B, Rumsey J, Grady C, Rapoport J. Cerebral metabolic landscape in autism, intercorrelations of regional glucose utilization. Arch Neurol 1988;45:749–756.

Ho HH, Lockitch G, Eaves L, Jacobson B. Blood serotonin concentrations and fenfluramine therapy in autistic children. J Pediatr 1986;108:465–469.

Jacobson JW, Janick MP. Observed prevalence of multiple developmental disabilities. Ment Retard 1983;21:87–94.

Kanner L. Autistic disturbances of affective contact. Nerv Child 1943;2:217–250.

Landau WV, Kleffner FR. Syndrome of acquired aphasia with convulsive disorder in children. Neurology 1957;7:523–530.

Lockyer L, Rutter M. A five to fifteen year followup study of infantile psychosis: IV. Patterns of cognitive abilities. Br J Soc Clin Psychol 1970;9:152–163.

Minshew N, Payton J, Wolf GL, Latchaw RE. ^{1}H NMR imaging of autistics: implications for neurology. Ann Neurol 1986;20:417.

Nass R, Gazzaniga MS. Cerebral lateralization and specialization in the human central nervous system. In: Plum F, ed. Handbook of physiology: the nervous system V. Baltimore: American Physiologic Society, 1987.

Nass R, Pietrucha D. Pervasive developmental disorder variant of epileptic aphasia. J Child Neurol 1990;5:327–328.

Opitz JM. X-linked mental retardation 2. Alan R. Liss, New York:1986.

Paul R. Natural history. In: Cohen DJ, Donnellan AM, Paul R, eds. Handbook of autism and pervasive developmental disorders. New York: Wiley and Sons, 1987.

Payton J, Minshew N. Early appearance of partial complex seizures in autism. Ann Neurol 1987;22:408.

Prior MR, Bradshaw JL. Hemisphere functioning in autistic children. Cortex 1979;15:73–81.

Prior MR, Tress B, Hoffman WL, Boldt D. Computed tomographic study of children with classic autism. Arch Neurol 1984;41:482–484.

Rapin I, Allen D. Developmental language disorders: nosologic considerations. In: Kirk U, ed. Neuropsychology of language, reading and spelling. New York: Academic Press, 1983.

Rapin I, Allen D. Syndromes in developmental dysphasia and adult aphasia. In: Plum F, ed. Language, communication and the brain. New York: Raven Press, 1988.

Rapin I, Mattis S, Rowan A, Golden G. Verbal auditory agnosia. Devel Med Child Neurol 1977;19:192–207.

Rapin I. Disorders of higher cerebral function in preschool children. Am J Dis Child 1988;142:1178–1182.

Ritvo ER, Freeman BJ, Scheibel AB, et al. Lower purkinje cell counts in the cerebella of four autistic subjects: initial findings of the UCLA-NSAC autopsy research report. Am J Psychiatry 1986;43:862–866.

Ritvo ER, Freeman BJ, Geller E, Yuwiler A. Effects of fenfluramine on 14 outpatients with the syndrome of autism. J Am Acad Child Psychiatry 1983;22:549–558.

Ritvo ER, Freeman BJ, Yuwiler A, et al. Fenfluramine therapy for autism: promise and precaution. Psychopharmacol Bull 1986;22:133–140.

Ritvo ER, Garber H. Cerebellar hypoplasia and autism. N Engl J Med 1988;319:1152.

Rosenbloom R, Campbell M, George AE, et al. High resolution CT scanning in infantile autism: a quantitative approach. J Am Acad Child Psychiatry 1984;23:72–77.

Rumsey JM, Hamburger SD. Neuropsychological findings in high-functioning men with infantile autism, residual state. J Clin Exper Neuropsychol 1988;10:201–221.

Schain RJ, Yannet H. Infantile autism. J Pediatr 1960;57:560–567.

Sherman M, Nass R, Shapiro T. Brief report: regional cerebral blood flow in autism. J Autism Devel Disord 1984;14:439–446.

Soper HV, Satz P, Orsini DL, et al. Handedness patterns in autism suggest subtypes. J Autism Devel Disord 1986;16:155–167.

Steg JP, Rapoport JL. Minor physical anomalies in normal, neurotic, learning disabled, and severely disturbed children. J Autism Child Schizophr 1975;5:299–306.

Strayhorn JW, Rapp N, Donina W, Strain PS. Randomized trial of methylphenidate for an autistic child. J Am Acad Child Adolesc Psychiatry 1988;27:244–247.

Tsai L. Pre-, peri- and neonatal factors in autism. In: Schopler E, Mesibov G, eds. Neurobiological issues in autism. New York: Plenum Press, 1987.

Tsai L, Stewart M. Etiological implication of maternal age and birth order in infantile autism. J Autism Devel Disord 1983;13:57–65.

Vilensky JA, Damasio AR, Maurer RG. Gait disturbances in patients with autistic behavior. Arch Neurol 1981;38:646–649.

Wing L. Asperger's syndrome: a clinical account. Psychol Med 1981;11:115–129.

Wing L, Atwood A. Syndromes of autism and atypical development. In: Cohen DJ, Donnellan AM, Paul R, eds. Handbook of autism and pervasive developmental disorders. New York: Wiley and Sons, 1987.

Wing L, Gould J. Severe impairments of social interaction and associated abnormalities in children: epidemiology and classification. J Autism Devel Disord 1979;9:11–29.

Witt-Engerstrom I, Gillberg C. Rett syndrome in Sweden. J Autism Devel Disord 1987;17:149–150.

Chapter 6

Tourette's Syndrome and Other Tic Disorders

Gerald Erenberg, MD

Tourette's syndrome and other tic disorders were once considered to be rare events of no major medical interest. More recently, there has been a dramatic increase in the public and scientific interest in them. Tics are the most common form of movement disorder in childhood. It has been estimated that up to 24% of children will experience tic movements at some time. Tourette's syndrome, the most serious tic disorder, must be seen in the context of its cardinal manifestation—tics.

Tics are involuntary, sudden, rapid, recurrent, purposeless, nonrhythmic, stereotyped motor movements or vocalizations. As is true for many movement disorders, the specific involuntary movement is often more easily recognized than precisely defined. Tics can be described by their anatomic location, frequency, number, intensity, duration, and complexity. Tics are generally considered involuntary, but they may be accompanied by a premonitory sensory urge. Persons with tics often describe the need to perform the action as irresistible, analogous to a person's need to breathe, even when told to hold their breath for as long as possible.

Tics can typically be suppressed for brief periods of time, which range from seconds to minutes. They increase in frequency and intensity when the person is under any form of mental or physical stress. Alternatively, some persons manifest their tics in the most obvious way when they are in a relaxed situation, such as quietly watching television. Tics are reduced or even disappear during sleep. They also tend to be at a low level when the person is placed in a novel or highly structured situation, and this explains why tics are often not seen when the patient is in the doctor's office. When tics are present over long intervals of time, their severity waxes and wanes. The specific form of tic may also be triggered by environmental stimuli. The cough that begins when the patient has an upper respiratory infection may continue for long periods as an involuntary vocal tic. New tics may also come about because of imitation of a normal occurring event such as hearing a dog bark.

Most researchers now believe that all persons with any form of a tic disorder are individuals with a genetic predisposition to this disorder. The genetic expression varies. The fullest expression of a tic disorder, Tourette's syndrome, is estimated to affect one in every 2500 persons. This makes Tourette's syndrome and related tic disorders an important neuropsychiatric condition, especially since many of these individuals have associated behavioral problems.

THE SPECTRUM OF TIC DISORDERS

The diagnosis of tics is a clinical one, and no biologic markers are known. Children with tic disorders are generally placed into one of three diagnostic categories, as listed in the *American Psychiatric Association Diagnostic and Statistical Manual of Mental Disorders, 3rd Edition, Revised (DSM III-R):* (1) transient tic disorder; (2) chronic motor or vocal tic disorder; (3) Tourette disorder.

These categories are based on the types of tics as well as their duration. Certain features are common to all three categories. They all begin before age 21, are more common in males, and include tics that occur many times a day. Motor and vocal (phonic) tics may be classified as either simple or complex. Simple motor tics typically begin with brief bouts of transient tics involving the face or head, and there is often a rostral-caudal progression, with tics of the face, head, and shoulders appearing earlier and in a higher proportion of patients than motor tics of the limbs or trunk. Simple motor tics are sudden, brief, meaningless movements such as eye blinking, facial grimacing, nose twitching, lip pouting, neck jerking, shoulder shrugging, and abdominal tensing. In contrast, complex motor tics are of longer duration and appear more purposeful. Examples include rolling the eyes upwards or side to side, thrusting out an arm, squatting, hopping, jumping, writhing, and assuming dystonic postures. Other varieties of complex tics may include imitating gestures or movements of other people (echopraxia) or the performance of obscene gestures (copropraxia). Included in the admittedly broad rubric of complex motor tics are movements that seem compulsive and ritualistic, such as smelling an object, touching their own or someone else's body, and following a complex pattern of walking, such as hopping on every third step. Complex motor tics are rarely present in the absence of simple motor tics.

Vocal tics may occur in isolation, but they occur more commonly in persons who also have motor tics, and they usually appear after the onset of motor tics. As is true for motor tics, vocal tics are classified as simple or complex. The range of possible vocal symptoms is extraordinary, and virtually any noise or sound has the potential of evolving into a tic. Examples of simple vocal tics include common and natural vocalizations such as throat clearing, sniffing, grunting, coughing, snorting, lip noises, hissing, and syllable sounds such as "uh", "ee", and "bu".

Complex vocal tics involve linguistically meaningful words, phrases, or sentences that may be shouted out at inappropriate times. During conversation, vocal symptoms may interfere with the smooth flow of speech and resemble stammering or stuttering. Vocal tics can include repeating the sounds or words of another person (echolalia), repeating one's own sounds or words (palilalia), and involuntary use of obscene language (coprolalia). As with motor tics, vocal tics may also develop a ritualistic quality, such as the need to repeat certain phrases a specific number of times or until it has been said in an exactly correct manner.

A *transient tic disorder* consists of single or multiple motor and/or vocal tics that occur for at least 2 weeks, but for no longer than 12 consecutive months. The most common forms of tics are eye blinking, facial movements, throat clearing, or sniffing. By definition, these tics disappear permanently after being present for less than 1 year.

A *chronic tic disorder* consists of either motor or vocal tics, but not both, lasting for more than 1 year. This disorder, which is similar to Tourette's syndrome, may consist of a single type of tic only, but there also may be a changing pattern of motor or vocal tics. The tics are often less severe and less bothersome than in Tourette's syndrome.

Tourette's syndrome is the diagnosis reserved for those children who have both multiple motor and vocal tics that have been present for more than 1 year. The tics range in severity from mild to severe. Since the diagnosis of Tourette's syndrome is based, in part, on the presence of symptoms for more than 1 year, children seen earlier in their course cannot be diagnosed with certainty until a sufficient period of time has passed.

DIFFERENTIAL DIAGNOSIS

The nomenclature used in describing movement disorders is entirely clinical, and no adequate anatomic, biochemical, or physiologic classification is in existence. Tics must be differentiated from other movement disturbances that can occur in childhood, including myoclonus, tremor, dystonia, chorea, athetosis, spasms, dyskinesias, and mannerisms. In the usual case, the identification of a tic disorder is generally straightforward when made in the context of the overall history and examination. But a difficult aspect of making the correct diagnosis is frequently in determining which of the categories of tic disorders best applies to the individual child.

The diagnosis of Tourette's syndrome in children with various developmental disorders may be difficult, because peculiar motor movements and language distortions are common in mental retardation, autism, or psychosis. Children with these disorders often have complex stereotyped movements, compulsive behavior, odd vocalizations, echolalia, echopraxia, or coprolalia. A further confounding factor is introduced when patients are treated with neuroleptic drugs, since both persistent and transient Tourette's syndrome have been reported following withdrawal of chronic neuroleptics. However, careful attention to the history of ever-changing motor and vocal tics usually allows a distinction between Tourette's syndrome and the manneristic behavior otherwise present in developmentally handicapped persons. It is possible that the tics of Tourette's syndrome and the manneristic behavior of developmental disorders may represent a common clinical expression of underlying central nervous system dysfunction.

The differentiation between tics and a seizure disorder should rarely be a problem. On occasion, however, the possibility of myoclonic seizures or complex partial seizures with automatisms is raised. Patients with tics retain consciousness when they have their movements, but an electroenceophalogram (EEG) should be performed if there is any doubt.

Sydenham's chorea, the neurologic manifestation of rheumatic fever, occurs in the same age group as do tic disorders, and its choreiform movements can easily be mistaken for tics. Close attention to the history, examination for the presence of other signs of rheumatic fever, and the long-term course of Sydenham's chorea should allow a correct diagnosis to be made. Sydenham's chorea leads to the subacute onset of emotional lability and declining school performance coincident with the onset of the involuntary movements. The chorea may occur as the sole manifestation of rheumatic fever, but it may be associated with carditis and arthritis. Even if untreated, Sydenham's chorea is self-limited and spontaneously disappears over several months. Recurrences of Sydenham's chorea are possible, but these repeat episodes tend to be years apart.

Wilson's disease can lead to involuntary movements that are diverse in nature but can mimic tics. The usual patient begins to manifest neurologic symptoms after the age of 10 years. On the other hand, the most common age of onset for tics is between the ages of 5 and 10 years. Persons with Wilson's disease may have disorders of other systems, including hepatic dysfunction, hemolytic anemia, or dementia and impulsive behavior.

Other disorders that may be confused with a tic disorder include tardive dyskinesia, chronic amphetamine abuse, posthemiplegic chorea, cerebral palsy, Lesch-Nyhan syndrome, heavy metal poisoning, torsion dystonia, the neuro-acanthocytosis syndrome, and subacute sclerosing panencephalitis. Each of these is a rare entity and, fortunately, has many features that are clinically different from those of a tic disorder.

EVALUATION OF THE CHILD WITH A TIC DISORDER

Diagnosis must be based on the history and physical examination, since there are no diagnostic laboratory studies. A complete past medical history is obtained to determine whether there has been any medical event that might have led to tics or other neurologic disorders. This history should include detailed questioning regarding prenatal events, birth history, head injuries, episodes of encephalitis or meningitis, poisonings, and medication or drug use, especially amphetamines. In addition, the developmental, behavioral, and academic histories are important. These include a detailed listing of developmental milestones, estimate of cognitive level, and history of learning problems. Specific questions must be asked about the possibility of attentional problems, mood lability, irritability, depression, anxiety, simple rituals, and obsessive worries and thoughts.

The age of onset of the involuntary movements, their pattern of waxing and waning, and their exact form must be documented. Questions are asked regarding the possibility of associated sensory urges, suppressibility, and factors associated with worsening or improvement. A detailed family history of tics is critical. In addition to searching for other family members with tics, questions must also be asked about others in the family with a history of attentional problems, hyperactivity, learning problems, obsessive-compulsive behaviors, or any other form of mental health disturbance.

Except for the tics, physical and neurologic examinations are normal in persons with Tourette's syndrome or any other form of a tic disorder, although the presence of soft signs has sometimes been emphasized. Soft signs generally reflect the maturity and degree of development of the central nervous system. Unfortunately, each person testing for soft signs seems to have developed his or her own examination battery, and standards for scoring are not uniform. There is a high incidence of both false-positive as well as false-negative findings, and most pediatric neurologists now believe that soft signs are not a reliable or important part of the evaluation of persons with a tic disorder. Since tics can be suppressed during the time that the child is in the office, no tics may be seen during the interview and examination. Nevertheless, the history can be considered reliable if the description is typical for tics.

In the usual child with a tic disorder, laboratory testing is unnecessary. All clinically available tests will be normal in children with tic disorders, and laboratory testing is ordered only when other causes for involuntary movements must be considered. Electroencephalograms are normal, although some reports have described minor, nondiagnostic abnormalities. An EEG is useful only in cases where the movements possibly represent myoclonic or complex partial seizures. Computerized tomography (CT) scans and magnetic resonance imaging (MRI) scans are normal in persons with tic disorders. The patient with possible Wilson's disease should have serum copper and ceruloplasmin checked, but the best screening test is actually a slit-lamp examination for Kayser-Fleischer rings. Patients suspected of having Sydenham's chorea should have an electrocardiogram (ECG) and streptococcal antibody determination. Psychological testing does not diagnose Tourette's syndrome, but it may identify associated conditions such as learning disabilities or attention deficits.

The typical child with a tic disorder may be assessed and treated entirely by the child psychiatrist. Although a neurologist need not see every child, a neurologist may be helpful if there are unusual features or if there are suspicions of an alternative neurologic cause for the involuntary movements.

TOURETTE'S SYNDROME

The disorder now known as Tourette's syndrome was first described by Georges Gilles de la Tourette in 1885. Tourette's syndrome was considered a medical curiosity until the 1970s, when the number of diagnosed cases increased rapidly. This increase corresponds to the time when treatment first became available and thinking shifted toward the disorder's being of neurologic origin.

As previously described, Tourette's syndrome is the form of tic disorder characterized by a changing pattern of multiple motor *and* vocal tics that persists for more than 1 year. The tics begin before age 21 and wax and wane in intensity. They are characterized by a continuing pattern of change in which old tics disappear and new tics develop. When the tics first begin, there may be periods of up to several months in which they disappear completely. As with all forms of tic disorders, the intensity of the tics increases under stress and decreases or disappears during sleep.

Either motor or, less often, vocal tics may be the initial manifestation. Most patients initially become symptomatic between the ages of 5 and 10 years. The exact age of onset is often difficult for parents to recall, but the median age seems to be approximately 7 years. The tics may begin abruptly with multiple tics that continue with no symptom-free periods. Typically, however, the onset consists of a single tic that lasts only a few weeks. Minor transient tics then come and go until the time when they last longer and become more intense. During this early phase, children are typically seen by various medical specialists, depending on the type of tic. If the child has an eye blinking tic, he or she may be seen by an ophthalmologist. If the child has recurrent sniffing or coughing, an allergist or otolaryngologist may be consulted. Another frequent outcome is for the child to be referred to a mental health professional for treatment of a presumed emotional problem, since an increase in tics is often associated with anxiety. All mental health providers must be aware of Tourette's syndrome, since they will frequently be involved in the evaluation of children with tics.

The first motor tic almost always involves the face and most often consists of eye blinking. Other early motor tics may also involve the neck and shoulders. Vocal tics can occur independently or in association with motor movements. Coprolalia is certainly the most disruptive form of involuntary vocalization. Although stressed in original report and fixed in the public's conception, coprolalia actually occurs in less than one-third of patients. Hence, coprolalia is far from necessary for the diagnosis of Tourette's syndrome.

Although Tourette's syndrome has been reported in all races, ethnic groups, and socioeconomic classes, it occurs much more frequently in white than in black persons. Initial reports revealed a high percentage of patients to be of Ashkenazi Jewish or Eastern European origin. However, more recent studies have shown that the percentage of patients with Jewish or Eastern European background is not unusually high. Tourette's syndrome is predominantly a disorder of males, and the male-to-female ratio is 4:1. Since there has been increasing publicity about Tourette's syndrome in the lay press and television, many cases are now being diagnosed by parents, relatives, or friends. In the past, the correct diagnosis was often delayed because of lack of physician awareness, a tendency for physicians to relate unusual activities to psychological problems, and a belief that coprolalia is necessary for diagnosis.

The symptoms of Tourette's syndrome can be mild, moderate, or severe, depending on their frequency, complexity, and the degree to which they cause impairment or disruption of the child's schoolwork, play, and family life. The symptoms, frequency, and severity can vary greatly over time. Children may suppress their symptoms while at school, but their tics may become quite severe when they return home.

This is often a source of great wonderment to parents, who cannot believe that their child's teacher does not notice the multitude and severity of tics that they witness at home.

The etiology of Tourette's syndrome is unknown. Most theories have implicated abnormalities of neurotransmitters, including serotonin, catecholamines, acetylcholine, and gamma-aminobutyric acid. These are attractive theories, since systems relying on neurotransmitters send projections to the substantia nigra and the striatum. Noradrenergic mechanisms have been suggested by the observation that clonidine, a drug that inhibits noradrenergic functioning by stimulation of an autoreceptor, may improve tic symptoms. Involvement of noradrenergic systems has also been suggested by the known exacerbation of symptoms by stress and anxiety.

Most theories, however, have centered on the potential role of dopamine abnormalities because dopamine blockers ameliorate the symptoms. Studies that have measured cerebrospinal fluid homovanillic acid, the metabolic end-product of dopamine metabolism, have shown conflicting results. Many have found decreased levels, leading to the possibility of hypersensitivity of postsynaptic dopamine receptors. In addition, Tourette's syndrome can be precipitated at times by the administration of psychostimulant drugs that increase the release of dopamine. Alternatively, recent studies, including autopsy reports, have raised the possibility that the neurochemical disorder is based on abnormalities in the endogenous opioid system.

There is now conclusive evidence based on systematic studies of Tourette's syndrome families that this is a genetic disorder, and an extensive search is in progress for the genetic marker. Current evidence indicates that this is an autosomal-dominant disorder. When one parent is a carrier or has Tourette's syndrome, there is a 50% chance that each child will receive the genetic vulnerability from that parent. However, not every child who inherits the gene will develop symptoms of the disorder, and this indicates incomplete penetrance. The penetrance is higher in males than in females. There is a 99% chance of males but only a 70% chance of females showing some clinical expression of the gene.

The gene for Tourette's syndrome also exhibits variable expression, which means that different symptoms occur in different people. These symptoms may include various combinations of involuntary movements and associated behavioral disabilities. The possibilities include full-blown Tourette's syndrome, chronic tic disorder, or, according to some authors, obsessive-compulsive disorder. Many individuals with Tourette's syndrome also have attention deficit hyperactivity disorder, but the question of whether this is an expression of the Tourette's syndrome gene is still controversial. There are also differences between males and females in the form of expression of the Tourette's syndrome gene. Males are more likely to have Tourette's syndrome or chronic tics, while females are more likely to have an obsessive-compulsive disorder. The severity of symptoms in a child cannot be predicted based on the severity of symptoms in the affected parent.

Genetic factors, however, cannot explain the presence of Tourette's syndrome in all patients. Perhaps 10 to 15% of patients with Tourette's syndrome do not acquire the disorder genetically. Tics have occasionally been described as having an acquired cause such as may occur after carbon monoxide poisoning, head trauma, or encephalitis. With or without a genetic predisposition, the course and severity of an individual person's Tourette's syndrome is affected by environmental factors, which can include emotional stresses, physical problems related to illness or abnormal birth processes, or the exposure to medication such as the psychostimulants.

ASSOCIATED CONDITIONS

Although Tourette's syndrome is a chronic disorder, it does not lead to any health problems or physical deterioration. At times, however, the motor tics may be severe enough to lead to local pain. Persons with this disorder have no shortening of their life span, and many persons have now been described who have Tourette's syndrome and are in their 70s and 80s.

The relationship between a patient's emotional life and his or her tics is deeply intertwined, but it is no longer believed that these emotional factors are the *cause* of Tourette's syndrome. Complex relationships exist between emotions and tics even in children whose day-to-day behavior is not out of the ordinary. For children with Tourette's syndrome, the severity of their tics often seems to be a barometer of their emotional state. Many patients exhibit a worsening of their symptoms at exciting times such as holidays, birthdays, or the beginning or ending of school. Once a patient enters a phase of increasing tics, a process may be triggered that takes several months before it has run its course.

A variety of associated behavioral and learning difficulties beset many children with Tourette's syndrome. These features have placed Tourette's syndrome on the border between neurology and psychiatry, and its explains the concept that Tourette's syndrome is a neuropsychiatric disorder. Associated behavior and learning difficulties can be present in children with mild tics as well as in those whose involuntary movements are severe. For many children, the associated behavioral and learning problems cause more difficulties in everyday life than do the tics. Even if tic control is achieved, there is not necessarily a corresponding improvement in the other aspects of the disorder.

The most common associated behavioral difficulties in childhood are of the types considered under attention deficit hyperactivity disorder. These include short attention span, distractibility, impulsiveness, and motor restlessness. It is important to note that the problems with attention deficits and hyperactivity usually precede the onset of tics. Therefore, many children have already been seen for medical attention because of their parents' concern regarding behavioral problems, even before the tics have emerged. Up to 50% of all children with Tourette's syndrome have attention difficulties, and these problems tend to increase and worsen as the tics develop and become more prominent. As with all of the associated behaviors, it is likely that the true incidence is lower than reported because of ascertainment bias. The incidence is quite high for those who come to medical attention, but family and epidemiologic studies have indicated that most *mild* cases do not have associated behavioral difficulties and do not come to clinical attention.

Obsessive-compulsive behaviors are frequent findings in persons with Tourette's syndrome. An estimated 30 to 40% of persons with Tourette's syndrome have such symptoms, and many of the complex motor and vocal tics could be considered obsessive-compulsive symptoms and not actual tics. As opposed to attention difficulties, which usually precede tics, obsessive-compulsive behaviors generally occur after the tics have been present for several years. They tend to worsen and may even occur first during adolescence or early adult life. Obsessive-compulsive symptoms range from mild to severe, and their importance can increase at the same time that the tics are becoming less of a problem.

Other behavioral characteristics, which occur in approximately 30% of children, include high levels of anxiety, fearfulness, emotional lability, low frustration tolerance, impulsivity, and aggressiveness. These tend to coexist with attention difficulties, and they frequently lead to temper outbursts that include screaming, hitting, biting, and threatening others. In general, the exact relationship between these behaviors and Tourette's syndrome is uncertain.

Physicians are frequently asked whether these aggressive behaviors are tics, involuntary in nature, or whether they can be controlled by the individual. This is a most difficult question to answer, but this situation is best conceived as being one in which patients exhibit emotional patterns that have been shaped by their neurologic disorder, but over which control can be achieved, even though with much greater difficulty than in the usual person. The feeling of being out of control is quite frightening to the children themselves as well as to their families.

Children with Tourette's syndrome often have difficulty in school, and many have repeated grades or are in special education programs. Their actual tics are disruptive in the classroom and lead to the mistaken belief that the movements or noises are being purposefully done to disrupt the classroom or to draw negative attention. Some children react to their emotional burden of having uncontrollable motor tics and noises by becoming depressed or aggressive. Those with attention difficulties may perform poorly because of their short attention span, distractibility, and poor organization. In addition, many children have true underlying learning disabilities as well.

Several studies have verified the presence of learning disabilities on psychological and neuropsychological testing, although the distribution of full-scale IQ scores is within the average range. No single pattern of cognitive dysfunction has been identified, but there is a tendency for Tourette's syndrome patients to have deficiencies on tests that require visual-spatial and visual-motor skills. Difficulties with handwriting, along with difficulties in performing well on timed tests, are other common problems. A final concern is the negative effect that medication treatment may impose on a child's ability to learn. All children with Tourette's syndrome should have psychoeducational testing if they are experiencing learning problems.

TREATMENT

No cure exists for Tourette's syndrome or any other tic disorder. Potential treatments are symptomatic, and there is no evidence that early treatment alters the natural course of the disorder. Many treatments have been unsuccessful,

including hypnotherapy, behavior therapy, psychotherapy, psychoanalysis, lobotomy, thalamotomy, and shock therapy. Medications that have been tried include sedatives, antidepressants, stimulants, antiparkinsonian drugs, antipsychotic drugs, and anticonvulsants. The spontaneous waxing and waning of symptoms make it particularly difficult to assess any treatment program and to design adequate studies.

The decision about whether or when to treat an individual patient depends on the degree to which the tics or other symptoms of Tourette's syndrome are interfering with the child's normal development or ability to function productively. If medication treatment is chosen, it is imperative that an initial decision be reached as to which of the symptoms of Tourette's syndrome requires treatment, since medications that ameliorate tics often do not improve associated behavioral difficulties. In fact, most patients with milder forms of Tourette's syndrome or chronic tics never require medication treatment.

Education, Coping, and Adapting

The initial approach to treatment is to explain the disorder fully to the child and the child's family. Even though Tourette's syndrome has become widely known, many lay persons have not heard of this disorder. Virtually all children with Tourette's syndrome have, at some time, been accused of voluntarily doing these mysterious acts. The involuntary nature of the condition must be stressed. Parents and children react to the diagnosis of Tourette's syndrome in a manner that reflects their individual personalities, their abilities to cope with uncertainty and stress, and the availability of social and medical support. Some families initially react with relief that there has finally been a medical diagnosis for the child's problems. Others react with anger and disbelief, and there may be a strong tendency to deny the diagnosis. This is made easier by the fact that the symptoms typically wax and wane, allowing the family to temporarily believe that their child is now cured because of the lessening or the disappearance of symptoms.

Others who might be involved in the child's everyday life also benefit from information on Tourette's syndrome and its various manifestations. The potential associated problems with short attention span, hyperactivity, impulsiveness, or learning disabilities must be brought to the attention of school personnel. A sensitive teacher can be of great help in fostering self-worth and self-esteem by showing that the child is accepted and respected, even with the difficulties. Special arrangements might be necessary in the classroom to help overcome a child's problems with learning disabilities, poor handwriting skills, or difficulty with taking timed tests.

Improved understanding can be helped through the services provided by the Tourette Syndrome Association, an active public support group with a national as well as many regional offices. The Tourette Syndrome Association can share in the education of families by speaking with them directly as well as by sharing their publications for the public-at-large as well as for patients and their families. Referring a family to a local Tourette Syndrome Association group is often helpful, but individual or family therapy may also be necessary. It is particularly difficult to deal with families who have previously been for counseling in a situation in which the true cause of the disorder was not appreciated.

Medication

The clinician should not attempt to begin medication treatment at the initial visit. The first several months should be used, if possible, to help establish a baseline of symptoms and to determine what difficulties are present in addition to the tics. This time is also used for helping educate the family about the disorder and helping them cope with the impact of the diagnosis. It often becomes apparent that the child's tics are mild and of little functional significance.

These children do not require medical treatment, and their families can be reassured that medication is available if the tics worsen in the future. The severity of the individual person's symptoms tends to become apparent within 2 to 3 years of the initial appearance of tics.

When symptoms are severe enough to require treatment with medication, the decision to start treatment must be agreed upon by the child, family, and physician. Whether the treatment is being aimed at tics or at behavioral symptoms, certain basic principles apply to all medications. Patients are always started on the smallest possible dose of medication to help determine the individual person's sensitivity. The dosage is increased gradually with attention to both the development of side effects and the improvement in symptom control. Increasing dosages slowly usually results in fewer and milder side effects. It may take several weeks of treatment before the beneficial effect of the medication is noted, and it is important to avoid discontinuing medication prematurely when symptoms do not respond immediately. Once an effective medication is found, the lowest effective dosage is maintained, but it is necessary to change the dosage periodically to keep up with the natural fluctuation of symptoms.

Medication To Suppress Tics

Haloperidol (Haldol), a dopamine-blocking agent, remains the best known and most widely used medication in the treatment of Tourette's syndrome and other tic disorders. Haloperidol is able to reduce tics in 70% of treated patients; however, more than 50% of those who receive this medication complain of side effects, and only 25% report significant improvement without any side effects. Hence, less than 50% of treated patients continue haloperidol for an extended period. Because therapeutic and toxic dosages are close, the best strategy is to keep the total dosage at an amount that decreases symptoms by approximately 75%.

Pimozide (Orap) and fluphenazine (Prolixin) are alternative neuroleptic drugs also thought to be effective because of their ability to block dopamine receptors. These two agents appear to have a somewhat lower incidence of side effects, but the list of possible reactions is similar with all three drugs. The most common short-term side effects include excessive fatigue, intellectual dulling, dysphoria, increased appetite and weight, memory problems, personality changes, parkinsonian symptoms, and anticholinergic symptoms.

The possibility of tardive dyskinesia exists with long-term use of dopamine receptor blockers. Tardive dyskinesia has occurred infrequently and has disappeared in all cases with discontinuation of the medication. School phobias may appear during the first weeks of neuroleptic treatment, even with low doses. Despite the improvement of tic symptoms, the anxiety about going to school can be disabling. This phobic behavior may continue for months unless recognized as a drug side effect, and the behavior will disappear within weeks after the medication has been discontinued.

The dosage of neuroleptic drugs required for the treatment of tics is considerably less than that for those used to treat psychoses. Treatment should begin with very small amounts such as 0.25 mg of haloperidol or 1 mg of pimozide taken once a day at bedtime. When the dosage is increased slowly on a weekly basis, dystonic reactions are rare. Most children are treated adequately by a dosage of 1.5 to 3.0 mg of haloperidol each day. The usual dosage of pimozide for children is 4 to 10 mg each day. Some physicians prescribe antiparkinsonian drugs prophylactically, but it is unknown whether they are beneficial. Initial reports on pimozide indicated the possibility of ECG abnormalities in the form of Q-T prolongation. Further investigations with larger numbers of patients have not justified these concerns, but follow-up ECG studies are still being advised by the manufacturer.

The problems associated with the use of neu-roleptic agents have led to a search for alternative medications. Clonidine (Catapres), an alpha-adrenergic agonist most frequently used for the treatment of hypertension, is an alternative medication. Although it is relatively free of severe side effects, reports on the effectiveness of clonidine have varied. Some studies have indicated that up to 62% of treated patients respond favorably, but one study found clonidine to be no more effective than placebo.

Clonidine is started at 0.05 mg once a day, and this is increased by 0.05 mg a day on a weekly basis until there is improvement or until tolerance is reached. Clonidine is best taken in small doses three or four times each day because of its relatively short half-life. A transdermal patch needing to be changed only once a week is available, but most children rapidly develop a dermatitis. Because of the lowered incidence of side effects, many clinicians begin medication treatment with clonidine and reserve the use of neuroleptic agents for refractory cases. Sedation is the most common side effect, while orthostatic hypotension and dizziness can occur at higher dosages. Tardive dyskinesia has not been reported. In addition to reducing motor and vocal tics, clonidine may also improve attention problems or lead to a feeling of calmness. In general, the neuroleptic agents do not improve the behavior problems associated with Tourette's syndrome.

Combinations of medications are sometimes used when a single agent is only partly effective. The combination of a neuroleptic and clonidine has been used for patients whose symptoms are not fully controlled on one of these agents alone, or in those patients who are having serious side effects when the medication is being used in high dosage. Smaller doses of both medicines are generally employed when the drugs are combined. Clonazepam (Klonopin) is a benzodiazepine that has also been used in combination with clonidine or a neuroleptic, but there is not yet strong evidence that this agent is effective in Tourette's syndrome.

Behavior-Modifying Medications

Many children require medications for attention deficit hyperactivity disorder whether or not they require treatment for tics. The relationship between Tourette's syndrome and psychostimulant medications has been a controversial one. A number of case reports and small series have suggested that psychostimulant medication may precipitate Tourette's syndrome or may increase the number of tics in individual patients. This purported effect is shared by all of the available stimulant agents, including methylphenidate, pemoline, and dextroamphetamine. The mechanism is postulated to be that these agents augment dopaminergic activity in the central nervous system.

The basic questions remain, "Do stimulants for the treatment of restless, poorly attentive behavior precipitate tics or Tourette's syndrome in persons who are genetically predisposed, or do these drugs cause the disorders in persons who are not predisposed and would otherwise have remained symptom-free?" The majority of clinicians believe that these agents have the potential for increasing or inducing tics in some, but not all, persons who are already destined to have Tourette's syndrome. If a child receiving such a drug develops tics, it is agreed that every attempt must be made to discontinue the medication. Unfortunately, discontinuing the stimulant agents often leads to major problems in the child's school and home adjustment.

Alternative medications for attention deficit hyperactivity disorder include clonidine and the tricyclic antidepressants. Tricyclic antidepressants do not appear to increase the natural pattern of tics, and these agents may also reduce emotional lability and obsessive-compulsive behaviors. If no medications other than the psychostimulants seem able to help a desperate behavioral situation, many pediatric neurologists will treat with a combination of a stimulant drug and a neuroleptic agent.

Obsessive-compulsive behaviors may also require treatment independent of treatment of other aspects of Tourette's syndrome. Tricyclic antidepressants may be used for this purpose, and the most effective agent appears to be clomipramine (Anafranil). Newer heterocyclic antidepressants such as fluoxetine (Prozac) are also frequently helpful, as shown by early studies in the use of this agent in persons with both Tourette's syndrome and obsessive-compulsive behaviors. The dosage range is between 20 and 80 mg per day, and several weeks may pass before positive effects are noticed. Combinations of low doses of neuroleptics and either fluoxetine or a tricyclic antidepressant can be used and may be helpful for individual patients. No serious interactions have been reported, but patients should be monitored carefully since there has not yet been extensive experience with combination therapy.

LONG-TERM COURSE AND PROGNOSIS

When a child with tics is initially evaluated, it is not possible to offer a definite prognosis. The tics may be transient or may become chronic, and they may be mild or severe. In addition, there may or may not be associated behavioral and learning difficulties. To complicate matters, individual components of Tourette's syndrome may follow opposite courses. Symptoms of attention deficit disorders tend to begin in the preschool years, peak in the early to middle school years, and become less prominent during adolescence. The motor and vocal tics often begin in the early school years and reach their peak during adolescence, after which they may begin to subside. On the other hand, the obsessive-compulsive behaviors most frequently begin in the later school years and then peak during late adolescence or early adulthood.

Because adolescence is a difficult time of life for almost everyone, it is not surprising that many persons with Tourette's syndrome experience great difficulties during this time. While some patients with Tourette's syndrome have an increase in their tic symptomatology during those years, it is equally important to understand that the same tics present at a younger age may become intolerable because of social pressures.

In contrast to classic descriptions of Tourette's syndrome's inevitably being a lifelong disorder, recent studies have found that up to 73% of patients report that their tics decreased markedly or mostly disappeared as they entered the latter years of adolescence or the early adulthood years. However, there may not be a proportionate improvement in the associated behavior difficulties. Moreover, some patients experience an exacerbation of tics during later adulthood, even when there had been a remission during the earlier adult years.

The life adjustments of Tourette's syndrome patients have not been adequately studied. Certainly, the severity of the tics is not the only factor that predicts a person's long-term adjustment and outcome. Rather, as preliminary information indicates, the associated behavioral or emotional problems are more likely to determine social adjustment, vocational status, and marital outcome. Since the majority of patients with Tourette's syndrome are children and adolescents, they may adapt and cope more effectively because of early diagnosis, treatment, and better understanding on the part of parents, teachers, the general public, and physicians.

REFERENCES

Cohen DJ, Bruun RD, Leckman JF, eds. Tourette's syndrome and tic disorders: clinical understanding and treatment. New York: John Wiley and Sons, 1988.

Erenberg G, Cruse RP, Rothner AD: The natural history of Tourette syndrome: a follow-up study. Ann Neurol 1987;22:383–385.

Kurlan R: Tourette's syndrome: current concepts. Neurology 1989;39:1625–1630.

Pauls DL, Leckman JF: The inheritance of Gilles de la Tourette's syndrome and associated behaviors: evidence for autosomal dominant transmission. N Engl J Med 1986;315:993–997.

Shapiro AK, Shapiro ES, Young JG, Feinberg TE. Gilles de la Tourette syndrome, 2nd ed. New York: Raven Press, 1988.

Stefl ME. Mental health needs associated with Tourette syndrome. Am J. Public Health 1984;74:1310–1313.

Resource
Tourette Syndrome Association
42-40 Bell Boulevard
Bayside, New York 11361

Chapter 7

MOVEMENT DISORDERS

Robert E. Burke, MD

Movement disorders include those abnormalities of motor control that are not primarily due to weakness or sensory loss. They are classified into three main groups: (*1*) the *dyskinesias,* which consist of a variety of abnormal involuntary movements, such as tics, dystonia, chorea, and tremor; (*2*) *parkinsonism,* which consists of a paucity of spontaneous movements typically in association with rigidity; and (*3*) the *ataxias,* which are characterized by imbalance, poor coordination, and other signs of cerebellar disease.

This chapter describes important varieties and causes of movement disorders among these three groups. Within each group, disorders are presented according to their clinical phenomenology, rather than their etiology, because the major emphasis is on how to recognize the conditions. The main focus is on how these conditions present, and particularly on the psychiatric or behavioral features that may lead to psychiatric referral. The most important diseases in the differential diagnosis of each movement disorder are discussed, and there is an outline of the appropriate diagnostic evaluation.

In addition to the sections organized by clinical phenomenology, separate sections on Wilson's disease and neuroleptic-induced movement disorders are included. These disorders are important because they are treatable and especially likely to be seen by the child psychiatrist. In addition, Wilson's disease and neuroleptics give rise to such a variety of movement disorders that they are best discussed separately. Tics are probably the most common movement disorder of childhood and are of such importance to the practicing child psychiatrist that they are considered in a separate chapter devoted to the subject (see Chapter 6).

THE DYSKINESIAS
Dystonia

CLINICAL FEATURES

Of the dyskinesias presenting in childhood, dystonia is one frequently misdiagnosed as psychogenic (Lesser and Fahn, 1978). Some of the reasons for this misdiagnosis are that the clinical features of dystonia are not widely known, it often occurs in the absence of other neurologic signs that would indicate its organic basis, and its features can vary tremendously during the examination. In spite of its name, dystonia is not an abnormality of muscle tone. It is a type of involuntary movement that tends to be twisting and sustained. As it becomes more severe, dystonia can lead to persistent postural deformities. However, many neurologists and psychiatrists have the misconception that it always leads to a state of severe, generalized postural abnormalities—the condition of whole-body contortion as often depicted in textbooks of neurology—but these cases are the minority and are observed later in the course. Earlier, when these patients are more mildly affected and more likely to be referred to a psychiatrist, the manifestations can be quite subtle.

Before 8 years of age, children are likely to present with dystonia affecting the foot. Typically, they develop posturing of the foot during walking. The foot typically assumes an equinovarus posture: inverted and plantar flexed. Other abnormal movements, such as sustained plantar flexion of the foot or sustained dorsiflexion of the toe, may be seen. It is important to realize that the involuntary movement may occur only on walking; the dystonia may be absent at rest, or with running, or with walking backward. Some of these children have been misdiagnosed as "psychogenic" because they have been unable to walk forward without the use of crutches and yet can walk backward or run forward normally.

At an older age, children are more likely to present with involvement of the hands, trunk, or neck, although it should be realized that dystonia is quite variable as to age and site of onset. Dystonia of the hand commonly presents as a sustained, abnormal posturing during writing. The fingers press overly tightly on the pen; the fist is clenched with strong contraction of forearm agonist and antagonist muscles; the wrist is forcibly either extended or flexed; the arm abducts and lifts the elbow off the writing surface. Eventually, these abnormal involuntary movements interfere with many hand movements. Sometimes, when children with dystonia attempt to resist or overcome the sustained involuntary movements, they develop superimposed rapid, jerking, or even oscillatory movements. Since many neurologists conceive of dystonia as purely slow, twisting movement, they may misdiagnose these rapid movements as chorea, myoclonus, or tremor.

Dystonia of the trunk may present as scoliosis or an excessive lordosis. When it affects the head and neck, dystonia may cause rotation (torticollis), flexion (anterocollis), or extension (retro-collis). As described for the foot and hand, the severity and pattern of involvement may vary according to the particular activity, and there may be superimposed rapid, jerking movements. In children, dystonia is less likely to affect the face, but it may if there is a later age of onset. The patterns of involvement include sustained eye closure (blepharospasm); facial grimacing; sustained jaw closure or opening (oromandibular dystonia); or strained speech (spasmodic dysphonia).

The following history illustrates a typical case of a child with dystonia:

A 6-year-old girl with a normal birth and development, and without a history of neurologic or psychiatric illness, sprained her ankle while playing soccer. The parents brought her to their pediatrician the following day, who diagnosed a sprain, and recommended bed rest, analgesics, and hot soaks. After a week, the pain had subsided, and the child attempted to return to school. There was no pain on walking, but the child noted that her foot was clumsy; it tended to in-toe, and there was a tendency to walk on the lateral edge of the sole. The clumsiness gradually became worse over 2 weeks' time, and twice the child tripped by catching her toe on a curb. The parents brought the child to their pediatrician, who found no evidence of soft tissue injury and no evidence of a fracture on X-ray. She was referred to an orthopedist for further management. On examination, she had equinovarus posturing of the foot when she walked, but there was no posturing when the foot was at rest. Examination of the foot and ankle were normal, and X-rays were normal. The orthopedist told the parents that there was no orthopedic abnormality, and he suspected that the foot problem might be an "attention-getting device." He recommended a bandage support and physical therapy.

However, the posturing of the foot became progressively worse, and the child started to use crutches. The orthopedist then referred the child to a psychiatrist for a presumed "conversion reaction." The psychiatrist observed that the child appeared happy and well-adjusted and, in fact, appeared to have "la belle indifference." On the promise of a reward with a piece of candy, the child could be coaxed to walk considerably better, at least briefly. The psychiatrist initially concurred that the foot problem was an attention-getting device but referred the child to a pediatric neurologist for a diagnostic evaluation of any possible organic cause.

The pediatric neurologist found a normal general neurologic exam; there was no abnormality of tone, no weakness, normal reflexes, and no sensory loss. He also noted that the child could walk backward normally. Lumbosacral spine films and a computed tomography (CT) scan of the head were normal. An electromyogram (EMG) showed concomitant contraction of the anterior tibialis and gastrocnemius muscles, which was interpreted as voluntary cocontraction of those muscles. The pediatric neurologist was convinced that an organic basis had been ruled out. Over the subsequent 2 years, the child developed involvement of the other leg and trunk, and she became wheelchair-bound.

This fictional case illustrates several points. Often, an injury early in the course is a "red herring" that leads to a negative orthopedic evaluation and futile attempts at therapy by casting or physical therapy. Second, the ability of suggestion to relieve dystonia transiently and the dystonia's disappearance with rest or an alternate motor act (such as walking backward) frequently lead to a misdiagnosis. Finally, the general neurologic and laboratory studies are always negative or normal in the primary dystonias and do not exclude organicity. Dystonia is a clinical diagnosis.

DIFFERENTIAL DIAGNOSIS

The causes of dystonia are classified into two major groups: (1) In the *primary* dystonias (also called idiopathic torsion dystonia, or "dystonia musculorum deformans"), the child has only dystonia. There is no intellectual decline, weakness, sensory loss, or pathologic reflexes. Also certain exclusion criteria have been met: (*a*) there must be no history of birth asphyxia or developmental delay, and (*b*) there must be no prior history of stroke, significant head injury, encephalitis, or treatment with neuroleptics. The primary torsion dystonias may be familial or sporadic (Table 7.1). (2) The *secondary* dystonias (or symptomatic dystonias) are those due to identifiable causes such as injuries and particular inherited or degenerative disorders (Table 7.1).

Table 7.1.
Etiologic Classification of the Dystonias[a]

Primary torsion dystonias (or idiopathic torsion dystonias)
Familial
Torsion dystonia in Ashkenazic Jews (autosomal-dominant)
Torsion dystonia in non-Jews (autosomal-dominant)
Levodopa-responsive dystonia (may also be sporadic)
Sporadic
Secondary dystonias (or symptomatic dystonias)
Perinatal asphyxia (including delayed-onset dystonia)
Head injury
Encephalitis
Stroke
Brain tumor
Antipsychotic drugs (e.g., phenothiazines, butyrophenones)
Huntington's disease
Wilson's disease
Juvenile parkinsonism

[a] This is a partial list. For a more complete review, the reader is referred to the review by Calne and Lang (1988).

Usually the secondary dystonias are associated with abnormalities on the neurologic examination in addition to the dystonia. However, there are exceptions; birth asphyxia or antipsychotic drugs can cause chronic dystonia that is indistinguishable from primary dystonia.

DIAGNOSTIC EVALUATION

In all patients, a complete history must be taken concerning the perinatal period, development, prior neurologic illnesses, and exposure to antipsychotics and other drugs. Not only should a verbal family history be taken but also as many first-degree relatives as possible must be *examined*. In many instances of childhood-onset familial dystonia, a simple verbal family history is negative, but examination reveals torticollis or writer's cramp in a first-degree relative. A detailed neurologic examination of the affected child must be performed; if there are any abnormalities other than dystonia, then one is dealing with a secondary dystonia, which requires an extensive evaluation (Calne and Lang, 1988). If, however, there is only dystonia on exam, then one is likely to be dealing with a primary dystonia, and only a few laboratory studies must be done to definitively exclude any secondary etiology. We recommend the following studies: (1) A serum ceruloplasmin determination and a slit-lamp examination of the cornea to evaluate for Kayser-Fleischer rings to exclude Wilson's disease; (2) an imaging study of the brain (either computed tomography with and without contrast or a magnetic resonance image (MRI) to exclude structural etiology (e.g., tumor, stroke, or prior asphyxial injury); and (3) a lumbar puncture. The cerebrospinal fluid (CSF) is always normal in the primary dystonias, and any CSF abnormality necessitates a more thorough evaluation for secondary dystonias.

TREATMENT

The initial medical trial should be with levodopa-carbidopa (Sinemet), gradually increased up to a dose of 25/100 three times a day. In a small percentage of patients with levodopa-responsive dystonia, a dramatic relief is observed (Nygaard et al., 1988). If there is not such a response, then this unique variant of primary dystonia has been excluded, and the levodopa should be tapered off and stopped. Then a prolonged trial of anticholinergic drugs should be started, beginning with low doses and gradually increasing. Approximately 70% of children with primary dystonia show a response to anticholinergic medications (Burke et al., 1986). If anticholinergic drugs fail to provide adequate relief, other medications that may be helpful include baclofen, carbamazepine, and clonazepam. Cryothalamotomy is primarily indicated in unilateral cases that cannot be controlled by medication.

Chorea

CLINICAL FEATURES

Choreic involuntary movements can affect any part of the body. They are abrupt in onset and brief. Their timing and location are random and therefore characteristically *unpredictable*. The movements tend to occur steadily, one after another, and are therefore said to be "flowing." In mild chorea, the movements are slight and infrequent, consisting of, for example, a flick of the finger or toe, or a sudden elevation of the eyebrows. As the movements increase in severity, whole limbs may be moved across joints and the gait may become lurching due to jerks of the torso.

Chorea is distinguishable from dystonia in two major respects: dystonic movements are *sustained* and they tend to occur *predictably* in the same location in an individual patient. For example, a child with equinovarus posturing of the right foot when walking will predictably show that type of movement in that location.

Early, mild chorea can be difficult to differentiate from mild intermittent tics. Both can be simple movements, abrupt in onset, and brief. Often helpful is the subjective report given by patients with tics that they experience an "urge" to move before the tic, and the movement relieves the "inner tension" that builds up. In addition, patients with tics report that they can suppress the movements, at least briefly, while choreic patients cannot. Patients with chorea can briefly grunt or sniff in conjunction with choreic torso movements, so these simple sounds do not reliably make a diagnosis of tics. More complex vocalizations, such as barks, whistles, or formed words do not occur in chorea and are indicative of a tic disorder. As these two movement disorders increase in severity, they become easier to differentiate. In tics, complex, stereotyped movements occur, such as kicking, squatting, or hand shaking; such complex movements do not occur in chorea. As chorea increases in severity, the movements occur "non-stop," one flowing into another, whereas tics tend to occur in abrupt flurries interspersed with periods devoid of any involuntary movements.

Early mild chorea may also be difficult to differentiate from some milder forms of myoclonus, such as minipolymyoclonus, observed in children with neuroblastoma (discussed below). The most distinguishing feature of myoclonic movements is that they lack the "flowing" quality of chorea.

DIFFERENTIAL DIAGNOSIS

Of the major causes of chorea in childhood (Table 7.2), one of the most common is *dyskinetic cerebral palsy (CP)*. Dyskinesias occur as the predominant neurologic disturbance in approximately 15% of children with static encephalopathy in the post-kernicterus era (Hagberg and Hagberg, 1984). While there is much controversy about the proportion of the static encephalopathies that are due to adverse perinatal events (Nelson and Ellenberg, 1986), the dyskinetic form seems to be particularly related to such events (Hagberg and Hagberg, 1984). Chorea in the setting of CP usually is not difficult to diagnose because there is a clear history of either an abnormal birth or a developmental delay. The neurologic exam is abnormal usually not only for involuntary movements but also for intellectual impairment, spasticity, or cerebellar abnormalities. In addition, chorea in dyskinetic CP is usually not "pure"; it occurs with athetosis and dystonia. Dystonia, in fact, is the most common and disabling involuntary movement of dyskinetic CP.

Sydenham's chorea (SC) is a neurologic complication of infection with group A streptococci, usually pharyngitis. In the postpenicillin era, SC

Table 7.2.
Causes of Chorea in Childhood[a]

Dyskinetic cerebral palsy
Sydenham's chorea
Chorea gravidarum
Huntington's disease
Wilson's disease
Drugs (both therapeutic drugs and drugs of abuse: oral contraceptives, neuroleptics, anticonvulsants, amphetamines, methadone)
Systemic illnesses: systemic lupus erythematosus, thyrotoxicosis, hypoparathyroidism
Neuroacanthocytosis

[a] This is a partial list.

has become rare. Nevertheless, the child psychiatrist may be called upon to evaluate children with SC because frequently they present with behavioral disturbances, including emotional lability, irritability, restlessness, or confusion. The chorea is usually bilateral, but in 20% of cases it is unilateral. It is sometimes associated with weakness. The diagnosis can be made with high probability if there is a positive throat culture, a rising antistreptolysin-O titer, clinical evidence of acute rheumatic fever, or rheumatic heart disease. However, because chorea often occurs months after the streptococcal infection, none of these evaluations may be revealing. In addition, only about a third of these patients develop rheumatic heart disease, so the cardiac examination may be unrevealing as well, making the diagnosis impossible to prove. The prognosis is good, and the duration of the chorea is limited to weeks or months. However, on rare occasions it persists for more than a year, and occasionally it recurs. However, the mental and behavioral changes are usually present only during the acute phase of the illness. A prior episode of SC often precedes the occurrence of chorea during pregnancy (*chorea gravidarum*) or during the use of birth control pills. A diagnosis of SC necesssitates penicillin prophylaxis against recurrent streptococcal infection.

Huntington's disease (HD), an important cause of chorea, is inherited as an autosomal-dominant illness with complete penetrance—50% of the offspring of affected individuals will inherit the gene and they will ultimately manifest the disease. Usually HD presents in middle age (30 to 40 years), but approximately 10 to 15% of cases present before age 20. HD is a neurologic illness that is especially likely to result in psychiatric referral because there are frequent alterations of intellect, affect, or personality. Although all patients develop dementia, a variety of psychiatric or behavioral disturbances may precede the dementia, including depression, mania, paranoid ideation, and aggressive or sexually inappropriate behavior.

HD not only presents with chorea, but in some cases, particularly in patients 20 years of age or younger, it may present as an akinetic/rigid variant. Children with this form are more likely to have the father as the affected parent. In this form, also called the "juvenile form," the illness may resemble parkinsonism, with slowness of movement and increased muscle tone. Dystonia may also predominate. Hence parkinsonism or dystonia that develops in childhood can be due to HD as well as to Wilson's disease or other causes. Young HD patients may also have seizures. Most patients at some point in their course develop abnormalities of eye movement, including slow saccades and poor visual fixation. The juvenile form is more rapidly progressive than the adult form.

The diagnosis of HD rests on recognition of the progressive deterioration in mentation, the characteristic abnormalities of motor control, and, above all, a history in successive generations of HD or neurologic or psychiatric disease. In particular, the physician must inquire with some detail into the causes of death. Since suicide occurs with high frequency in HD families, it must be viewed as suggestive when considering HD (Farrer, 1986). The only studies that may be helpful are CT or MRI scans, which may help confirm the diagnosis if they reveal the characteristic caudate atrophy. Although DNA markers for the HD gene locus on chromosome 4 currently offer the promise of permitting prenatal and preclinical identification of gene carriers within a family, the abnormal gene itself has not been identified and characterized. There is not, as yet, a biochemical marker that permits a diagnosis of HD in isolated individuals.

While symptomatic therapy for choreic movements and psychiatric disturbances is available, there is no intervention that alters the relentless progression, and the disease generally leads to death in 10 to 15 years. The choreic movements can be suppressed with either dopamine receptor blocking drugs, such as the phenothiazines or butyrophenones, or with a dopamine depletor,

such as reserpine. Antipsychotic drugs can also be useful in treating psychiatric symptoms.

HD must be distinguished from Wilson's disease, which may also cause alterations in mentation and chorea. However, Wilson's is inherited as an autosomal-recessive illness (see below). HD must also be distinguished from neuroacanthocytosis, a rare illness that causes a variety of neurologic findings, including chorea and caudate atrophy. Patients with neuroacanthocytosis generally have other involuntary movements besides chorea, such as tics, dystonia, and self-mutilating oral dyskinesias. This diagnosis is made by finding acanthocytes in a Wright's-stained blood smear.

A variety of drugs are capable of inducing chorea. As mentioned above, oral contraceptives have been reported to induce a recurrence of chorea in young women with a prior history of Sydenham's chorea or other medical causes of chorea. To be discussed further below are the movements induced by neuroleptic drugs: tardive dyskinesia (which differs in some important respects from true chorea) and withdrawal emergence syndrome, a true chorea usually observed in children. The anticonvulsants phenytoin (Dilantin) and carbamazepine (Tegretol) have also been reported to induce chorea. Drugs of abuse have also been reported to induce chorea, including amphetamines (Rylander, 1972) and methadone (Wasserman and Yahr, 1980).

The child psychiatrist should be aware that systemic lupus erythematosus and thyrotoxicosis, either of which may cause changes in personality or psychiatric symptoms, may present with chorea.

EVALUATION

Diagnostic evaluation of a patient with chorea requires a detailed history of the family and of drug use. In the neurologic exam, particular attention must be given to evaluation of the mental status and the eye movements. Blood studies should be obtained to evaluate for the conditions listed in Table 7.2: antistreptolysin-O titer, a sedimentation rate, antinuclear antibodies, thyroid function, serum calcium and serum ceruloplasmin. A blood smear should be examined for acanthocytes. If the patient is a young woman, a pregnancy test should be obtained. A throat culture should be obtained, and an echocardiogram performed to evaluate for valvular disease. A CT or MRI scan should be performed to evaluate for atrophy of the caudates and any evidence of long-standing cerebral injury as may be observed in CP. A slit-lamp examination for Kayser-Fleischer rings should be performed.

TREATMENT

Whether and how to treat chorea depend very much on the cause and are beyond the scope of this chapter. Underlying medical illnesses are treated in their own right. Sydenham's chorea may not require treatment if it is mild and remits spontaneously. There is some evidence that adrenocorticosteroids shorten the duration of chorea (Dr. A. Chutorian, personal communication). In severe cases the chorea can be suppressed with reserpine, which depletes brain dopamine, or with a dopamine receptor blocker, such as haloperidol. Similarly, in HD the chorea can be suppressed by either reserpine or haloperidol. Often, however, in HD the chorea is more a cosmetic problem that does not require treatment; it is the mental deterioration and late appearance of dystonia that impose disability.

Myoclonus

CLINICAL FEATURES

Myoclonus is a sudden, shock-like involuntary movement. Of all the movement disorders, it is the most difficult to encapsulate briefly because it has a variety of presentations, can be due to lesions located throughout the neuraxis, and has many different causes. Myoclonus may be focal (affecting a single body region, such as the arm), segmental (affecting structures innervated by a single spinal level), or generalized. When generalized, it may be synchronous (all movements occurring simultaneously) or asynchronous.

Myoclonus must be distinguished from chorea and tics, which also may present as sudden, brief movements. As stated earlier, chorea typically flows, with movements occurring one immediately after another. However, myoclonic movements usually occur intermittently, punctuating an otherwise quiet appearance. Tics also occur intermittently, but they are preceded by a subjective urge to make the movement and are suppressible. In addition, tics may be complex motor acts, such as squatting and kicking, whereas myoclonic movements are simple, such as a shock-like arm extension. Finally, whereas myoclonic jerks may be induced by a stimulus (such as a loud noise or sudden touch), tics and chorea rarely are.

DIFFERENTIAL DIAGNOSIS

Myoclonus may occur as a normal, physiologic phenomenon (Table 7.3). Children and adults,

Table 7.3.
Causes of Myoclonus in Childhood[a]

Physiologic myoclonus (sleep; anxiety)
Essential myoclonus
Childhood myoclonic epilepsies
    Lennox-Gastaut syndrome
    Infantile spasms
Myoclonus associated with seizures or cerebellar signs.
    Myoclonus epilepsy with ragged red fibers (MERRF)
    Lafora body disease
    Sialidosis
    Neuronal ceroid lipofuscinosis
    Ramsay Hunt's syndrome
Symptomatic myoclonus
    Viral
        Subacute sclerosing panencephalitis (SSPE)
        HIV (primary or secondary to opportunistic infection)
    Metabolic
        Renal failure
        Nonketotic hyperglycemia
    Other causes of brain injury
        Hypoxia
        Trauma
        Stroke
Opsoclonus-myoclonus

[a] This is a partial list.

as they are falling asleep, experience myoclonic jerks (hypnic jerks). Anxiety may also cause occasional myoclonic jerks.

When myoclonus occurs in the absence of other neurologic signs and without identifiable cause, it is referred to as "essential myoclonus." In general, essential myoclonus begins in childhood or adolescence and often does not progress. While often reported in families, sporadic cases may occur.

Certain seizure disorders of childhood, including infantile spasms and the Lenox-Gastaut syndrome, produce myoclonic movements. A detailed discussion of these and related disorders is presented in the chapter on epilepsy (Chapter 8) in this book.

A number of metabolic or degenerative diseases may present in adolescence with myoclonus associated with seizures or cerebellar signs, or both. There continues to be controversy over how best to classify these disorders, given our incomplete understanding of them (Andermann et al., 1989; Harsden and Obeso, 1989). Myoclonus epilepsy with ragged red fibers (MERRF) appears to be a distinct entity due to an abnormality of cytochrome c oxidase, which is partly encoded by mitochondrial DNA. As an abnormality of mitochondrial DNA, this condition displays maternal inheritance (i.e., the disease is transmitted only through the mother), because the mother's ovum provides all of the mitochondria for the formation of the zygote; the sperm provides none. In many cases a diagnosis can be made by a muscle biopsy demonstrating "ragged red fibers," accumulations of abnormal mitochondria stained red on trichrome stain.

Many times an extensive evaluation of a child presenting with myoclonus and ataxia does not reveal a specific diagnosis, and the diagnosis of Ramsay Hunt's syndrome is made, recognizing that this undoubtedly includes a heterogeneous group of disorders (Marsden and Obeso, 1989).

Since there are a large number of symptomatic myoclonias—those due to identifiable causes— only a few are mentioned. Subacute sclerosing panencephalitis (SSPE), due to a measles-like virus infection of the brain, typically presents in children between 5 and 15 years of age, often with personality change and intellectual deterioration. Eventually, myoclonic jerks appear. The myoclonus has been described as "slow" or sustained. Diagnosis is supported by a characteristic abnormal pattern on the EEG consisting of periodic, paroxysmal bursts of synchronous high-voltage activity, often associated with clinical myoclonus. Elevated levels of antibodies to measles in serum and CSF support the diagnosis. Until the introduction of mass measles vaccination, which seems to prevent SSPE as well as measles, SSPE was one of the most common causes of dementia in late childhood.

Opsoclonus-myoclonus is a distinctive clinical syndrome in which generalized, asynchronous myoclonic movements are associated with chaotic involuntary eye movements. The myoclonus is often aggravated by movement or startle. This syndrome usually follows a viral encephalitis, but in a significant proportion of cases it is a remote effect of an underlying neuroblastoma, which therefore must be investigated by assay of urinary catecholamines and their metabolites.

Myoclonus may also be observed as a complication of acquired immunodeficiency syndrome (AIDS), either as a consequence of central nervous system opportunistic infection or as a direct consequence of primary viral infection (Nath et al., 1987).

There is such a variety of causes of myoclonus that a child with myoclonus requires an extensive neurologic evaluation that often includes muscle biopsy, lumbar puncture, and an extensive metabolic assessment. The treatment, of course, depends on the cause. A benzodiazepine, clonazepam, is often effective for a number of causes of myoclonus.

Tremor

CLINICAL FEATURES

Tremor is a regular, oscillatory involuntary movement. Each tremor can be characterized by its frequency in cycles-per-second (Hertz, or Hz) and classified clinically into three broad categories, depending on the circumstances in which it appears (Table 7.4). *Rest tremors* are present when the limb is still and there is no voluntary muscle activity. The most common cause of resting tremor is parkinsonism. This tremor is usually 4 to 5 Hz. *Action or postural tremors* are elicited when the patient voluntarily contracts muscles, as in holding the hands prone in extension. This category includes essential tremor and enhanced physiologic tremor, and it is the main focus of this chapter. *Intention tremor* is a slow (2 to 4 Hz), large-amplitude oscillation observed as the limb approaches the destination in target-directed limb movements, such as in finger-to-nose tests. It is due to disease of the cerebellum or its outflow pathways.

A rapid (6 to 12 Hz) tremor present with action or on posture holding is due either to essential tremor or enhanced physiologic tremor,

which can be clinically identical. Essential tremor is a neurologic disorder characterized by action tremor in the absence of other neurologic signs. Approximately 30% of patients have a positive family history (Findley, 1988). Although essential tremor is more common in older age groups, it can present in adolescence. It generally begins as a tremor of the hands. Although it may begin unilaterally and be more prominent on that side throughout its course, it almost always is bilateral ultimately. Essential tremor also commonly affects the head or the voice, and it may affect these alone. The head may either shake from side to side ("negative tremor") or nod anterior to posterior ("affirmative"). The legs are rarely affected.

Everyone has a normal, physiologic tremor at a frequency of 7 to 12 Hz. This tremor has several causes, including mechanical resonating effects of the heartbeat, and synchronization of motor units in the spinal reflex arc. In a number of settings, usually associated with enhanced circulating catecholamines, physiologic tremor can become clinically noticeable and bothersome to the patient. Anxiety is an important cause. A number of medical conditions, which may present with anxiety or other psychiatric symptoms and which often are associated with enhanced physiologic tremor, include thyrotoxicosis, pheochromocytoma, and hypoglycemia.

A variety of medications induce action tremor. Many medications, such as the sympathomimetics and bronchodilators used for treating asthma, caused augmented catecholamine effects and thereby induce enhanced physiologic tremor. Among drugs used for treating psychiatric illness, lithium is particularly likely to induce action tremor.

EVALUATION

In the evaluation of a child with tremor, the neurologic exam must focus on circumstances that elicit the tremor. Careful attention must be paid to possible signs of parkinsonism and cerebellar disease. In essential and enhanced phys-

Table 7.4.
Tremor in Childhood[a]

Tremor at rest
   Parkinsonism (4 to 5 Hz)
Action or postural tremor
   Essential tremor (5 to 8 Hz)
   Enhanced physiologic tremor (7 to 12 Hz)
      Stress induced
         Anxiety
      Metabolic
      Thyrotoxicosis
         Pheochromocytoma
         Hypoglycemia
      Drugs:
         Epinephrine
         Terbutaline and other sympathomimetics
         Theophylline and related compounds
         Lithium
         Amphetamines
         Adrenocorticosteroids
         Alcohol withdrawal
         Sodium valproate
         Phenothiazines
      Wilson's disease (may also be present at rest)
Intention tremor
   Cerebellar disease (2 to 4 Hz)

[a] This is a partial list.

iologic tremor, the neurologic exam, other than for the presence of tremor, should be normal. Like the other movement disorders, diagnosis of these tremors is clinical and not based on laboratory studies. The EMG, for example, is not of great diagnostic use in the evaluation of essential tremor; it may show co-contraction of agonist and antagonist muscles, or it may show alternating contraction of these muscle groups. If an action tremor is diagnosed clinically, it is appropriate to evaluate for possible causes of enhanced physiologic tremor by measuring thyroid hormone levels, a fasting blood glucose, and urinary catecholamine metabolites.

TREATMENT

Enhanced physiologic tremor is managed by treating the underlying cause. Essential tremor is initially treated with a beta-blocker, usually propranolol, in gradually increasing doses up to 2 to 4 mg/kg/day in children. It is estimated that 50 to 75% of patients respond initially, although many lose benefit with time (Findley, 1988). Propranolol is probably acting primarily at a peripheral beta-2 receptor, but central effects have not been excluded (Findley, 1988). If propranolol is not beneficial, primidone may be. It must be started in low dose (25 to 50 mg) to minimize the likelihood of initial toxicity (sedation, ataxia, and nausea).

Stereotypies

Stereotypies tend to be repeated, complex and patterned involuntary movements that resemble purposeful movements. Examples include head and trunk rocking in mentally retarded children, and repeated leg crossing/uncrossing in akathisia. In their complexity and repetition, these movements demonstrate intact motor control.

In recent years, attention has been brought to Rett's syndrome. This condition, which occurs only in girls, is distinguished by a peculiar and unique stereotypy of the hands that resembles repetitive wringing or washing. The child psychiatrist must be aware that this disease may present as autism. The clinical features have been described in detail by Hagberg and coworkers (1983), and there is now a consensus on diagnostic criteria (Rett Syndrome Diagnostic Criteria Work Group, 1988) for this poorly understood condition. These girls have normal pre- and perinatal histories, and they develop normally until ages 6 to 18 months. They then regress intellectually, socially, and, most characteristically, in motor skills. They lose skilled hand movements and develop the peculiar hand wringing movements that bring the hands up to their chests and occasionally into their mouths. In addition, they develop gait ataxia.

Their intellectual decline is characterized by loss of any previously acquired language function and is accompanied by acquired microcephaly and seizures. The change in social behavior resembles autism; these children lose interest in other people and develop inappropriate smiling or laughing. Laboratory tests are unrevealing, except that the EEG may show background slowing with superimposed high-voltage slow waves. Sleep recordings often show paroxysmal activity in the form of repetitive spike-wave complexes. There is no treatment that stops progression of the disease or controls the stereotypies.

NEUROLEPTIC-INDUCED MOVEMENT DISORDERS

Although neuroleptics have an important role in the management of many psychiatric disturbances of childhood and adolescence, most literature about the neurologic complications of these medications is based on observations made in adults. In adults, five types of movement disorders are observed, and although these also occur in the pediatric group, the incidence of each probably differs from that observed in adults. The major types of reactions, listed in the order of their usual appearance during the course of therapy, include: acute dystonic reactions, acute akathisia, parkinsonism, the tardive dyskinesias, and neuroleptic malignant syndrome. The withdrawal emergence syndrome (WES), which has been considered by some authorities to be a form of tardive dyskinesia, occurs only in children.

Acute Dystonic Reactions

Although acute dystonic reactions are said to occur in 2 to 5% of patients, the figure may be higher in children. Among children with intravenous metoclopramide (a dopamine receptor antagonist antiemetic) prior to cancer chemotherapy, 27% experience dystonic reactions (Kris et al., 1983). In addition, acute dystonia tends to be more severe in the pediatric group. Whereas in adults the reactions often occur in cranial muscles (face, tongue, neck), in children the reactions tend to involve limbs and trunk. Severe back arching, which may be mistaken for meningismus, may occur. Virtually diagnostic of the acute dystonic reaction is oculogyric crisis, a sustained upward or lateral deviation of the eyes. Acute dystonia responds readily to anticholinergics (e.g., benztropine) or antihistaminics (e.g., diphenhydramine).

Acute Akathisia

Acute akathisia is the most common neurologic side effect of neuroleptics in adult populations (Ayd, 1971), but its incidence in the pediatric group is unknown. The clinical manifestations of akathisia are often subtle, and it is frequently unrecognized or misdiagnosed. It is characterized by a subjective state of restlessness, but many times patients use vague terms in describing what they are feeling: e.g., "jittery", "about to explode", or "like I'm jumping out of my skin." Obtaining a clear subjective report is especially difficult in children. The subjective state of akathisia often is so tormenting that it has been associated with suicide attempts and aggressive behavior, and it has been misdiagnosed as anxiety, agitated depression, or psychosis. The motor signs of akathisia are also frequently missed by the unprepared eye because they are complex, stereotyped movements that resemble purposeful acts. They most frequently affect the legs and include crossing/uncrossing the legs and marching in place. Movements of the arms also occur, and include repetitive rubbing of the face, smoothing the hair, and scratching. Acute akathisia does not respond as well to anticholinergics as does acute dystonia or parkinsonism, and it may require a reduction in neuroleptic dose. There are several recent reports that beta-adrenergic receptor antagonists, such as propranolol, may be effective.

Parkinsonism

Neuroleptics are capable of inducing all of the four cardinal signs of parkinsonism: tremor at rest, bradykinesia (slowness of movement), rigidity, and postural instability. In a young patient who develops parkinsonism, an evaluation for Wilson's disease must be performed, including a serum ceruloplasmin and a slit-lamp exam. In general, neuroleptic-induced parkinsonism responds to dosage reduction and/or anticholinergics.

Tardive Dyskinesia

Most psychiatrists are well aware of the oral-buccal-lingual form of tardive dyskinesia, the most common neuroleptic-induced dyskinesia in adults, that consists of repetitive chewing, lip-smacking, and tongue-popping movements. Many are not aware that neuroleptics can also induce a persistent dystonic form of tardive dyskinesia, called *tardive dystonia* (Burke et al., 1982). This particular disorder seems to be a more common form of tardive dyskinesia in young patients, particularly young men. Although a significant number of the patients whom we reported had a static encephalopathy, it is unknown whether such preexisting brain damage predisposes to this condition (Burke et al., 1982). Unlike oral-lingual tardive dyskinesia, tardive dystonia frequently is quite disabling. Tardive dystonia frequently affects the muscles of the face and neck. Retrocollis, a sustained backward pulling of the neck, commonly is observed. As in acute dystonic reactions, tardive dystonia is likely to have a widespread distribution in younger patients, who often have sustained extension of the arms and arching of the back. The legs are not commonly involved, and they are never involved in isolation.

The diagnostic evaluation of a patient who develops persistent dystonia during neuroleptic treatment consists of obtaining a CT or MRI to exclude a structural cause and performing an evaluation for Wilson's disease. If these studies are negative and the neurologic examination reveals only dystonia, then tardive dystonia is the appropriate diagnosis. However, if other neurologic abnormalities are present, then evaluation for the many secondary causes of dystonia must be performed, and neurologic consultation must be obtained. The treatment of tardive dystonia consists initially of discontinuing neuroleptics, if possible, because a certain percentage of these patients will undergo a spontaneous remission. If that is not possible, or if the dystonia persists in spite of discontinuation of antipsychotics, then the patient can be treated with either anticholinergics or a dopamine depletor, such as reserpine (Kang et al., 1986).

Another form of tardive dyskinesia is tardive akathisia, essentially a persistent akathisia with symptoms and signs similar to those observed in acute akathisia. This form of tardive dyskinesia is less common in the pediatric age group (Burke et al., 1989).

Withdrawal Emergence Syndrome

Withdrawal emergence syndrome (WES) occurs almost exclusively in children. It is observed in children who have been treated chronically with neuroleptics and who then undergo an abrupt discontinuation of the drug. They develop a generalized chorea that mimics Sydenham's chorea or Huntington's disease. In addition, the children become ataxic. Generally, WES either remits spontaneously or, if necessary, can be suppressed by reintroduction of neuroleptics followed by very gradual tapering and withdrawal.

Neuroleptic Malignant Syndrome

The rarest but most life-threatening neurologic complication of antipsychotic drugs is neuroleptic malignant syndrome (NMS). This condition may arise at any time during neuroleptic treatment. It consists of high fever without infectious cause, alteration in mental status, and either parkinsonian rigidity or severe dystonia. The fever and the severe muscle spasms frequently lead to an elevation of serum enzymes indicative of muscle injury (CPK, SGOT, LDH), and myoglobin may appear in the urine. The myoglobinuria may lead to renal failure and death. Treatment must be provided in an intensive care unit to monitor vital signs, control temperature, provide intravenous hydration, and monitor urine output. Neuroleptics must be stopped. A number of reports indicate that the direct-acting muscle relaxant dantrolene sodium is effective in preventing progressive muscle injury. There also are reports that bromocriptine, a direct-acting dopaminergic agonist, is beneficial.

WILSON'S DISEASE

An evaluation for Wilson's disease is indicated if a patient has, in addition to psychiatric symptoms, any neurologic signs, particularly a movement disorder, whether or not the patient is taking neuroleptics. Wilson's disease is a rare, autosomal-recessive disorder of copper metabolism that is treatable, but fatal if untreated. The longer it goes undiagnosed and untreated, the more likely it is to cause irreparable brain damage. Wilson's disease must always be kept in mind, because it has protean psychiatric, neurologic, and medical presentations.

The psychiatric presentations of Wilson's include adolescent adjustment problems, anxiety, mania, depression, and psychosis. The ability of Wilson's to mimic many common psychiatric disturbances often leads to a delay in diagnosis. A typical example, which has been published (Francone, 1976) and summarized previously (Cartwright, 1978), illustrates these problems. A 24-year-old woman developed nervousness and a tremor. She was treated with tranquilizers. She then became depressed and attempted suicide. An antidepressant was prescribed. She then developed psychotic symptoms, was diagnosed to have acute schizophrenia, and treated with electroshock. She was referred to an internist for abnormal liver function tests, which were attributed to chlorpromazine. A neurologist attributed several neurologic signs, including dystonia, tremor, and bradykinesia, to chlorpromazine. Ultimately, duuring a psychiatric admission for "hysterical neurosis, conversion type," a physician noted Kayser-Fleischer rings and a diagnosis of Wilson's was made almost 4 years after onset. The patient was treated with penicillamine and had resolution of all psychiatric symptoms and many of her neurologic signs (Francone, 1976). One of the key lessons to be learned from this woman's misfortune is that one must not assume neurologic signs are due to neuroleptics until Wilson's has been excluded, a point also emphasized earlier in relation to the diagnosis of tardive dystonia.

Wilson's disease also presents with a variety of neurologic signs, but usually there is evidence of a movement disorder: tremor, dystonia, parkinsonism, ataxia, or chorea. Often tremor is reported at the onset. The tremor may be present at rest, as in parkinsonism; however, its amplitude may be markedly increased on action or posture-holding. A pronounced abduction movement of the arms at the shoulder joint while holding the forearms flexed across the chest has been called a "wing-beating tremor." Another, more constant, feature of neurologic involvement in Wilson's disease is dysarthria, which can progress to total anarthria.

The most common mode of presentation in childhood is with liver disease. Patients may present with either chronic hepatitis or an acute fulminant hepatitis. Additional medical abnormalities due to Wilson's include hemolytic anemia, osteoporosis, and renal tubular acidosis.

The appropriate screening procedure include a determination of the serum ceruloplasmin, which in the disease is lower than normal (higher than 20 mg/dl), and an examination of the cornea by slit lamp for Kayser-Fleischer rings, which are due to deposition of copper in Descemet's membrane. A Kayser-Fleischer ring is almost universally observed in neurologic Wilson's disease, and many times it can be seen at the periphery of the cornea during bedside examination. If these screening procedures indicate a diagnosis of Wilson's disease, then confirmatory studies should be performed, including determination of a 24-hour urine copper and a liver biopsy for copper content, both of which are elevated.

Wilson's disease, once diagnosed, must be treated promptly with a chelating agent such as penicillamine. Because Wilson's is inherited as a recessive disease, the physician also has a responsibility to examine and evaluate siblings of the affected child.

PARKINSONISM

CLINICAL FEATURES

There are a small number of children who present with classic signs of parkinsonism and no other neurologic abnormalities, who have no identifiable causes of secondary parkinsonism, and who therefore have primary parkinsonism. In a recent review, individuals with the onset of parkinsonism before the age of 40 years were grouped into those with onset before age 21 years and those with onset between 21 and 40 years. Patients with onset before 21 years always had a positive family history for parkinsonism (Quinn et al., 1987). This form of parkinsonism may be distinct from idiopathic Parkinson's disease, but its pathology has yet to be defined. Inidividuals with early-onset parkinsonism frequently present with dystonic features. Parkinsonism consists of any combination of four cardinal neurologic signs: tremor at rest, rigidity, bradykinesia, and postural instability. As stated earlier, a parkinsonian rest tremor is slow (4 to 5 Hz), and, unlike essential tremor, is suppressed by action. It is frequently distal, resulting in alternating flexion of the thumb and index finger, giving rise to the term *"pill-rolling" tremor*. Many times the tremor becomes more noticeable as the patient walks with arms at the side. The tremor may be asymmetric. Unlike essential tremor, Parkinsonian rest tremor often affects the legs. The area around the mouth may also be affected, but generally the head itself does not shake, as it does in essential tremor.

The muscle rigidity of parkinsonism is detected by moving the patient's limb passively at a joint. The neck is rotated; the arm is flexed and extended at the elbow and wrist, the leg at the knee and ankle. Rigidity is felt by the examiner as a resistance to the movement; in parkinsonism the rigidity is felt equally in flexion and extension and is often called "lead pipe rigidity." The steady resistance of lead pipe rigidity may be associated with a regular, repetitive catch in the resistance, called "cogwheeling," which is due to a superimposed tremor. Parkinsonian rigidity must be distinguished from spasticity, in which resistance is much more pronounced at the initiation of passive movement, and more in one direction than the other (e.g., more in extension of the elbow than in flexion).

Bradykinesia is slowness of movement and a decrease in the amount of spontaneous movement. Bradykinesia can be subtle and easily overlooked if not sought. In the face, there is a loss of the normal range of expression, and the patient develops "poker face" and a staring expression. Bradykinesia of truncal and limb movements is seen during walking as a diminished swing of the arms and a tendency to turn "en block." Slowness of movement can be further demonstrated on examination by slowness in tasks requiring rapid repetition, such as finger or toe tapping. Bradykinesia can make a patient look depressed, as it mimics the psychomotor retardation commonly observed in depression. One must carefully search for the other signs of parkinsonism in such a patient to be certain that one is, in fact, dealing with depression and not parkinsonism.

The most debilitating feature of parkinsonism is postural instability, which leads to significant injuries from falls. Frequently, Parkinson patients relate a history of unexplained or easily provoked falls. On examination, a slight backward pull on the patient will demonstrate a propensity to fall (and the examiner must therefore be ready to catch the patient) in spite of normal leg strength, cerebellar testing, and position sense.

DIFFERENTIAL DIAGNOSIS
A few of the causes of parkinsonism in the pediatric age group are listed in Table 7.5. As mentioned earlier, a variety of dopamine receptor blocking drugs (antipsychotics, antiemetics) or depleting drugs (reserpine) can induce all of the signs of parkinsonism. Lithium may do so as well. Both Wilson's and Huntington's disease may present as parkinsonism in the pediatric population, although often there are associated cognitive or personality changes.

EVALUATION
Parkinsonism in children is so unusual that one must always be suspicious that there has been

Table 7.5.
Some Causes of Parkinsonism in Childhood

Primary parkinsonism
  Familial
  Sporadic
Secondary causes of parkinsonism
  Drug-induced
    Neuroleptics
    Lithium
  Wilson's disease
  Huntington's disease
  Neuroacanthocytosis
  Hydrocephalus
  Encephalitis

ingestion of a neuroleptic or antiemetic medication. A detailed family history is important in relation to several possible etiologies, including Wilson's disease, Huntington's disease, neuroacanthocytosis, and the inherited forms of primary parkinsonism. It is important to realize that parkinsonism is a clinical diagnosis, made independently of laboratory tests. The laboratory evaluation for possible etiologies should include a serum ceruloplasmin, a blood smear for acanthocytes, and either a CT or an MRI scan to evaluate for hydrocephalus and caudate atrophy.

TREATMENT

In its early stages, parkinsonism should be treated with the selective monoamine oxidase B inhibitor deprenyl. There is firm evidence in adult populations that deprenyl slows the progression of the disease (Parkinson's Study Group, 1989), and it seems reasonable to expect that it would also do so in younger patients. When symptomatic therapy becomes necessary, either anticholinergics or amantadine are used initially. Eventually, the use of levodopa is required, although unfortunately, patients with an earlier onset seem especially prone to the development of fluctuations in response and dopa-induced dyskinesias (Gershanik, 1988).

THE ATAXIAS

CLINICAL FEATURES

Cerebellar disease in childhood presents with a variety of neurologic signs related to disturbances in motor coordination and balance. Usually these signs clearly indicate a neurologic basis of an illness, but occasionally they are misinterpreted as psychogenic. Quite often, cerebellar disturbances in children first become apparent as a gait disturbance. The stance becomes broadbased, walking becomes uncertain and reeling, and falls frequently result. Cerebellar disease also causes signs at other levels of the neuraxis. The eye movements are often affected, demonstrating instability of fixation, overshooting the visual target (ocular dysmetria), and nystagmus. The speech disturbance in cerebellar disease is characterized by loss of normal rhythm, inappropriate slowing or pauses, and fluctuations in volume. In the arms, there is loss of accuracy in approaching a target (dysmetria) and an intention tremor.

DIFFERENTIAL DIAGNOSIS

Many of the acquired causes of cerebellar disease in childhood present with a subacute onset, whereas the metabolic and degenerative etiologies present with chronic progression. One of the most common causes of subacute ataxia in childhood is postviral cerebellar ataxia. This syndrome can be observed after any of the childhood exanthematous diseases, but it is most common after varicella. Generally, it develops just as the child begins to recover from the acute exanthematous phase, presenting as ataxia. Less commonly, nystagmus or speech disturbance occurs. Fortunately, this disease is almost always self-limited and requires no treatment. Children may recover as rapidly as within 1 week, but the usual duration is about 2 months.

A number of causes of acute ataxia must be considered in the differential diagnosis. Acute labyrinthitis causes a disturbance of balance and falling. Usually it can be distinguished from cerebellar ataxia by the presence of severe subjective vertigo with nausea and vomiting. A variety of drugs, if accidentally ingested by a child, may cause ataxia, including alcohol, sleeping medications, minor tranquilizers, and anticonvulsants. Rarely, multiple sclerosis may present with the rather sudden onset of ataxia. All children presenting with ataxia must be evaluated neuroradiologically for the possible presence of brain tumor in the posterior fossa, the most common location in children. Possible tumor types include cerebellar astrocytoma, medulloblastoma, and ependymoma.

A considerable number of metabolic and degenerative neurologic diseases of childhood may present as slowly progressive ataxia, but the child psychiatrist need only be aware of the more common causes and the rare, but potentially treatable, causes. The most common type of inherited ataxia in childhood is Friedreich's ataxia, which is an autosomal-recessive condition. Friedreich's presents before age 25 years, and in addition to signs of ataxia on examination, there is also absence of the deep tendon reflexes. Pes cavus (a high foot arch) is characteristic. Many patients eventually also develop pyramidal tract signs (weakness of the legs with Babinski signs) and loss of distal joint and position sense. In about two-thirds of cases, there are abnormalities on the electrocardiogram, most commonly T-wave or conduction abnormalities. Since the primary underlying biochemical deficit in Friedreich's is unknown, the diagnosis must be made on the basis of these clinical criteria.

Two causes of slowly progressive ataxia in childhood that must be considered, because they are treatable, are Wilson's disease and abetalipoproteinemia. Wilson's has been discussed. Abetalipoproteinemia is an autosomal-recessive disorder in which there is impaired ability to synthesize apoprotein B, which functions in transporting lipids. As a result of the deficiency, there are low levels of serum lipids, including cholesterol, and poor absorption of fat-soluble vitamins. As a result of inadequate absorption of vitamin E, these patients develop ataxia, loss of reflexes, and loss of position sense. Treatment with large doses of vitamin E arrests the symptoms and in some cases improves them (Harding, 1987).

Further differential diagnosis of the progressive ataxias in childhood is lengthy and pediatric neurologic consultation is mandatory. Unfortunately, there is no pharmacotherapy that relieves the signs and symptoms of ataxia.

REFERENCES

Andermann F, Berkovic S, Carpenter S, Andermann E. The Ramsey Hunt syndrome is no longer a useful diagnostic category. Mov Disord 1989;4:13–17.

Ayd FJ. A survey of drug-induced extrapyramidal reactions. JAMA 1961;175:1054–1060.

Burke RE, Fahn S, Jankovic J, Marsden CD, Lang AE, Gollomp S, Ilson J. Tardive dystonia: late-onset and persistent dystonia induced by antipsychotic drugs. Neurology 1982;32:1335–1346.

Burke RE, Fahn S, Marsden CD. Torsion dystonia: a double-blind, prospective trial of high-dosage trihexyphenidyl. Neurology 1986;36:160–164.

Burke RE, Kang UK, Jankovic J, Miller LG, Fahn S. Tardive akathisia: an analysis of clinical features and response to open therapeutic trials. Mov Disord 1989;4:157–175.

Calne DB, Lang AE. Secondary dystonia. Adv Neurol 1988;50:9–13.

Cartwright GE. Diagnosis of treatable Wilson's disease. N Engl J Med 1978;298:1347–1350.

Farrer LA. Suicide and attempted suicide in Huntington disease: implications for preclinical testing of persons at risk. Am J Med Genet 1986;24:305–311.

Findley LJ. Tremors: differential diagnosis and treatment. In: Jankovic J, Tolosa E, eds. Parkinson's disease and movement disorders. Baltimore: Urban & Schwarzenberg, 1988:243–262.

Francone CA. My battle against Wilson's disease. Am J Nurs 1976;76:247–249.

Gershanik OS. Parkinsonism of early onset. In: Jankovic J, Tolosa E, eds. Parkinson's disease and movement disorders. Baltimore: Urban & Schwarzenberg, 1988:191–204.

Hagberg B, Aicardi J, Dias K, Ramos O. A progressive syndrome of autism, dementia, ataxia, and loss of purposive hand use in girls: Rett's syndrome: report of 35 cases. Ann Neurol 1983;14:471–479.

Hagberg B, Hagberg G. Prenatal and perinatal risk factors in a survey of 681 Swedish cases. In: Stanley F, Alberman E, eds. Epidemiology of the cerebral palsies. Philadelphia: JB Lippincott, 1984:116–134.

Harding AE. Vitamin E and the nervous system. CRC Crit Rev Neurobiol 1987;3:89–103.

Kang UJ, Burke RE, Fahn S. The natural history and treatment of tardive dystonia. Mov Disord 1986;1:193–208.

Kris MG, Tyson LB, Gralla RJ, et al. Extrapyramidal reactions with high-dose metoclopramide. N Engl J Med 1983;309:433.

Lesser RP, Fahn S. Dystonia: a disorder often misdiagnosed as a conversion reaction. Am J Psychiatry 1978;153:349–352.

Marsden CD, Obeso JA. The Ramsay Hunt syndrome is a useful clinical entity. Mov Disord 1989;4:6–12.

Nath A, Jankovic J, Pettigrew LC. Movement disorders and AIDS. Neurology 1987;37:37–41.

Nelson KB, Ellenberg JH. Antecedents of cerebral palsy. N Engl J Med 1986;315:81–86.6.

Nygaard TG, Marsden CD, Duvoisin RC. Dopa-responsive dystonia. Adv Neurol 1988;50:377–384.

The Parkinson's Study Group. Effect of deprenyl on the progression of disability in early Parkinson's disease. N Engl J Med 1989;321:1363–1371.

Quinn N, Critchly P, Marsden CD. Young onset Parkinson's disease. Mov Disord 1987;2:73–92.

The Rett Syndrome Diagnostic Criteria Work Group. Diagnostic criteria for Rett syndrome. Ann Neurol 1988;23:425–428.

Rylander G. Psychoses and the punding and choreiform syndromes in addition to central stimulant drugs. Psychiatr Neurol Neurochir 1972;75:203–212.

Wasserman S, Yahr MD. Choreic movements induced by the use of methadone. Arch Neurol 1980;37:727–728.

Chapter 8

EPILEPSY

A. David Rothner, MD

INTRODUCTION

Epilepsy, which is the tendency to have recurrent seizures, is a *sympton* of central nervous system (CNS) dysfunction. All seizures are due to excessive and paroxysmal neuronal discharge: the cerebral event is primary, and all seizures result in sudden disturbance of function. They usually have a recognizable offset and conclusion. The episodes may range from simple attacks of staring to tonic-clonic convulsive movements. The basic physiology of the epileptic event is traceable to an unstable cell membrane. Changes in factors affecting the cell membrane alter the seizure threshold (Brown and Feldman, 1983).

Each year, 50 per 100,000 people in the United States are diagnosed as having epilepsy. The onset of epilepsy is highest among people younger than 20 years. The prevalence of epilepsy in preschool children is approximately 1.5 per 1000; in school children through age 17, 5 per 1000. Boys are more likely than girls to have epilepsy, and the disorder is more prevalent in nonwhites (Hauser and Hesdorffer, 1990). Certain types of seizures are more common in certain age groups. Infantile spasms (IS) occur between the ages of three months and two years. The Lennox-Gastaut syndrome (LGS) with myoclonic seizures and mental retardation usually begins after age 1 and before age 10. Absence, or petit-mal, seizures occur in the early school years. Juvenile myoclonic epilepsy begins in ad-olescence. Grand mal, or tonic clonic, seizures can occur at any time.

CLASSIFICATION

The epilepsies have recently been reclassified according to both an International Classification (Table 8.1) and a classification of epileptic syndromes (Dreifuss, 1989). The main differentiation of the epilepsies depends upon the localization of the focus. In *partial seizures*, the discharge arises in a focal area of the cerebral cortex. In *primarily generalized seizures*, both hemispheres are affected simultaneously—presumably from a subcortical central focus.

Approximately 50% of children with epilepsy can be categorized as having an epileptic syndrome. This additional category may indicate a clinical profile, prompt a specific therapy, and suggest a prognosis. The seizures associated with these epileptic syndromes are age-related and may reflect developments in the CNS.

Partial Seizures

Aproximately 45% of seizures occurring in childhood are partial seizures. The most important types of partial seizures are the following: simple partial seizures, the benign focal or Rolandic seizures, and complex partial seizures, which are also known as temporal lobe or psychomotor seizures. All begin in a specific area of the brain that may have an underlying struc-

Table 8.1.
Simplified Classification of the Epilepsies

Partial
    Simple (no impaired consciousness)
      Motor
      Sensory
    Complex (impaired consciousness)
    Secondarily generalized
Generalized
    Tonic-clonic
    Absence
    Myoclonic

tural lesion. Also, partial seizures may spread and become secondarily generalized.

During a partial seizure or focal seizure, consciousness is not lost. The simple partial seizure may be either motor or sensory. A simple partial seizure with motor signs consists of recurrent clonic movements of one part of the body without loss of consciousness. This motor activity may cease or spread ipsilaterally in a Jacksonian march or spread to the other hemisphere and result in a secondarily generalized tonic-clonic seizure. A simple partial sensory seizure consists of paresthesias or pain in a single part of the body. It may spread ipsilaterally or become secondarily generalized. Most partial seizures last approximately 1 to 2 minutes and consciousness is not lost. The location of the abnormal focus of neurons determines the exact nature of the seizure (Wyllie et al., 1989).

Benign focal epilepsy of childhood (BFEC), also called Rolandic epilepsy, is the most common focal epileptic syndrome seen in children less than age 15 (Lerman and Kivity, 1975). BFEC is a genetic disease—a family history is found in 9 to 68% of patients—focal brain pathology is not usually seen.

The syndrome can be divided into four groups based on Rolandic (central temporal) sharp waves on the electroencephalogram (EEG) and the presence or absence of neurologic deficits and characteristic seizures: (1) Rolandic sharp waves with neither neurologic deficit nor seizures; (2) Rolandic sharp waves with neurologic deficit but

no seizures; (3) Rolandic sharp waves with both neurologic deficit and seizures, and (4) Rolandic sharp waves with seizures but no neurologic deficit. The first and fourth groups are most commonly encountered. The electrical manifestations of this disorder, which may be seen in up to 10% of children with migraine (Kinast et al., 1982), are age-related and peak between the ages of 4 and 11 years.

Children with BFEC may exhibit either generalized tonic-clonic seizures or facial seizures preceded by somatosensory aura affecting the tongue, cheek, lips, gum, and face. This aura is followed by jerking of the mouth, face, and lips that may spread to the hand or arm ipsilaterally. Salivation and speech arrest occur. The children retain consciousness and have no postictal confusion. The usual seizure lasts between 30 seconds and 3 minutes and occurs during sleep. Most of these children do not need anticonvulsants. BFEC is considered a benign epileptic syndrome and the prognosis for spontaneous remission of the seizures is excellent.

Illustrative Case A:
A 6-year-old girl had been entirely well prior to the onset of her spells. Her mother reported that for the preceding 2 weeks, almost nightly, about 2 hours after falling asleep, the child moaned. She found her child sitting up in bed, drooling, and unable to speak. Twitching of the right face lasting 2 minutes followed. There was no loss of consciousness. The child later said she remembered everything and that the spells were preceded by tingling and numbness of the right side of her face and tongue. The neurologic examination was normal. An EEG demonstrated left-sided Rolandic spikes. MRI was negative. Treatment with carbamazepine 200 mg twice daily completely eliminated the spells.

Complex partial seizures (CPS) are distinguished from simple partial seizures and BFEC by alteration of consciousness (Kotagal et al, 1987). These seizures are often preceded by an aura, such as an abnormal or unpleasant sensation, a bad taste, or strange odor. The aura is followed by staring and altered consciousness,

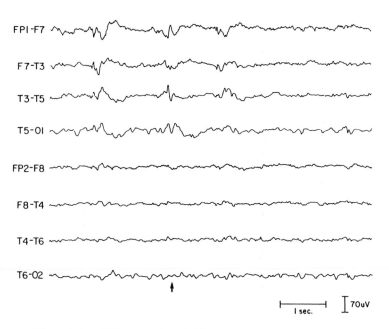

FPI-F7

F7-T3

T3-T5

T5-OI

FP2-F8

F8-T4

T4-T6

T6-O2

I sec.   70uV

Figure 8.1.   EEG as seen in a child with complex partial seizures.

usually without falling. Abnormal movements, called automatisms, which follow, may consist of picking, rubbing, lip-smacking, or swallowing. The spells last about 2 minutes and are followed by confusion, drowsiness, and amnesia for the event. The EEG may show sharp waves or spikes from the temporal region (Fig. 8.1). CPS may become secondarily generalized and result in a bilateral tonic-clonic seizure.

Generalized Seizures

TONIC-CLONIC SEIZURES

Primarily generalized tonic-clonic seizures, also known as grand mal and major motor seizures, involve both hemispheres simultaneously from the onset. They are the most dramatic of all seizures—involving immediate loss of consciousness, falling to the ground, and tonic extension and stiffening of muscles. Abdominal and chest muscles contract, and the "epileptic cry" occurs. Inhibition of respiration causes cyanosis. Jerking of all extremities in a symmetrical fashion, which represents the clonic phase of the attack, is usu-

ally associated with incontinence of urine and feces and oral trauma. The attack usually lasts 2 to 5 minutes and is followed by somnolence and confusion. In the postictal period, children usually have severe headaches and muscle aches and pains.

Absence

Absence, or petit-mal seizures, which are another form of primarily generalized seizures, occur frequently in early school-age children who are otherwise well (Sato et al., 1982). Usually having no aura, the child simply stops what he or she is doing, stares ahead, and has impaired consciousness for 10 to 20 seconds. In a variety of this seizure, the child may stare and flutter the eyelids. Although automatisms may occur, there is no falling or incontinence. Consciousness is immediately regained. The attacks occur frequently—as many as 20 to 30 times daily. They may be provoked by stress and exercise. The electroencephalogram shows a characteristic 3-Hertz (Hz) spike-and-wave pattern (Fig. 8.2). In some of the children, the attacks disappear

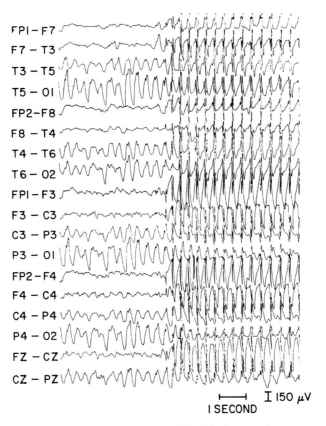

Figure 8.2.   EEG as seen in a child with absence seizures.

spontaneously during adolescence, but in others they may be replaced or become associated with generalized tonic-clonic seizures.

Illustrative Case B:
A 7-year-old boy had been well until 3 weeks prior to his appointment, when he developed brief lapses of attention that occurred several times daily, including mealtimes. His examination was normal. Hyperventilation for 3 minutes resulted in cessation of the overbreathing, staring, and fluttering of the eyelids. The child did not recall the spell. An EEG showed generalized spike-wave discharges at a frequency of 3 Hz. Treatment with ethosuximide 250 mg three times a day caused the spells to disappear. After 3 years of treatment, his mother discontinued the medication.

One year later the child returned, having experienced a brief nocturnal generalized tonic-clonic seizure. Reevaluation was unremarkable except for

an EEG that showed both generalized 3-Hz spike-wave activity and generalized spikes. Treatment with sodium valproate resulted in remission of the seizures.

Absence seizures must be differentiated from complex partial seizures. Consciousness is lost or altered in both syndromes. In absence seizures the attacks occur 20 to 30 times per day, but in CPS they occur once or twice per day to several times per week. The absence attacks last 10 to 20 seconds, while the CS attacks last 2 to 3 minutes. After an absence, consciousness is immediately regained, whereas after CPS the child is usually confused and drowsy. In absence, the EEG abnormality is a generalized 3-Hz spike-and-wave discharge, whereas in CPS there are sharp waves or spikes in the frontal or temporal lobe. The treatment for absence is ethosuximide or sodium valproate, whereas the treatment for complex partial seizures is carbamazepine, phenytoin, or phenobarbital.

JUVENILE MYOCLONIC EPILEPSY

Juvenile myoclonic epilepsy is being recognized with increased frequency in adolescents (Asconape and Penry, 1984). These children, who are otherwise well, present with either a generalized tonic-clonic seizure or episodes of myoclonic jerks that usually occur in the morning. These myoclonic jerks may cause the boy or girl to drop or throw things. The neurologic examination is usually normal, but the child's EEG shows generalized polyspikes. This disorder lasts throughout the child's entire life and is best treated with sodium valproate.

Illustrative Case C:

A 14-year-old boy had been perfectly well until the day prior to his visit, when he experienced a 4-minute generalized tonic-clonic seizure associated with urinary incontinence and tongue biting. He acknowledged later that on many mornings during the prior 2 months he had had severe arm tremors that resulted in his dropping or throwing things. His examination was normal. His EEG demonstrated generalized polyspike activity as well as a photoconvulsive response to photic stimulation. MRI scan was negative. Treatment with sodium valproate resulted in dramatic cessation of both the arm tremors and the convulsions.

"Minor Motor" Seizures

The so-called "minor motor" seizures usually occur in the context of mental retardation and mixed seizures that include infantile spasms (IS), atonic seizures, akinetic seizures, tonic seizures, and myoclonic seizures (Markand, 1977). IS is relatively uncommon—occurring in approximately 1 in 3500 children—and has its onset between the ages of 3 months and 1 year (Lacy and Penry, 1976). Initially the spells appear to be a normal startle reaction but evolve to a typical salaam jack-knife seizure with sudden flexion or extension of the arms and legs. The spasms occur in clusters, especially when the child is awakening or falling asleep. The seizures last from 1 to 3 seconds and are associated with an hypsarhythmic EEG. This characteristic EEG pattern consists of a chaotic mixture of irregular high-voltage slow spike-and-wave discharges combined with multifocal sharp waves, burst supression, and an abnormal background rhythm.

In idiopathic IS, the child appears normal prior to the attacks and no etiology is found. In symptomatic IS the child's development may be delayed prior to the onset of seizures and an etiology is frequently found. IS may result from a variety of developmental or acquired brain abnormalities that require an extensive evaluation, including metabolic testing and neuroimaging. IS is difficult to control, and standard anticonvulsants generally are not helpful. Useful medications include adrenocerticotropic hormone (ACTH), valproic acid, and the benzodiazepines. Although the prognosis is related to the child's developmental level at presentation, seizure control, and etiology, 90% of children with IS will be moderately or markedly retarded at followup. Many will eventually suffer from a chronic, intractable, mixed seizure disorder.

The term *myoclonic seizures* includes akinetic seizures, atonic seizures, tonic seizures, and myoclonic seizures (Markand, 1977). These seizures usually occur in the first decade of life. The incidence is approximately 1 per 1000 children. When myoclonic seizures occur in the context of a mixed seizure disorder, including generalized seizures and mental retardation, the term *Lennox-Gastaut Syndrome* is used. The EEG is usually disordered and shows slow spike-and-wave or multifocal spike discharges. The myoclonic seizures have similar characteristics: brevity—the seizures last only a matter of seconds; frequent repetition—these seizures occur multiple times per day; and an association with mental retardation. The physical examination of affected children is usually abnormal. Like IS, this disorder may result from a variety of causes, including degenerative disorders, and an extensive evaluation is necessary. It is also refractory to treatment. Although phenobarbital, phenytoin, primidone, and carbamazepine have all been used with varying success, other medications, such as valproic acid, ACTH, and benzodiazepine, may be more effective. In addition, a ketogenic diet or a corpus callosotomy may benefit some children. Nevertheless, the prognosis is poor for seizure control and normal intellectual development.

FEBRILE SEIZURES

In children between the ages of 6 months and 6 years, simple febrile seizures or brief generalized seizures associated with a rise in temperature are common and once serious illnesses such as meningitis have been ruled out, require no ongoing treatment (Hirtz and Nelson, 1983). Current recommendations include no prophylactic treatment as long as no additional neurologic problems are present. However, if the child has an abnormal developmental history, a family history of epilepsy, prolonged or a focal febrile seizure, repetitive seizures during the same illness, or seizures secondary to a central nervous system infection, the likelihood of epilepsy in later years is increased.

STATUS EPILEPTICUS

Status epilepticus is a medical emergency consisting of continuous seizures or multiple prolonged seizures without consciousness being regained (Rothner and Erenberg, 1980). When generalized tonic-clonic status epilepticus occurs, it is a life-threatening situation for which intravenous medications and intensive support are needed. If prolonged, this status may be followed by neurologic residual.

Status epilepticus can also occur in other forms of epilepsy (Rothner and Erenberg, 1980). For example, generalized absence status eilepticus, or spike-wave stupor, is characterized by a variable degree of clouding of consciousness ranging from simple confusion to immobility and mutism with no tonic-clonic or myoclonic activity.

Since certain "automatic" functions can still be carried out, this situation may be confused with a psychiatric disorder. It occurs most frequently in children who have preexisting absence epilepsy. The EEG shows generalized, symmetric spike-wave discharges between 1 and 5 Hz. The disorder can usually be treated effectively with intravenous diazepam followed by ethosuximide, valproic acid, or both. The prognosis in these children is usually good because severe underlying CNS abnormalities are rarely present.

Complex partial status eilepticus, which is rare, produces confusion, immobility, inability to follow requests, hallucinations, and automatisms. An EEG, which helps distinguish this entity from generalized absence status epilepticus, typically reveals continuous focal slowing or spike discharges arising from the temporal lobe. The disorder may result from a variety of causes. The prognosis depends on the underlying temporal lobe abnormality. If no serious injury has occurred, the prognosis is good once the status has been arrested.

THE EVALUATION
(Rothner, 1984)

History

The history is the most important factor in determining whether the child has true epilepsy or other paroxysmal nonepileptiform disorder that mimics seizures. Questioning must be directed to both the child, parents, and anyone else who has observed episodes. The initial aspect of the history includes data concerning the seizure itself as well as any precipitating factors. Important questions include: (1) the type or types of seizures observed; (2) their frequency and duration; (3) precipitating factors and times of occurrence; (4) the presence of an aura; (5) a description of the ictal activity, and especially whether it was focal, generalized, tonic-clonic, or staring; and (6) the condition during the postictal state, such as incontinence, oral trauma, confusion, fatigue, headache, and muscle spasm.

The history must also include factors that determine whether the child is seizure prone, such as cerebral palsy, mental retardation, delayed development, or prior encephalopathic events, such as head injury, febrile seizure, or CNS infection. Further questioning must include data concerning a family history of epilepsy and use of medications, street drugs, or alcohol.

Examination

The mental status examination is easily carried out in school-aged children possessing adequate speech and comprehension. The child's spontaneous speech, activity, cooperation, awareness, and response to external stimuli should be noted. Orientation to time, place, and person should be recorded. Memory, reading, mathematic calculations, and repetition are useful adjuncts to the mental status examination. The general physical examination follows and should include a careful search for any other organ abnormality that may result in secondary CNS dysfunction. Dysmorphic features should be noted, since they may indicate a coexisting anomaly of the CNS. The vital signs are important. Fever may indicate an infectious process, and hypertension an underlying renal or vascular disorder. Cardiac murmurs, wheezing, organomegaly, or mass lesion indicate underlying medical problems that may secondarily affect the nervous system. In critically ill children, a stiff neck may indicate meningitis or a subarachnoid hemorrhage. The skin should be examined closely and may yield useful information. Striae may indicate previous use of steroids or an adrenal disorder; petechia, an underlying blood dyscrasia; café-au-lait spots, neurofibromatosis; hypopigmented macules, tuberous sclerosis; and facial vascular abnormalities, vascular abnormalities of the brain.

The neurologic examination follows, and it begins with examination of the head. The head circumference should be determined. It may show microcephaly that is associated with CNS maldevelopment or retardation. Macrocephaly

may be familial, secondary to hydrocephalus, or associated with neurofibromatosis. A bruit over the head or neck may indicate an arteriovenous malformation. The child's gait may reflect difficulties with balance or weakness, or even hysteria. The fundi must be adequately visualized, but if the child is uncooperative this examination may be postoned until the end of the examination. The physician should search for hemorrhages, papilledema, optic atrophy, and retinal scarring. The cranial nerves should function symmetrically. Any asymmetry indicates an underlying neurologic abnormality. The inability to move one or both eyes completely laterally may indicate a sixth nerve palsy, a nonspecific sign of intracranial pressure. Abnormalities of the lower cranial nerves, incoordination, or ataxia indicates a posterior fossa lesion. Strength, tone, reflexes, and sensory function must be carefully noted. If asymmetry is apparent, a CNS disorder is suspected.

The Differential Diagnosis

Epilepsy is a symptom of neurologic dysfunction with many etiologies. Prior to ordering any laboratory tests, a differential diagnosis should be formulated because the type of testing depends on the suspected etiology. In an otherwise healthy child with a single generalized seizure, determination of the serum glucose, calcium, electrolytes, complete blood count, EEG, and neuroimaging may be all that is needed. In the acute situation, a prolactin level frequently aids in differentiating a psychogenic seizure from an epileptic tonic-clonic seizure. In a child with a focal seizure in which underlying cerebral lesion is suspected, MRI scanning is preferable to CT scanning (Fig. 8.3). In a child with a progressive neurologic disorder, additional specialized testing may be needed. Answers to the following questions are needed prior to ordering laboratory tests: (1) Does the child have seizures or some other paroxysmal disorder simulating seizures? (2) If the child does have seizures, are they focal

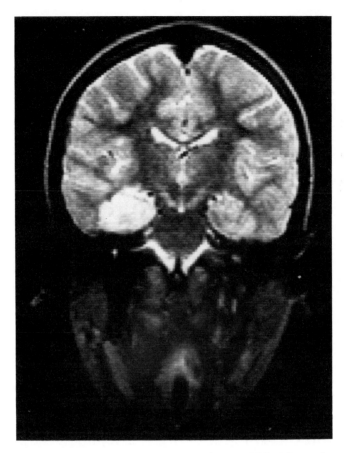

Figure 8.3.   MRI scan showing lesion in the temporal lobe in a child with complex partial seizures.

or primarily generalized? (3) Does the child have a progressive neurologic disorder or symptoms of increased intracranial pressure?

Among the most common etiologies are congenital malformations. Other conditions that predispose children to seizure disorders are chromosomal abnormalities, structural malformations, such as agenesis of the corpus callosum, or migrational abnormalities, such as heterotopias. In utero infections, including the "Torches"—Toxoplasmosis, Rubella, Cytomegalic inclusion disease, Herpes, and Syphilis—often cause neurologic impairment and seizures. Congenitally acquired HIV infection may cause seizures and progressive neurologic deterioration. Acquired CNS infection, such as menin-

gitis or encephalitis, may be associated with seizures either acutely or following resolution of the infection. Notably, the acute onset of focal seizures in association with an abnormal mental status can be caused by herpes simplex encephalitis. Since this infection may be treated, rapid diagnosis is critical.

Seizures may occur at the time of head trauma or afterward. Although accidental trauma is common in childhood, the battered child syndrome must always be suspected when evaluating a traumatized child. Toxins that may injure the CNS occur with great frequency in our environment. Lead poisoning, more common in the past, may cause seizures in the toddler who eats paint peelings or plaster chips. Accidental or purposeful ingestion of medications, especially tranquilizers, may result in seizures. In adolescents who are substance abusers, alcohol, cocaine, amphetamines, and barbiturates may all result in seizures.

Endocrine disorders should be suspected of causing seizures. Hypoglycemia, hypocalcemia, and electrolyte imbalance all predispose to seizures. Neoplasms are an uncommon cause for seizures in children but are more common in adolescents. The most common location is the temporal lobe, and this area is best imaged using MRI with injection of gadolinium. Disorders of the vascular system, including migraine, vasculitis, and vascular malformations, may result in seizures. If the child has seizures and coma in the context of acidosis, hyperammonemia, or hypoglycemia, a metabolic disorder should be suspected and specialized specific testing may be rewarding. If the child has seizures and a progressive loss of abilities or neurologic regression, a degenerative disorder should be suspected and specialized tests are required for diagnosis. The neurocutaneous syndromes such as tuberous sclerosis, neurofibromatosis, and Sturge-Weber syndrome are frequently associated with epilepsy.

PAROXYSMAL NONEPILEPTIFORM DISORDERS

Many children suspected of having epilepsy may have pseudoseizures or some other paroxysmal nonepileptiform disorder (PNED) (Rothner, 1989) (Table 8.2). Some authors have suggested that up to 20% of children suspected of having epilepsy do not have it. A properly obtained history and video-EEG monitoring are the keys to the diagnosis. In a child presenting with recurrent paroxysmal spells that are not easily classified, video-EEG and polysomnographic monitoring should be considered. PNEDs occur frequently and are not readily responsive to antiepileptic drugs. Identifying the specific nature of these spells is important to avoid unnecessary laboratory tests, anticonvulsant drugs with their

Table 8.2.
Paroxysmal Nonepileptiform Disorders

Cardiovascular
  Breath-holding spells
  Mitral valve prolapse syndrome
  Cardiac dysrhythmias
Nocturnal/sleep-related events
  Pavor nocturnus
  Narcolepsy/cataplexy
  Somnambulism/somniloquy
Migraine disorders
  Common disorders
  Classical migraine
  Complicated migraine
    Ophthalmoplegic migraine
    Hemiplegic migraine
Migraine variants
  Paroxysmal vertigo
  Confusional migraine
  Basilar artery migraine
  Paroxysmal torticollis
Movement disorders
  Paroxysmal choreoathetosis
  Tourette's syndrome/tics
  Shudder attacks
  Startle disease
  Spasmus nutans
Psychologic disorders
  Pseudoseizures
  Episodic rage
  Munchausen's syndrome by proxy
  Daydreaming/attention-deficit disorder
  Hyperventilation
Gastrointestinal disorders
  Gastroesophageal reflux
  Recurrent abdominal pain
  Cyclic vomiting

attendant risks and side effects, and the psychologic and economic stigmata of epilepsy.

LABORATORY EVALUATION

Routine laboratory studies, including a complete blood count, urine analysis, chemistry profile, and sedimentation rate, should be performed to exclude systemic disorders. These tests also provide the baseline of the child's hematologic, renal, and hepatic status, which are needed before prescribing certain anticonvulsants.

The EEG is fundamental in the diagnosis and treatment of children with epilepsy. It may be useful in determining the location of the discharge and the type of seizure disorder. It may also be useful in differentiating pseudoseizures from true epilepsy. A normal routine, 1-hour EEG does not exclude a diagnosis of epilepsy, because many children with well-controlled seizure disorders or infrequently occurring seizures have a normal EEG. Moreover, the presence of spikes, sharp waves, or "an epileptiform EEG" suggests, but is not "proof," that the child has a clinically active seizure disorder. Up to 2% of normal children may have spikes or sharp waves on their EEGs without having epilepsy, and an additional 20% may show nonspecific EEG abnormalities.

The more frequent the seizures, the more likely the EEG is to be abnormal. Activating techniques, such as hyperventilation, sleep deprivation, sleep recordings, photic stimulation, extra electrodes, and prolonged recording times may detect EEG abnormalities not observable on routine recordings. Hyperventilation, which is necessary in evaluating the child with absence seizures, frequently provokes a clinical seizure. Photic stimulation is frequently abnormal in adolescents with juvenile myoclonic epilepsy. Prolonged video-EEG monitoring is useful in evaluating children with spells of unknown etiology, psychogenic seizures, "difficult-to-diagnose" seizure disorders, and nocturnal disturbances, and in those who are candidates for epilepsy surgery (Luders et al., 1989). When specific abnormalities such as sharp waves, spikes, polyspikes, and spike-and-wave discharges are noted, epilepsy is likely.

Neuroimaging must be performed in any child with focal neurologic symptoms, focal seizures, focal neurologic signs, progressive neurologic symptomatology, or increased intracranial pressure. Both computed tomography (CT) and magnetic resonance imaging (MRI) may reveal congenital malformations, hydrocephalus, abscesses, hemorrhage, neoplasms, calcification, atrophy, and stroke. Although CT is safe, rapid, and accurate, more useful information is obtained from MRI. This technique converts beamed magnetic waves into electrical signals using a giant magnet. It does not involve ionizing radiation, as does the CT scan. It is frequently able to reveal abnormalities not visible on CT scans, such as ones in the craniocervical region, pituitary gland, and temporal lobes, which are frequently associated with complex partial seizures.

Positron-emitted computed tomography (PET) uses signals from positron-emitting particles to create a three-dimensional computer image, measure cerebral blood flow, and depict brain metabolism. PET is helpful in understanding the etiology and pathogenesis of seizures. It has proved most useful in evaluating children with complex partial seizures for epilepsy surgery. An interictal area of hypometabolism correlates well with a seizure focus. However, it is not a routine diagnostic test in the evaluation of epileptic children.

A lumbar puncture (LP) is useful in determining the presence of an infection, subarachroid hemorrhage, increased intracranial pressure, a neoplasm, or a degenerative disorder. Except in the suspicion of an acute infection, such as meningitis or encephalitis, an LP should be preceded by either a CT or MRI scan. In an acute infection, in which a delay in treatment may be fatal, the LP should be done without delay. In the presence of increased intracranial pressure secondary to a space-occupying mass lesion, an LP is contraindicated because it may cause herniation. An LP is not routinely performed in a child with a seizure disorder who is otherwise healthy.

In children with cognitive dysfunction or emotional illness associated with epilepsy, psychologic testing can be helpful (Louick and Boland, 1978). Testing instruments can be grouped into four general areas: (1) cognitive and developmental, (2) academic, (3) neuropsychologic and perceptual, and (4) emotional and personality. In addition, rating scales and checklists can be used to evaluate adaptive skills, behavioral tendencies, attention deficit disorder, and similar difficulties. The most commonly used cognitive instruments are the Stanford-Binet Scale and the Wechsler Intelligence Scale for Children, Revised (WISC-R). Commonly used academic testing instruments include the Woodcock-Johnson Psychoeducational Battery, the Wide Range Achievement Test-Revised, and the Peabody Individual Achievement Test. Perceptual instruments include the Bender-Gestalt and the Halsted-Reitan Battery. Emotional factors and personality are frequently evaluated using the Children's Perception Test, the Personality Inventory for Children, and the Minnesota Multiphasic Personality Inventory (MMPI). The Rorschach and Projective Drawing Tests are also useful. Among the self-administered checklists or rating scales are the Yale Children's Inventory, the Conner's parent and teacher questionnaires for attention deficit disorder, the Child Behavior Checklist for behavioral problems, and the Vineland Adaptive Behavior Scale for adaptive behavior.

These tests may be useful in determining the presence of an underlying neurologic deficit, a neurodegenerative disorder, or stressful circumstances that are precipitating PNED. They are also useful in determining the cognitive and behavioral effects of antiepileptic medication.

Other laboratory tests, including chromosome analysis, tissue biopsy, lysosomal enzyme testing, and specialized metabolic testing, may be useful in specific neurologic disorders associated with seizures. Unusual historical information, such as exposure to toxins, or atypical physical findings, such as an unusual body odor or abnormal hair, may dictate the need for other, less frequently ordered tests.

SPECIAL CONSIDERATIONS FOR PSYCHIATRIC CONSULTATION

There are special considerations that must be addressed when a psychiatrist is evaluating chil-

dren with psychiatric symptoms who may have an underlying or associated neurologic problem (Rivinus et al., 1975).

Autism is a biologically based disorder that usually appears before the age of 2.5 years. It is characterized by abnormalities in social and interpersonal behavior and language. Children frequently perform repetitive body movements and exhibit obsessive-compulsive behaviors. Epilepsy develops in 23% of autistic children by age 19 years.

A search for the underlying biologic basis of autism should be undertaken (Golden, 1988). Fragile-X and Rett's syndromes, two particular causes of autistic behavior, should be considered. Other potential causes are other genetic factors, chromosomal abnormalities, residua of infectious diseases, metabolic disorders, structural abnormalities, and intoxications. Approximately 33% of children with autism are severely to moderately mentally retarded; 38% are mildly to moderately retarded; and 29% are in the borderline to normal range. Major treatment modalities used are special education and psychologic treatments. Antiepileptic drugs should be used when indicated; other medications to control hyperactivity or abusive behavior may also be helpful. The evaluation of the autistic child with seizures is similar to the evaluation of other children with seizure disorders.

Schizophrenia typically has its onset in children beyond the age of 7 years (Massie, 1978). Both mental deficiency and seizures are rare in childhood schizophrenia. Unless overt neurologic symptoms are present, a search for an underlying organic condition is usually unrewarding. It should be noted that the occurrence of a schizophreniform psychosis in children with complex partial seizures is well-recognized (Perez and Trimble, 1980). This association occurs more commonly in adults than in children. It is more likely to be caused by complex partial seizures with a structural temporal lobe abnormality than in children with mesial temporal sclerosis. The seizure disorder is usually present prior to the development of behavioral or psychiatric problems. It has been suggested that psychiatric abnormalities are more common in children with left temporal lobe dysfunction (Waxman and Geschwind, 1975).

Depression is common in children and adolescents (Kashani et al., 1981). Metabolic encephalopathy, which may mimic depression, can be caused by abnormalities in serum electrolytes, calcium levels, cortisol production, and thyroid function, or by drug abuse. Also a blunted affect may result from medications for epilepsy, migraine, and attention deficit disorder. Tricyclic antidepressants may increase the likelihood of seizures, but only to a minimal degree in a predisposed individual.

Migraine is a familial disorder affecting up to 5% of individuals by age 15 (See Chapter 11). The episodic nature of this disorder, its occasional association with altered consciousness, atypical movements, and other neurologic symptoms, as well as its association with EEG abnormalities have caused it to be confused with epilepsy (Rothner, 1986). The paroxysmal nature of this disorder, its association with headache, nausea, and vomiting, as well as a positive family history usually allow the clinician to separate this disorder from epilepsy. It is well-recognized that academic stress, family disharmony and diet may all play a role in increasing the frequency of migraine. Children with migraine may respond to counseling and biofeedback as well as to medication. Tricyclic antidepressants are useful both in pure migraine as well as in the mixed headache syndrome, which includes daily headaches and intermittent migrainous headaches. If migrainous headaches are associated with neurologic symptoms or signs, albeit transiently, neurologic evaluation, including neuroimaging, is indicated

Psychogenic seizures are frequent in adolescents and may be difficult to diagnose (Wyllie et al., 1990). This disorder is heralded by clinical events that resemble epileptic seizures but are not associated with abnormal cortical-electrical discharges. Most young children seem to have a subconscious component to the episode so that psychogenic seizures are not entirely volitional; however, in some cases the behavior appears to be intentional. Correct diagnosis is mandatory to reduce unnecessary exposure to antiepileptic medication.

Psychogenic seizures should be suspected when the attacks are frequent despite careful medical management, when the attacks have atypical or bizarre clinical features, and when the EEGs are repeatedly normal. Some children have obvious psychologic problems with clear secondary gain; in other cases the emotional etiology is less clear. Video-EEG recording of a typical episode is helpful in making the definitive diagnosis so that firm recommendations regarding discontinuation of antiepileptic medication and pursuit of psychiatric treatment take place. Typical episodes may resemble epilepsy and include thrashing movements, limb-jerking, and staring, with or without unresponsiveness. Many children with pseudoseizures have lack of injury, lack of incontinence, and lack of postconvulsive stupor in the presence of convulsive movements. On many occasions the spells are exacerbated by stress. Current data indicate that the majority of young children with psychogenic seizures do not have concurrent epilepsy. Psychiatric treatment and discontinuation of antiepileptic medication result in a good outcome in the majority of children.

Illustrative Case D:
A 17-year-old girl had experienced two febrile seizures at ages 16 and 21 months. Her maternal uncle was retarded and had seizures. At the age of 15 years, she began having "spells" that consisted of 2 to 3 minutes of a frightened feeling followed by slumping to the floor and thrashing. There was no oral trauma and no incontinence. Her EEG showed normal variants: generalized slowing with hyperventilation, mild asymmetry of her posterior rhythms, and sharp waves maximal at the vertex during drowsiness. Phenytoin was prescribed.

She continued to have one to two spells weekly at school and was asked to stop attending, since her spells were traumatic to the other students. Phenobarbital was added to the phenytoin, but the spells continued. Finally, she was monitored with video-EEG. Her spells were found not to be associated with EEG evidence of seizures. Also a serum prolactin level obtained 10 minutes after an episode did not rise. She was tapered off her medication and improved with psychiatric intervention.

Episodic dyscontrol, aggression, and/or rage is a syndrome characterized by sudden episodic outbursts of verbal abuse and physical violence for either no reason or in response to minor provocations. It may be associated with altered behavior for which the child may be amnesic. During the outburst, the child may seem to be out of contact with reality and unresponsive. The child may have a preexisting neurologic disorder, such as epilepsy, or a coexisting psychiatric disorder. In all children, a combined neurologic and psychiatric evaluation should be undertaken. A diligent search for an underlying seizure disorder should take place. Prolonged EEG recordings may be useful. Toxicology screening to detect substance abuse is mandatory. When no underlying, treatable neurologic condition is noted, treatment with anticonvulsants, propranolol, tranquilizers, and lithium have all been advocated, but there are few data to substantiate a best treatment (Jenkins and Maruta, 1987).

The *hyperventilation syndrome* is characterized by a constellation of symptoms occurring at rest or after exercise that includes light-headedness, vertigo, paresthesias, dizziness, visual disturbances, headache, shortness of breath, and even loss of consciousness, although it is not usually associated with convulsive movements (Perkins and Joseph, 1986). The disorder most frequently occurs in adolescent females and is aggravated by stress. Children may have preexisting psychologic symptoms. The paroxysmal nature of the symptom and its association with loss of consciousness may result in an erroneous diagnosis of epilepsy. The EEG is normal or shows generalized slowing. Immediate treatment involves rebreathing from a paper bag and reassurance.

Simple *syncope*, or fainting, is a common cause of loss of consciousness in school-aged children and adolescents (Beder et al, 1985). The loss of consciousness is secondary to decreased cerebral perfusion. Common precipitants include rising from the recumbent position, prolonged standing, pain, and fright. Children frequently exhibit light-headedness, pallor, and graying of their vision prior to loss of consciousness. The loss of consciousness is usually brief and is only infrequently followed by convulsive movements. Many children are dizzy and fatigued after the spell. No evaluation is indicated in the usual case of infrequent syncope; however, if syncope is prolonged, recurrent, severe, or associated with bradycardia a diagnostic evaluation is indicated. The spectrum of diseases resulting in syncope ranges from benign to life-threatening conditions. The evaluation consists of history, physical examination, electrocardiogram (ECG), EEG, echocardiogram, and Holter monitoring. Antiepileptic drugs are of no value.

Pavor nocturnus, or *night terrors*, is a common disorder occurring most frequently in children between 2 and 5 years (Fisher et al, 1973). The spells occur during non-REM sleep, usually within 2 hours of falling asleep, and are characterized by fear and unresponsiveness. Children seem to awaken, open their eyes, sit up, frequently run or walk about, and cannot be comforted. Sweating and tachycardia are present. The episodes last 1 to 2 minutes and may recur at a later time that same night. The frequency is variable, from nightly to infrequently. In most cases the event is not recalled in the morning, and this characteristic differentiates night terrors from nightmares. Night terrors must also be differentiated from benign focal epilepsy of childhood. During the night terror and between episodes, the EEG is normal. Anticonvulsant drugs are of no benefit. When spells are severe, occur nightly, or are potentially injurious, tricyclic antidepressants or benzodiazepines may be useful. If the clinical presentation is characteristic, sleep studies are not indicated. Since anxiety appears to increase the number of attacks, counseling may be indicated. Parents may be reassured to know that spontaneous resolution occurs within months in most children.

Munchausen syndrome by proxy is a term used to describe a condition in which the *parents* of children consistently give fraudulent information and fabricate signs, causing their children to undergo needless medical investigations and treatments over months to years (Asker, 1951). The "seizures" are usually bizarre and do not fit a traditional pattern. This condition should be suspected when parents insist that the child has organic problems and move from doctor to doctor, and when repeated examinations and investigations are negative. Unnecessary procedures and treatments must be avoided. Family and individual therapy may be useful.

MANAGEMENT

(Dodson, 1989; Pellock, 1989)

Once the results of the history, physical examination, and laboratory testing have been reviewed, a tentative diagnosis should be made. If the diagnosis is epilepsy, the type of seizure should be specified because effective treatment depends on the selection of the appropriate anticonvulsant drug and dosage. Factors predisposing to recurrent seizures such as sleep deprivation, extraneous medication, and alcohol should be removed. Child and parent education increases compliance with a therapeutic regimen. Information regarding the disorder itself, medications used to treat it, and their side effects must be shared. The parents should be allowed to play a role in deciding the timing of medication. A simple schedule also improves compliance. Written and videotaped information is a useful adjunct in improving compliance. At periodic intervals the history, physical examination, and anticonvulsant blood determinations should be repeated. The author believes that children on anticonvulsants should be seen a minimum of twice yearly. If the child's clinical course changes, seizures exacerbate, or side effects become apparent, reevaluation is manda-

tory. A balance between the therapeutic benefits and side effects of the medication must be maintained. Attempts should be made at monotherapy—use of a single drug at the appropriate dosage—to decrease side effects, decrease excessive costs, and increase the likelihood of seizure control. If seizures are not controlled wih high-dose monotherapy or if toxicity supervenes, alternative treatments using high-dose monotherapy with a second drug should be considered. Two drugs should not be used together until high-dose monotherapy with multiple single drugs has been tried and has failed. If two medications are used together, their side effects may be additive or supraadditive. Once initiated, medications should never be discontinued abruptly as this may precipitate status epilepticus. Special consideration should be given prior to use of anticonvulsant medication in women of childbearing age, since birth defects can occur in women taking anticonvulsants during pregnancy. When seizures appear to be refractory to the use of two medications, consultation is indicated. The major anticonvulsant drugs used in the treatment of epilepsy and their side effects are described in Table 8.3.

Phenobarbital was the first of the modern effective anticonvulsant drugs and was introduced in 1912. It may be effective in tonic-clonic-simple-partial and complex-partial seizures. Life-threatening toxicity is rare. Allergies may occur. Paradoxic hyperactivity and behavioral disorders are common in school-aged children and may occur in 30 to 40% of children. Hyperactivity, fussiness, lethargy, disturbed sleep, irritability, disobedience, stubbornness, and depressive symptoms are most common. In adolescents, drowsiness, sedation and impaired cognitive function are significant problems. It causes deficits on neuropsychologic tests and impairs short-term memory and concentration tasks. The medication can be given once or twice daily, and it should be noted that 2 to 3 weeks of therapy are needed before a steady-state therapeutic level is reached. In order to avoid side

Table 8.3.
Antiepileptic Drugs Used in Epilepsy

Drug	Half-Life (hours)	Time to Reach Steady State (days)	Therapeutic Range (µg/ml)	Usual Dose (mg/kg/day) Child	Usual Dose (mg/kg/day) Adult	Symptoms of Toxicity	Side Effects
Carbamazepine	8.5–25	4–6	6–12	20	20	Diplopia, nystagmus, ataxia, drowsiness	GI upset, liver dysfunction, low WBC count, aplastic anemia
Phenytoin	18–22	5–7	10–20	5–10	5	Diplopia, nystagmus, sedation, possible worsening of seizures, cognitive changes	Gum hyperplasia, hirsutism, acne, hepatic failure, neuropathy, lymphadenopathy, fetal hydantoin syndrome
Valproic acid	6–17	2–5	50–100	15–60	15–60	Nausea, vomiting, cognitive effects, tremor, sedation	Nausea, weight gain, alopecia, pancreatitis, liver failure teratogenicity
Primidone	6–8	2–3	8–12ᵃ	20	20	Sleepiness, ataxia, cognitive effects, dizziness, vertigo	Nausea, vomiting, skin rash, emotional changes
Phenobarbital	40–120	10–21	15–40	3–5	2	Sedation, cognitive effects, hyperactivity	Lethargy, serum-sickness reaction, leukopenia, Stevens-Johnson syndrome
Chlorazepate	40–50	10–13		—	0.6–1	Cognitive impairment, sedation	Blurred vision, headache, dry mouth, drowsiness, irritability

ᵃ Also, measure phenobarbital level.

effects, the author uses a low dosage initially at bedtime and increases the dose weekly until the seizures have ceased or side effects have supervened. Blood levels are determined routinely 2 to 3 weeks after the dosage has been optimized, if toxicity occurs, or if seizure control has not been achieved.

Primidone (Mysoline), introduced in 1954, is a congener of phenobarbital and has a similar spectrum of effectiveness. Since it is metabolized to phenobarbital, primidone is not used in combination with phenobarbital. Primidone has a relatively short half-life and causes lethargy. It must be administered three or four times daily. When monitoring blood levels, both primidone levels and phenobarbital levels should be measured. Behavioral side effects and cognitive side effects are similar to those caused by phenobarbital.

Phenytoin (Dilantin), which became available in 1938, was the first anticonvulsant to be discovered via planned and systematic screening in animals. It, too, is useful in the treatment of tonic-clonic, simple-partial, and complex-partial seizures. Chronic administration may lead to gingival hyperplasia and hirsutism. It causes behavioral problems less frequently than does phenobarbital. Among its adverse dose-related side effects are dizziness, nystagmus, ataxia, and diplopia. It causes deficits on neuropsychologic testing, including impaired attention, problem-solving ability, and visual-motor coordination. Depending on the preparation used, phenytoin can be given once or twice daily. Use of phenytoin suspension should be avoided. Ten to fourteen days of adminstration are necessary to reach a steady-state therapeutic level.

Carbamazepine (Tegretol) is effective in simple-partial, complex-partial, and tonic-clonic seizures. Carbamazepine is chemically related to the tricyclic antidepressants and, although definitive data regarding usage in these disorders are not available, it is actually being used in children and adolescents with behavioral and psychiatric abnormalities. Common side effects include diplopia, dizziness, drowsiness, and transient leukopenia. Rarely, carbamazepine may cause aplastic anemia and hepatotoxicity. Infrequently it causes difficulty sleeping, agitation, irritability, and emotional lability. However, many parents relate that their children's behavior has improved when they are placed on carbamazepine. It may also impair task performance on neuropsychologic testing, but to a lesser degree than with phenobarbital, primidone, and phenytoin. The half-life is short, approximately 12 hours, and it must be administered two to three times daily. In addition to determining anticonvulsant blood levels, periodic monitoring of blood counts and liver function is suggested. It takes 5 to 7 days to reach steady-state therapeutic levels.

Sodium valproate (Depakene or Depakote), used for epilepsy since 1978 in the United States, is effective not only for generalized tonic-clonic seizures and generalized absence seizures but also for myoclonic seizures and partial seizures. It appears to elevate the concentration of gamma-aminobutyric acid, an inhibitory neurotransmitter, in the CNS. This anticonvulsant must be taken two to three times daily. A steady-state level is reached within 5 to 7 days. Common side effects include gastrointestinal distress, tremor, and thinning of the hair. *In rare instances, especially in children under the age of 2, fatal hepatotoxicity has occurred.* Pancreatitis is another rare complication. Valproic acid may cause drowsiness, especially when it is used in combination with barbiturates. However, it does not usually cause behavioral problems and has minimal adverse effects on psychologic testing. Laboratory testing must be performed before starting the medication to determine whether hepatic function is normal. Therapy is initiated at 10 mg/kg divided into a two- or three-times-daily schedule and increased slowly to a maximum of 60 mg daily with weekly or biweekly increments of 10 mg/kg. Minor elevations of hepatic enzymes are common. Precipitous rise in hepatic enzymes requires discontinuation of the medication. Valproate-related thrombocytopenia is common, level-related, and treated by lowering the medication.

Ethosuximide (Zarontin) is useful in treating absence seizures, but it does not control coexisting major motor seizures. Because of its gastrointestinal irritation, ethosuximide is usually given three times per day. The most common side effects include nausea, vomiting, and anorexia. Behavioral and cognitive side effects are uncommon.

Other less frequently used anticonvulsants include diazepam, clonazepam, clorazepate, and acetazolamide. Other methods of treating epilepsy include the ketogenic diet and ACTH injections. Psychotherapy and counseling may be used to supplement anticonvulsant therapy in children whose seizures are aggravated by emotional problems. This is an adjunctive rather than primary, form of therapy. In children with focal seizures arising in a temporal lobe that are unresponsive to medication, surgical removal of portions of the temporal lobe can eliminate or reduce the frequency of seizures. Evaluation of such children is complex and should be undertaken only in major medical centers specializing in this form of therapy.

Anticonvulsants do not cure epilepsy but can control seizures in approximately 70% of children. All anticonvulsants alter cognition and behavior (Pellock, 1989) and produce some degree of drowsiness and sedation. The physician, child, and parents must be made aware of the adverse effects of anticonvulsant drugs on the recipient's behavior and learning. The adverse effects may be directly related to the level of medication; however, some children demonstrate idiosyncratic responses and demonstrate side effects even at low anticonvulsant levels. Many studies have shown that both behavior and cognitive function may improve after anticonvulsant medications have been changed, discontinued, or lowered.

The physician should consider clinical situations in which anticonvulsants should not be used. If a child has a single seizure and the recurrence risks are small, consideration should be given to not using anticonvulsant medication. In children with behavioral problems or headaches that are not clearly seizures, and despite the presence of an EEG abnormality, consideration should be given to avoiding anticonvulsants. Most of these children do not have epilepsy. Consider using the smallest amount of medication possible. Therapeutic levels are meant as guidelines. In some children who have seizure thresholds that are relatively high; control can be achieved on so-called "subtherapeutic levels," The level of the medication should be matched with the severity of the child's seizure disorder. If the child is doing well on subtherapeutic dosages, the medication dosage should not be raised.

If a child has been free of seizures for 2 to 5 years, the need for continued therapy with anticonvulsants should be reevaluated. Risk factors that may preclude successful discontinuation of medication include a persistently abnormal EEG, frequent seizures before control was achieved, a known structural lesion or neurologic disorder, mental retardation, the onset of seizures before 2 years of age, focal or complex partial seizures, or multiple seizure types. The decision to discontinue medication is a difficult one and must be individualized, since recurrence of seizures may involve job loss and driver's license revocation. If anticonvulsants are to be withdrawn, the child and family must be advised of the risk of recurrent seizures. The medication should be withdrawn slowly. The author prefers to withdraw a single medication at a time over a period of several months.

Because seizures disrupt and interfere with normal function, the child with epilepsy is subject to a wide variety of social, psychiatric, vocational, and psychologic problems (Vining, 1989). Attitudes of friends, neighbors, and employees intensify the difficulties that must be overcome. Control of seizures is the first step in the treatment of the whole child. Some pediatricians and neurologists work directly with their children toward rehabilitation, while others find that referral to psychologists, psychiatrists, or agencies such as the Epilepsy Foundation are useful. Children must be provided with contacts who can help them with their education and vocational planning. The goal of treatment is to make the child a fully-functioning member of society.

REFERENCES

Asconape J, Penry JK. Sime clinical and EEG aspects of benign juvenile myoclonic epilepsy. Epilepsia 1984;25:108.

Asher R. Munchausen's syndrome. Lancet 1951;1:339.

Beder SD, Cohen MH, Riemenschneider TA. Occult arrhythmias as the etiology of unexplained syncope in children with structurally normal hearts. Am Heart J 1985:109:309.

Browne TR, Feldman RG. Epilepsy. Boston: Little, Brown, 1983.

Dodson WE. Medical treatment and pharmacology of antiepileptic drugs. Pediatr Clin North Am 1989:36:421.

Dreifuss FE. Classification of epileptic seizures and the epilepsies. Pediatr Clin North Am 1989;36:265.

Fisher C, Kahn E, Edwards A, et al. A psychophysiological study of nightmares and night terrors. Arch Gen Psychiatry 1973;28:252.

Golden GS. Biological basis of autism. Int Pediatr 1988;3:110.

Hauser WA, Hesdorffer DC, eds. Facts about epilepsy. New York: Demos Publications, 1990;1.

Hirtz DG, Nelson KG. The natural history of febrile seizures. Annu Rev Med 1983;34:453.

Jenkins SC, Maruta T. Therapeutic use of propranolol for intermittent explosive disorder. Mayo Clin Proc 1987;62:204.

Kashani JH, Husain A, Shekim WO, Hodges KK, Cytryn L, McKnew DH. Current perspectives on childhood depression: an overview. Am J Psychiatry 1981;138:143.

Kinast M, Luders H, Rothner AD, Erenberg G. Benign focal epileptiform discharges in childhood migraine (BFEDC). Neurology 1982;32:1309.

Kotagal P. Rothner AD, Erenberg G, Cruse RP, Wyllie E. Complex partial seizures of childhood onset. A five-year follow-up study. Arch Neurol 1987;44:1177.

Lacy JR, Penry JK. Infantile spasms. New York: Raven Press, 1976.

Lerman P, Kivity S. Benign focal epilepsy of childhood. Arch Neurol 1975;32:261.

Louick D, Boland TB. Psychologic tests: a guide for pediatricians. Pediatr Neurol 1978;12:86.

Luders H, Dinner DS, Morris HH, Wyllie E, Godoy J. EEG evaluation for epilepsy surgery in children. Cleve Clin J Med 1989;56(suppl 1):S53–61.

Markand ON. Slow spike-wave activity in EEG and associated clinical features. Often called "Lennox" or "Lennox-Gastaut" syndrome. Neurology 1977;27:746.

Massie HN. The early natural history of childhood psychosis. Ten cases studied by analysis of family home movies of the infancies of the children. J Am Acad Child Psychiatry 1978;17:29.

Pellock JM. Efficacy and adverse effects of antiepileptic drugs. Pediatr Clin North Am 1989;36:435.

Perez MM, Trimble MR. Epileptic psychosis—diagnostic comparison with process schizophrenia. Br J Psychiatry 1980;137:245.

Perkins GD, Joseph R. Neurological manifestations of the hyperventilation syndrome. J Soc Med 1986;79:48.

Rivinus TM, Jamison DL, Graham PJ. Childhood organic neurological disease presenting as psychiatric disorder. Arch Dis Child 1975;50:115.

Rothner AD. Evaluation of the child with seizures. Cleve Clin Q 1984;51:267.

Rothner AD. The migraine syndrome in children and adolescents. Pediatr Neurol 1986;2:121.

Rothner AD. Not everything that shakes is epilepsy. The differential diagnosis of paroxysmal nonepileptiform disorders. Cleve Clin J Med 1989;56:S206.

Rothner AD, Erenberg GE, Status epilepticus. Pediatr Clin North Am 1980;27:593–601.

Sato S, White BG, Penry JK, et al. Valproic acid versus ethosuximide in the treatment of absence seizures. Neurology 1982;32:157.

Vining EPG. Educational, social, and life-long effects of epilepsy. Pediatr Clin North Am 1989;36:449.

Waxman SG, Geschwind N. The interictal behaviour syndrome of temporal lobe epilepsy. Arch Psychiatry 1975;3:1580.

Wyllie E, Friedman D, Rothner AD. Psychogenic seizures in children and adolescents: outcome after diagnosis by ictal video and electroencephalographic recording. Pediatrics 1990;85:480.

Wyllie E, Rothner AD, Luders H. Partial seizures in children. Clinical features, medical treatment, and surgical considerations. Pediatr Clin North Am 1989;36:343.

Chapter 9

BRAIN TUMORS IN CHILDREN

Patricia K. Duffner, MD, and Michael E. Cohen, MD

INTRODUCTION

Although brain tumors are the second most common malignancy in childhood, there are only approximately 1200 to 1500 newly diagnosed children with brain tumors in the United States each year. For this reason, most pediatricians will take care of a limited number of children with central nervous (CNS) malignancies in their professional lives. Although pediatricians should be able to recognize signs and symptoms of increased intracranial pressure, they may be less familiar with the neuropsychiatric aspects of central nervous system malignancies. Therefore, children may be referred to the child psychiatrist because of a variety of "psychological" complaints that in fact reflect structural disease of the CNS. The child psychiatrist, in turn, is in the position of evaluating children who may harbor unsuspected brain tumors. This chapter reviews general principles in the diagnosis and management of children with brain tumors, with an emphasis on signs and symptoms, neuroimaging, treatment, and long-term effects of therapy. Those neuropsychiatric symptoms that should prompt referral to a child neurologist are emphasized.

NONLOCALIZING SIGNS AND SYMPTOMS

As with other organic diseases of the nervous system, the clinical presentation of children with brain tumors is variable. It is the rare child with a CNS neoplasm who presents with a catastrophic onset. For the most part, the tempo and course of the disease are characterized by the insidious development of symptomatology and signs.

Nonfocal signs and symptoms such as irritability, lethargy, vomiting, anorexia, headache, and change in behavior may reflect increased intracranial pressure. Pressure may occur as a result of a mass growing within the intracranial cavity or may be the result of increased volume secondary to obstruction of the spinal fluid pathways. Early obstruction may be seen in tumors of the cerebellum. Midline cerebellar tumors commonly obstruct the outflow tract of the 4th ventricle. Conversely, pontine tumors, which are found on the basal surface of the brain, occlude the 4th ventricle only late in the course. Tumors of the cerebral hemisphere produce increased pressure by mass effect rather than by direct compromise of the spinal fluid pathway.

Some focal neurologic signs may reflect a nonspecific intracranial process. For instance, the abducens nerve, because of its long, free intracranial course and its proximity to bony structures, may become compressed as a result of increased intracranial pressure. The resultant complaint of diplopia and the finding of a lateral, rather than a lateralizing, rectus paresis, may reflect a generalized process. Therefore, it is called a "false" localizing sign.

The finding of papilledema should always suggest increased intracranial pressure. This important sign may not be present in infants and very young children, who can expand their cranial sutures, with resultant enlargement of the head, in an effort to accommodate increasing pressure. Early signs of papilledema are an increase in the blind spot (cecal), scotoma, and/or loss of color vision (dyschromatopsia) in the face of normal visual acuity. Visual loss and optic atrophy, unrelated to disease of the visual pathway, may reflect late manifestations of chronic increased intracranial pressure. Compromise of the visual axis is usually insidious. Therefore, signs of visual loss must be sought diligently, since most children will not offer visual complaints.

Although headaches may be a manifestation of an expanding mass lesion, most children with headaches do not have structural disease. Head pain is one of the most common nonspecific complaints a clinician is asked to evaluate (Barlow, 1982). The symptom spans all age groups. Most brain tumors become clinically apparent within 8 weeks of the onset of head pain and most assuredly within 4 to 6 months (Honig and Channey, 1982). Hence, clinical suspicion of a neoplasm associated with head pain is the greatest within the first 6 months of onset of symptoms. Chronic headaches of long duration are usually not associated with neoplasm.

The brain itself does not contain pain-bearing fibers. The origin of the head pain is secondary to either dural irritation of the 5th, 9th, and/or 10th cranial nerves or the upper cervical nerves, or it reflects distortion and stretching of arterial or venous channels. Therefore, tumors located in the posterior fossa are associated with occipital pain, whereas tumors in the middle and anterior fossa are associated with pain in the region of the ophthalmic division of the trigeminal nerve. A continuously focal headache, unlike generalized headache, is more likely associated with organic disease. This finding, in the absence of increased intracranial pressure, may suggest pathology underlying the focus of head pain or represent referred pain from a distant source. Headaches associated with increased intracranial pressure is more likely to occur in the early morning, shortly after awakening, or may wake the child from sleep. The pain is usually mild, but there may be increasing severity of pain over time. History of increased headache with coughing, straining, sneezing or other forms of Valsalva maneuvers is a reliable, but often neglected, symptom of increased intracranial pressure.

Vomiting is also a symptom commonly associated with brain tumors. The vomiting may be secondary to increased intracranial pressure or may reflect direct involvement of the area postrema of the 4th ventricle. Vomiting tends to occur early in the morning and then resolves as the day progresses. The vomiting does not have to be projectile to be significant. Persistent or recurrent vomiting should suggest intracranial pathology.

Even more than in adults, changes in affect, energy level, and/or motivation should be considered abnormal in a young child. The tendency of a child to be indifferent to playmates or to not want to continue previous play activity may suggest depression, but it is also a reliable sign of organic disease. Virtually the whole gamut of abnormalities seen in psychiatric disease has been associated with central nervous system tumors. Changes in mentation, delirium, and agitation may be nonspecific and reflect intracranial pressure. On the other hand, anorexia, bulimia, weight loss or gain, somnolence, failure to thrive, sexual precocity, or symptoms of an autonomic nature raise the suspicion of disease of the hypothalamic pituitary axis. The caveat resulting from these observations is that in the assessment of an acute or subacute psychiatric illness in a child, an organic etiology should be excluded.

LOCALIZING SIGNS AND SYMPTOMS

In addition to the nonlocalizing signs and symptoms discussed above, focal features suggest specific anatomic sites of involvement. Focal seizures may be the presenting symptom in a patient with a supratentorial mass lesion. In general, seizures occur more frequently with slower growing tumors such as oligodendrogliomas and low-grade astrocytomas rather than with the higher-grade tumors such as glioblastoma multiforme. Although most children with seizures do not have mass lesions, neoplasms should be suspected in those patients with long-standing seizure disorders who undergo changes in school performance or behavior, frequency or type of seizure, alteration on neurologic examination, or development of a slow wave dysrhythmia on electroencephalogram (EEG) (Page et al., 1969).

The more common signs and symptoms associated with supratentorial mass lesions include motor, sensory, and hemianopic defects. Compared with the catastrophic onset of hemiparesis in patients with cerebrovascular accidents, hemiparesis in patients with supratentorial tumors is usually subtle and slowly progressive. Sensory distortion of a cortical nature may be present in patients with parietal lobe tumors. However, the complete loss of pain and temperature and/or loss of vibration and position sense usually identified with either spinal cord disease or hysteria would be distinctly unusual in tumors of the cerebral hemispheres.

Signs and symptoms of midline CNS tumors include visual complaints and endocrinopathies. Visual loss may reflect either direct involvement of the optic nerves and/or chiasm or may be secondary to chronic papilledema and 2° optic atrophy. The presence of nystagmus in a young child, often associated with a chiasmatic mass, may erroneously be attributed to congenital nystagmus or spasmus nutans. Visual field abnormalities may be a sign of craniopharyngioma, chiasmatic tumor, or a lesion compressing the optic tracts or optic radiations (Fig. 9.1).

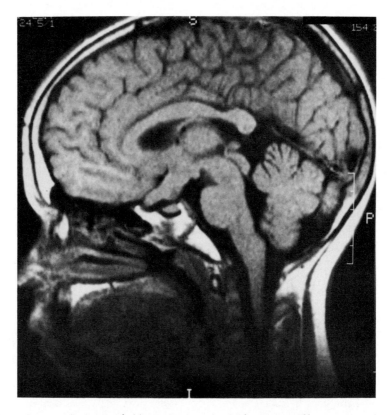

Figure 9.1.   Large optic nerve and chiasmatic tumor in child with neurofibromatosis and visual loss.

Endocrine dysfunction may include weight loss or weight gain. Weight loss is typical of the diencephalic syndrome of infancy in which, despite adequate intake, a young child with a hypothalamic glioma presents with a severe failure to thrive (White and Ross, 1963). In contrast, older children with lesions of the hypothalamus may develop increased weight gain, particularly if the satiety center in the hypothalamus is damaged. In general, organic causes of obesity are associated with a deceleration of linear growth, such as is seen in hypothyroidism and Cushing's disease. Hence, if increased weight is accompanied by deceleration in linear growth, referral to an endocrinologist is indicated.

Precocious puberty is another endocrinopathy that should raise the suspicion of central nervous system disease. Children with pineal region tumors tend to have excessive androgen effects. Therefore, minimal testicular enlargement will be found in the presence of a large penis; axillary, inguinal, and facial hair; and increase in both bone age and longitudinal growth. In contrast, males with precocious puberty secondary to hypothalamic lesions, tend to have large testes along with other signs of sexual precocity. These patients cannot be reliably distinguished clinically from children with idiopathic precocious puberty. In any case, children with inappropriately advanced sexual development should be evaluated by an endocrinologist. Referral to a neurologist generally will be forthcoming.

Children with tumors located in the cerebellum typically present with disorders of coordination. Tumors in the midline tend to be associated with truncal ataxia, whereas tumors located in the cerebellar hemispheres are more likely associated with appendicular ataxia. Scanning speech, hypotonia, pendular reflexes, and skew deviation of the eyes are less common signs of cerebellar disease. Patients with cerebellar tumors typically present with signs and symptoms of increased intracranial pressure secondary to obstruction of the 4th ventricle or aqueduct of Sylvius.

Children with tumors in the brainstem have the typical triad of cranial neuropathies, long tract signs, and cerebellar signs. However, because of the tumor's location in the basis pontis, the children usually do not present with signs and symptoms of increased intracranial pressure until late in the tumor's course.

Even in the absence of increased intracranial pressure, irritability and personality change are reported in children whose tumors are located in the supratentorial, midline, and posterior fossa regions. Change in school performance may be a nonspecific sign of a mass lesion or may reflect unsuspected seizures secondary to a supratentorial tumor.

In summary, children with brain tumors commonly present with nonspecific and nonlocalizing signs such as headache, vomiting, personality change, and double vision. Localizing signs generally suggest the specific anatomic site of involvement. However, there are some children with brain tumors who, despite minimal neurologic signs and symptoms, harbor extremely large mass lesions (Fig. 9.2).

Epidemiology

Brain tumors are the most common solid tumor in childhood, with an incidence in the United States of 2.4 per 100,000 children 0 to 15 years of age. The male-to-female ratio is approximately equal, although there is a slight predominance of males. Central nervous system neoplasms are found in all age groups, with a peak during the 5- to 9-year interval. The location of tumor varies with age. Infants in the first year of life tend to have supratentorial tumors, whereas children older than 3 years usually have tumors located in the posterior fossa. The most common brain tumors in children, regardless of age, are low-grade supratentorial astrocytomas and medulloblastomas. The next most common tumors in children less than 2 years old are ependymomas, primitive neuroectodermal tumors, and glioblastomas; in children 5 to 9 years old, cerebellar astrocytomas and brainstem gliomas tend to predominate.

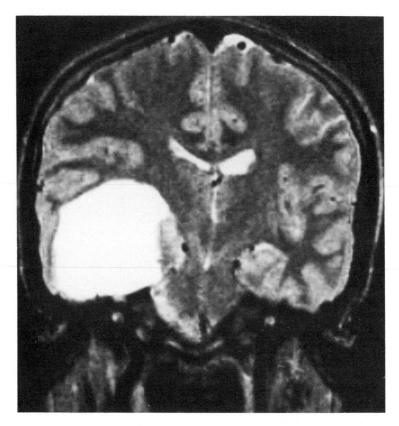

Figure 9.2.   Large temporal lobe anaplastic astrocytoma. Patient presented with a single seizure and normal neurologic exam.

The histopathologic distribution of malignant tumors in children less than 15 years of age is noted in Figure 9.3 (Duffner et al., 1986). The SEER Registry (Surveillance, Epidemiology, End Results) does not code for craniopharyngiomas, since they are considered to be benign. In other studies, craniopharyngiomas may represent 6 to 10% of the total.

There are several well-known genetic syndromes associated with the development of brain tumors. Neurocutaneous syndromes such as neurofibromatosis, tuberous sclerosis, von Hippel-Lindau disease, and the basal cell nevus syndrome are all associated with increased incidence of brain tumors. Other factors associated with an increased incidence of malignancies include low-dose radiation, immunosuppression, certain forms of chemotherapy, and environmental ex-

posure to aromatic hydrocarbons, triazenes, and systemic hydrazines (Cohen and Duffner, 1984).

Diagnostic Tests

The decade of the mid-1970s and 1980s has resulted in a profound change in diagnostic methodology. Prior to the advent of computed tomography (CT) scan and, more recently, magnetic resonance image (MRI) scanning, pneumoencephalography (i.e., the introduction of air via the ventricular or subarachnoid route) would outline the anatomy of the ventricular system. The presence of an intracranial mass was then implied by either distortion or alteration of ventricular anatomy or the findings of ventricular outflow obstruction. Not only was this methodology painful and rather barbaric, the end re-

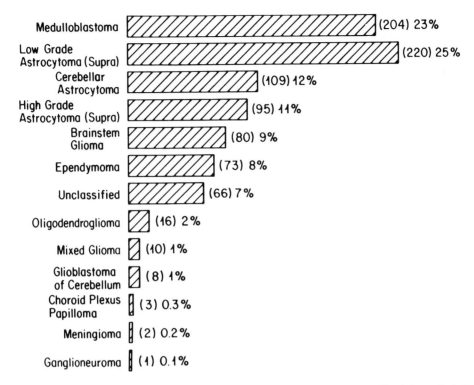

Figure 9.3. Distribution of tumor types in the SEER Registries (Surveillance, Epidemiology, End Results). (From Duffner PK, Cohen ME, Myers MH, et al. Survival of children with brain tumors: SEER Program 1973–1980. Neurology 1986;36:597, with permission.)

sult many times did not warrant the cost or the effort.

Similarly electroencephalography, although heralded in the early 1920s and 1930s as a major diagnostic tool, has been helpful in a limited way in the diagnosis of an intracranial mass. Alteration of waking patterns, depression of sleep spindles, or focal slowing has been associated with altered neurologic function and only inferentially has been associated with a mass. Unfortunately, the EEG has never fulfilled the promise of relating function to structure. At best, the EEG provides information regarding paroxysmal states such as seizures or abnormalities in frequency patterns from one hemisphere to the other. At its worst, the EEG may provide confusing and uninterpretable information. There are no specific patterns or electrical abnormalities that allow differentiation of tumors from metabolic or vascular states. The findings of slow waves, polymorphic delta, depression of rhythms, absence of sleep spindles, and diffuse delta and theta rhythms suggest functional alterations but need to be confirmed by more specific diagnostic methods.

Unlike air encephalography and EEG, arteriography continues to be an important part of the diagnostic armamentarium. This modality continues to define most clearly the vascular supply of the tumor and its primary feeding vessels. Identification of anatomic variants, new vessel formation, and vascularity of the tumor assists the surgeon in formulating an operative strategy. On occasion, the arteriogram may identify an arteriovenous malformation that previously had been mistaken for an intracranial neoplasm.

As with EEG and air encephalography, radionuclide scans have been replaced by other forms of neuroimaging such as CT or MRI. Perhaps more than any other methodology, CTs (for which the Noble Prize was awarded) and MRIs have represented major diagnostic advances in imaging brain tumors. Since the mid 1970s, the quality and resolution of CT scans has improved (Segall et al., 1985). Today's CT scans provide thin slices of brain with limited radiation. Scans can be obtained either in the axial or coronal plane and readily reconstructed in the sagittal plane. The new generation scanners allow definition of gray-white matter interfaces and relatively small or difficult-to-visualize intracranial structures, such as the basal ganglia, internal capsule, and red nucleus. CT scans, with judicious use of contrast, reveal abnormalities of the subarachnoid space or the intracranial vasculature. Cerebral edema, dilation and obstruction of the ventricular systems, and extraaxial fluid collections can readily be distinguished. CT scanning has progressed to the point that 90% of all intracranial neoplasms can be readily identified. However, because of the artifacts produced by the skull, areas such as the sella, parasella, and posterior fossa continue to be poorly defined by CT imaging.

Unlike CT scanning, magnetic resonance imaging provides superb resolution without radiation. Thin sections can be obtained in all three planes (i.e., axial, coronal, and sagittal). Further, there is unsurpassed definition of gray-white matter interfaces as well as small intracranial structures. The routine use of gadolinium as a contrast agent and the various paradigms of imaging available by variations in T1 and T2 weighting have made this the diagnostic procedure of choice. Although MRI allows superb definition of anatomic structures as well as the separation of pathologic from non-pathologic tissue, differentiation of edema from tumor continues to confound the ability to identify the margins of a tumor.

MRI angiography may limit the need for arteriography except in the most select cases. Similarly, MRI scanning has the potential to replace myelography in assessing disease of the spinal axis. To date, CT myelography is most accurately able to identify leptomeningeal metastases. However, MRI has the potential to allow accurate definition of spinal cord structures without invading the spinal subarachnoid space. Once the neuroradiologists are comfortable in delineating artifact from drop metastasis, MRI myelography may replace CT myelography. At this juncture in the history of diagnostic neuroimaging, the sensitivity of the techniques may be much greater than the specificity. For this reason, MRI and CT myelography are complementary.

SPECT (single photon emission computed tomography) and PET (positron emission tomography) scanning are enhancing the ability to define metabolic differences between normal and neoplastic tissue. SPECT scanning is particularly useful in establishing patterns of blood flow to the tumor, whereas PET is capable of differentiating normal from abnormal metabolism. The ability to overlay PET scans on MRI and CT scans raises the potential of being able to identify metabolism within specific altered structural anatomy.

Thus, technologic advances have virtually eliminated the difficulty in establishing the presence or absence of an intracranial mass lesion. The challenge for the physician of the future has turned to treatment rather than diagnosis.

Treatment

The treatment of patients with brain tumors consists of surgery, usually followed by radiation, and in some cases chemotherapy. Pediatric surgical mortality and morbidity has decreased significantly with the advent of improved anesthesia, the dissecting microscope, the cavitron, laser surgery, and the use of an intensive care unit. In contrast to Cushing's surgical mortality of children with medulloblastomas of 32%, modern treatment is associated with less than a 5% mortality. Complete surgical resection of some tumors (i.e., cerebellar astrocytomas, meningiomas, and craniopharyngiomas) may be associated with a definitive cure without further therapy. In other cases, surgical resection will relieve increased intracranial pressure, prevent shift of intracranial structures, and reestablish cerebrospinal fluid (CSF) integrity. Finally, even in those patients in whom only biopsy is possible, a tissue diagnosis can be established that will determine further therapy. Adjuvant therapy, such as radiation and/or chemotherapy, is most effective when the tumor burden is the least. Therefore, in most cases, debulking surgery is recommended. Bloom has shown that children with medulloblastomas treated with total surgical resection have significantly better rates of survival than do those treated with partial or subtotal resection (Bloom et al., 1990).

Radiation has been the standard treatment for most brain tumors in children and adults. The volume and dose of radiation is in a constant state of reexamination. *Volume of radiation* refers to the total amount of brain radiated and depends on the tendency for the tumor to seed throughout the neuraxis. Medulloblastomas and primitive neuroectodermal tumors, which tend to seed the CSF pathways, are treated with craniospinal radiation with a boost of radiation to the tumor bed. In contrast, patients with brainstem gliomas, which have a limited tendency to metastasize, are treated with radiation to the posterior fossa alone.

Standard radiation doses range from 4500 to 5500 centigrey (cGy). Hyperfractionation is a technique by which the total dose of radiation given over a defined period of time is increased beyond that of standard radiation without a concomitant increase in side effects. The dose per fraction is decreased but the number of fractions per unit of time is increased. Therefore, rather than the typical 150 cGy given in a single course in a 24-hour period, the dose per fraction is reduced to 110 to 120 cGy given twice a day. In this manner, the total dose of radiation is increased by 10 to 20% without theoretically increasing adverse effects (Freeman et al., 1988).

Since radiation affects both normal and abnormal cells, a variety of different techniques have been developed to limit the amount of radiation exposure experienced by normal tissue. One of these techniques is interstitial radiotherapy, in which radioactive pellets are placed directly into a cavity in the tumor bed. This provides high-dose radiation to the tumor bed and spares normal tissue. This approach is restricted to tumors that are relatively small in size and do not extensively invade surrounding tissue.

The use of chemotherapy in the treatment of pediatric brain tumors has increased in recent years. Chemotherapeutic drugs must be able to breach the blood-brain barrier. Properties that influence access of the drugs to the CNS include low molecular weight, non-ionizability at physiologic pH, high lipid solubility, and lack of plasma protein binding. Whereas the necrotic center of a tumor does not have an intact blood-brain barrier, the blood-brain barrier in the periphery of the tumor remains intact. This region of tumor is the most viable and has the greatest capacity for proliferation.

Despite these caveats, chemotherapy has been used effectively in an adjuvant fashion with radiation, or alone at the time of recurrence. Although the addition of chemotherapy to radiation has not statistically influenced survival rates of standard-risk children with medulloblastoma, adjuvant chemotherapy has been associated with significantly improved progression-free and overall survival rates in children with medulloblastomas who are considered to be high-risk. Hence, very young children and those with extensive disease have benefitted from adjuvant chemotherapy (Evans et al., 1990; Bloom et al., 1990).

There has also been wide experience using chemotherapy at time of recurrence. The most effective agents have been the nitrosoureas, cyclophosphamide, cisplatinum, and vincristine. These and other agents have shown efficacy in phase 2 studies (i.e., studies in which patients with recurrent tumors are treated with a single agent). Combination chemotherapy at the time of recurrence has been even more effective.

Because radiation of the young child's brain is associated with severe neurotoxicity, the Pediatric Oncology Group developed a treatment protocol in which postoperative chemotherapy was used to delay radiation in infants with malignant brain tumors. Infants less than 3 years of age were treated with cytoxan, vincristine, cisplatinum, and VP-16 for 12 to 24 months, depending upon age at diagnosis. Radiation has been delayed between 1 and 2 years in a significant percentage of patients. This is the first time that chemotherapy has been shown to have a first-line role in the treatment of malignant brain tumors.

In summary, the treatment of children with brain tumors consists of surgery, chemotherapy, and radiation. Although chemotherapy use is expected to increase over the next several years, radiation remains the standard treatment for brain tumors in children as well as adults. Unfortunately, none of these techniques is curative. Investigational treatments include biologic response modifiers, immunotoxins, and monoclonal antibodies.

Prognosis

Based on SEER Registry data, the 5-year survival of children with brain tumors of all types in the United States is approximately 50%. Survival rates vary according to tumor type. Hence, children with cerebellar astrocytomas have an anticipated 5-year survival of more than 90%, whereas those with brainstem gliomas have a 5-year survival of less than 20%. Survival rates of children with medulloblastomas have improved dramatically during the past 20 years, a result of improved surgery, radiation to the entire neuraxis, and increased radiation to the tumor bed. A select group of patients with medulloblastomas has 5-year survival rates approaching 70% (Hughes et al., 1988).

Survival rates vary according to age. Infants with malignant brain tumors have significantly worse survival rates than do other age groups. Hence, infants with ependymomas and medulloblastomas do worse than children of older ages with the identical tumor type. Despite advances in treatment, the prognosis for infants with brain tumors as well as those children with ependymomas, brainstem gliomas, glioblastomas, anaplastic astrocytomas, and primitive neuroectodermal tumors remains poor. In contrast, good survival rates can be expected with low-grade supratentorial astrocytomas, craniopharyngiomas, optic pathway tumors, meningiomas, "good risk" medulloblastomas, and cerebellar astrocytomas (Table 9.1).

ILLUSTRATIVE CASES
Supratentorial

D. L. presented at 6 years of age with grand mal seizures. She had a normal neurologic examination and normal EEG and brain scan. She was a good student and there were no interpersonal conflicts in the home. Seizures were fairly well controlled on Tegretol. At age 13 years she had a gradual personality change. She began acting out sexually, was failing in school, and was in constant conflict with her parents. Simultaneously, her seizures increased in frequency and character. Seizures that previously had been generalized tonic-clonic seizures were now characterized as staring followed by picking at her clothing and uttering nonsense syllables. Neurologic examination remained normal. She was diagnosed as having an "adolescent adjustment reaction." Despite therapeutic drug levels, she continued to have frequent seizures. A repeat EEG revealed a slow wave focus in the left temporal lobe. CT scan demonstrated a calcified mass in the left temporal lobe. The patient underwent a total resection of an oligodendroglioma. She has remained seizure-free without medication for 10 years and has had no further behavioral problems.

Table 9.1.
Common Brain Tumors in Childhood

Tumor Type	Treatment	Prognosis (5-year survival)
POSTERIOR FOSSA		
Cerebellar astrocytoma	Surgical resection	More than 90%
Medulloblastoma	Surgery + craniospinal radiation therapy ± chemotherapy	"Good risk," 70% "Poor risk, 30–40%
Brainstem glioma	± Biopsy Local radiation (hyperfractionation)	Less than 20%
MIDLINE TUMORS		
Craniopharyngioma	Surgery—total or partial resection ± RT	50–90%
Hypothalamic glioma	Biopsy + local radiation	50–70%
Germinoma	Surgery + radiation + chemotherapy	70–90%
SUPRATENTORIAL		
Oligodendroglioma	Surgery ± local RT	70%
Glioblastoma multiforme	Surgery + wide field RT (consider chemotherapy)	0–20%
Low-grade astrocytoma	Surgery ± local radiation	50–70%

Discussion

This patient had a seven-year history of seizures that had changed in character from generalized tonic-clonic to partial complex. In addition, she had a change in personality and school performance. Her original EEG, which had been normal, later revealed a slow wave focus suggesting structural disease. At surgery, an oligodendroglioma was found. Presumbly this tumor evolved from a preexisting hamartoma, or alternatively, the oligodendroglioma had remained indolent for many years. Although many of her personality characteristics were compatible with an adolescent adjustment reaction, there were enough warning signs present to suggest an organic cause for her psychologic dysfunction.

Posterior Fossa

Two years prior to evaluation, T.M. had been diagnosed as having anorexia nervosa. At the time of her initial presentation, her examination had been normal. Because of persistent somatic complaints, she was admitted for reevaluation to the Children's Hospital of Buffalo, where she complained of headache in the occipital area and neck that she spontaneously related to tension.

She had been told that her difficulty in swallowing was due to "globus hystericus." Complaints of dizziness and unsteady gait were found but were considered a form of astasia-abasia.

She was alert but emaciated. She had nystagmus in all planes of gaze, chronic papilledema, and decreased visual acuity. She had a left 9th nerve paresis with inability to elevate the palate. Cerebellar examination revealed left-sided dysmetria and pendular reflexes. A CT scan revealed a large cystic mass with 4th ventricular outflow obstruction. At surgery, a cystic cerebellar astrocytoma was completely removed. She is free of tumor 15 years later.

Discussion

This adolescent presented with weight loss and anorexia. Neurologic examination and radionuclide scanning were normal. Over time, her physical complaints were attributed by both her psychiatrist and herself to psychosomatic disease. The occipital headache and neck pain were due to irritation of the cervical roots secondary to incipient tonsillar herniation. The "globus hystericus" was due to bulbar dysfunction, and her "astasia-abasia" was secondary to a cerebellar

mass lesion. Once her initial diagnosis of anorexia nervosa had been made and despite a
plethora of symptoms, she never had a repeat
neurologic examination.

Midline

B.S. presented at 10 years of age with a history
of intermittent frontal headache occurring
throughout the day for the past 3 months. In
the 3 weeks prior to evaluation, the patient had
complained of nausea and nonprojectile vomiting. He was characterized as a good student, but
his grades had recently declined. There had been
some interpersonal conflicts at home. The father
was an alcoholic and the sister had run away
from home. Examination revealed a small youngster whose weight and stature were in the 5th
percentile for age. Visual acuity was 20/100 in
the right eye and 20/20 in the left eye, with
evidence of a right hemianopsia. A CT scan revealed a calcified mass obstructing the foramen
of Monro with 2° dilation of the ventricles. A
diagnosis of craniopharyngioma was suspected.
The patient underwent surgical resection with
total removal of the mass. The postoperative
course was uneventful except for the presence of
diabetes insipidus. This was readily controlled
with vasopressin. Over the next 1½ years, the
patient developed excessive weight gain, became
morbidly obese, and stopped fraternizing with
his friends. Whereas before the surgery he had
been an active youngster participating in sports
and involved in many school activities, following
surgery he became withdrawn, poorly motivated, and was no longer interested in social
intercourse. Despite multiple attempts at controlling his weight, he continued to be a compulsive eater. There was extensive catch-up
growth. Three years after surgery he was in the
75th percentile for height. He remained well
above the 95th percentile for weight, had
dropped out of school, and generally had an amo-
tivational syndrome.

Discussion

This patient had a rather characteristic course
for patients with craniopharyngiomas. He initially presented with growth retardation, headache, vomiting, and visual compromise. The
headache and the vomiting resulted from increased intracranial pressure secondary to obstruction of the foramen of Monro. The growth
retardation was a direct effect of the craniopharyngioma, either involving hypothalamic or
pituitary structures. Visual loss was secondary
to compromise of the left optic nerve and tract.
Despite total surgical removal of the tumor, the
patient developed diabetes insipidus and required replacement therapy with antidiuretic
hormone. The development of obesity and hyperphagia, diabetes insipidus, and abulia reflect
involvement of the hypothalamus and its projections to the frontal and limbic areas. Excessive
eating secondary to organic disease responds in
a limited way to psychotherapy using behavioral
therapy techniques. Abulia may occur for years
and eventually resolve. In patients with craniopharyngiomas, psychiatric manifestations occur as a result of the treatment. Cure rates for
this tumor following treatment are 80 to 90%.
Unfortunately morbidity (i.e., endocrinopathies, usually diabetes insipidus), visual loss, and
personality change approach 80%.

Long-Term Effects of Treatment

Children who receive cranial irradiation for leukemia, lymphoma, and brain tumors are at risk
for a variety of long-term effects of therapy. The
most important of these include adverse effects
on intelligence and endocrine function, leukoencephalopathy, and oncogenesis.

Intelligence

Radiation-induced dementia was first studied extensively in children with leukemia. Some children with leukemia receive cranial irradiation in

doses of 1800 to 2400 cGy to prevent CNS leukemia. Retrospective studies have shown that although IQs generally are normal, they are significantly lower than IQs of patients treated with chemotherapy alone. Moreover, many patients are learning disabled. Patients radiated for brain tumors, who receive much larger doses of radiation to the brain than do children with leukemia, are at greater risk for intellectual sequelae. Indeed, retrospective studies have revealed that 30 to 50% of children radiated for brain tumors have IQs lower than 70, whereas only 10 to 20% have IQs above 90. More recent prospective evaluations have shown a lower incidence of frank mental retardation, particularly in children beyond the age of 10 at the time of radiation, but almost all children have learning disabilities requiring special classes. These abnormalities may be progressive over time. The most severely affected children are infants and very young children. In a recent prospective study, children radiated before age 7 were reported to have a 25 point loss in IQ after cranial radiation (Packer et al., 1989). Several risk factors are associated with radiation-induced dementia. Patients who have evidence on neuroimaging or leukoencephalopathy and vasculopathy almost invariably are neuropsychologically impaired. Furthermore, patients with supratentorial rather than infratentorial tumors are more likely to have learning difficulties, as are those who receive whole brain versus local radiation (Ellenberg et al., 1987). Chemotherapy also plays a role in radiation-induced dementia. It is known that the combination of methotrexate and radiation can produce severe necrotizing leukoencephalopathy associated with intellectual deterioration. Whether other chemotherapeutic agents in the presence of radiation will also be associated with intellectual decline is not yet known. Focused prospective studies are needed in order to assess the role of the various risk factors.

At least one study has suggested that patients radiated for brain tumors may improve if placed in special educational classes (Mulhern et al., 1983). Hence, it is extremely important that those patients treated with cranial irradiation for leukemia, lymphoma, or brain tumors are followed longitudinally with IQ evaluations as well as achievement tests. If the patient shows intellectual decline or difficulty with learning, special educational help should be provided. Recognition that radiation-induced dementia may be progressive argues for close long-term follow-up, preferably on a yearly basis.

Endocrinopathy

The most common postradiation endocrinopathy is growth hormone deficiency. Approximately 80% of children radiated for brain tumors are growth hormone deficient and have abnormal longitudinal growth rates (Duffner et al., 1985). Radiation-induced growth hormone deficiency putatively relates to damage to the ventromedian nucleus of the hypothalamus, which produces growth hormone releasing factor. Since radiation to the posterior fossa extends as far anteriorly as the posterior clinoid, the port includes the ventromedian nucleus of the hypothalamus. Therefore, patients treated with either whole-brain radiation or radiation to the posterior fossa alone are at risk for the development of growth hormone deficiency. To complicate matters, patients who receive craniospinal radiation also have growth failure because of adverse effects on the vertebral bodies. Children radiated at 1 year of age may anticipate a 10 cm loss in ultimate adult height, whereas children radiated at age 10 may potentially lose 5½ cm of ultimate adult height (Shalet et al., 1987). A third factor contributing to growth failure in children with brain tumors is their tendency to develop precocious puberty and hence prematurely fuse their epiphyses. Therefore, although growth hormone replacement therapy will enhance growth, patients radiated for brain tumors may not reach their predicted adult height.

Another endocrine problem associated with radiation is hypothyroidism. Children who receive radiation to the cervical spine as part of craniospinal radiation may develop primary hypothyroidism, and those who receive whole-brain radiation may develop secondary or tertiary hypothyroidism. Poor school performance and poor growth may be due partly to undetected hypothyroidism.

Patients treated for brain tumors with spinal radiation and chemotherapy are also at risk for gonadal dysfunction. Boys treated with cyclophosphamide have normal pubertal maturation and normal libido but may develop oligo- or even azoospermia. Girls have less risk of gonadal dysfunction from cyclophosphamide. Conversely, girls often develop ovarian dysfunction secondary to spinal radiation, whereas males are

at less risk for testicular damage (Clayton et al., 1988).

Leukoencephalopathy

Leukoencephalopathy is a late complication of radiation treatment of the central nervous system, with and without the concomitant use of chemotherapy, especially methotrexate. The condition is characterized clinically by dementia, seizures, ataxia, focal motor deficits, and, at times, coma and death. Multifocal white matter destruction, particularly in the centrum semiovale and periventricular regions, is characteristic. There is loss of oligodendroglia and myelin (Price and Birdwell, 1975; Price and Birdwell, 1978). Leukoencephalopathy is identified on CT scan and MRI as enlarged ventricles and subar-

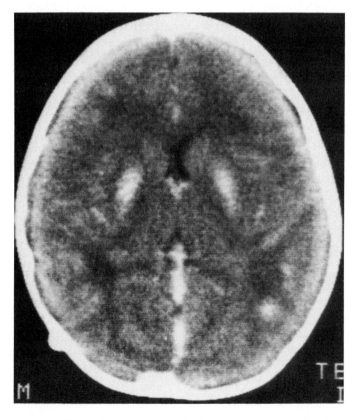

Figure 9.4. CT scan compatible with leukoencephalopathy in a patient treated with radiation and methotrexate for a brain tumor. Note basal ganglia calcification and areas of low density.

achnoid space, areas of calcification, particularly in the basal ganglia, and hypodense areas. On MRI there is a pattern of periventricular hyperintensity (PVH) (i.e., increased T2 weighted signals in deep white matter). PVH has a scalloped, symmetric appearance that extends to the gray-white matter junction (Packer et al., 1986) (Figs. 9.4 and 9.5).

Leukoencephalopathy was first reported in children with leukemia who were treated with a combination of methotrexate and radiation. With the advent of MRI, it is now recognized that children may develop leukoencephalopathy after treatment with radiation alone. Although there are rare patients with periventricular hyperintensity who do not have intellectual

dysfunction, the majority of patients suffer progressive intellectual declines. Hence, a child treated for leukemia, lymphoma, or brain tumor who develops insidious deterioration of IQ or school performance, personality change, and/or seizures may be developing leukoencephalopathy. Unfortunately, leukoencephalopathy is not amenable to treatment.

Oncogenesis

Oncogenesis is a particularly tragic sequela of cranial irradiation and some forms of chemotherapy. Oncogenesis implies that the second tumor is not the result of metastases but rather arises de novo and is of different histologic type. Radiation-induced tumors have occurred with

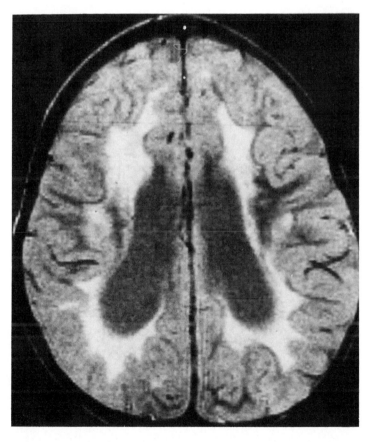

Figure 9.5. MRI of patient with leukoencephalopathy following treatment with radiation and methotrexate. Note symmetric scalloped increased T2 weighted signals. The T2 abnormalities do not extend from white into gray matter.

low-, moderate-, and high-dose radiation. The best example of low-dose radiation-induced tumors has come from the Israeli experience in which more than 10,000 patients were treated with radiation dosages as low as 500 cGy for tinea capitis. There was a seven-fold increase in neural tumors among radiated children compared with controls. Of these, meningiomas and gliomas were the most common (Ron et al., 1988).

Children with acute lymphocytic leukemia (ALL) treated with moderate-dose radiation for CNS prophylaxis are also reported to develop brain tumors. The types of tumors are predominately meningiomas and high-grade gliomas (Fig. 9.6). As might be anticipated, children treated with high-dose radiation for brain tumors are also at risk for second unrelated malignancies. In general, second primaries occur in intervals from 5 to 25 years following initial treatment. They usually occur within the radiation port.

Patients treated for brain tumors are also at risk for extracranial malignancies. Radiation to the thyroid gland, as part of craniospinal radiation, may be associated with the late development of thyroid cancer.

The literature on oncogenesis is steadily increasing as more children survive their primary

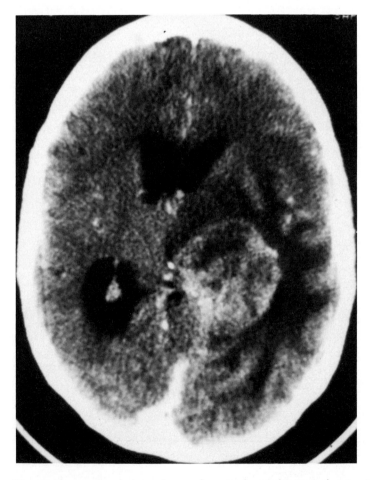

Figure 9.6.   An 18-year-old man treated at age 2 years for acute lymphoblastic leukemia with radiation and chemotherapy. At 16 years of age he was diagnosed with a meningioma and at 18 years of age he was diagnosed with a glioblastoma multiforme.

brain tumors. It is important to recognize that a second primary may not be of the same degree of malignancy as the original. Hence, a child who develops signs and symptoms suggestive of a mass lesion several years after the original diagnosis may have a benign meningioma rather than recurrence of the original primary. Surgical intervention in cases of doubt is recommended, since some of these second tumors may be far more amenable to treatment than the original.

When Should the Psychiatrist Refer a Patient to a Neurologist?

Personality change, declining school performance, apathy, and irritability are symptoms in children with virtually all types of brain tumors,

regardless of location (Table 9.2). Patients with brainstem gliomas as well as those with supratentorial glioblastomas may present with similar "emotional" complaints. In the 1930s, Cushing described a child with a cerebellar astrocytoma. In part he said, "attendance at school meanwhile may continue but the teacher soon notices that the child is listless, inattentive and the character of his work noticeably falls off." Minor behavior changes may indeed be the first sign of the child with a brain tumor. Behavior changes are soon associated with alterations in playtime activity, school behavior, and interpersonal relations. After this, nonspecific signs of increased intracranial pressure may develop. Later, more specific lateralizing signs relative to the site of the

Table 9.2.
Common Neuropsychiatric Symptoms According to Location

Tumor Location	Psychiatric Symptoms	Neurologic Symptoms	Commentary
Posterior fossa	Irritability Lethargy Apathy Somnolence Decreased school performance	Cranial neuropathies Long tract signs Increased ICP[a]	Medulloblastomas more likely have truncal ataxia, whereas cerebellar astrocytomas have appendicular ataxia. Both have increased ICP. Patients with BSG present with cranial neuropathies, long tract, and cerebellar signs. Increased ICP occurs late.
Midline	Eating disorders Sleep disorders Mood swings Lethargy Decreased school performance	Endocrinopathies Visual axis abnormalities Autonomic abnormalities Parinaud's syndrome Precocious puberty Increased ICP[a]	Craniopharyngiomas present with visual field abnormalities and increased ICP. Hypothalamic gliomas present with eating disorders and endocrinopathies. Pineal region tumors in males may present with precocious puberty and Parinaud's syndrome.
Supratentorial	Hallucinations Personality change Sensory distortion Decreased school performance	Focal motor Focal sensory Visual field abnormalities Seizures Increased ICP[a]	Psychiatric symptoms are more common in patients with slower growing tumors (i.e., oligodendrogliomas and low grade astrocytomas. GBM has a more truncated course, often with increased ICP.

[a] Neurologic signs of increased ICP: headache, diplopia, papilledema, VI nerve palsy.
Key:
  ICP = Intracranial pressure
  GBM = Glioblastoma multiforme
  BSG = Brainstem glioma

tumor will become apparent. Although psychiatric symptoms are common presenting symptoms in children with a variety of brain tumors, most patients have other signs and symptoms that help localize the true cause of the behavior difficulties.

Seizures

Brain tumors are an infrequent cause of seizures in children, since most seizures are idiopathic in childhood. However, those children with a long-standing history of seizures who develop change in personality, decrease in school performance, or loss of seizure control need reevaluation. There have been a number of patients identified with partial complex seizures in whom the initial CT scans have been negative but repeat CT or MRI has revealed structural abnormalities. Some of these have been diagnosed as gangliogliomas, oligodendrogliomas, hamartomas, or low-grade astrocytomas. Hence, it is possible that some long-standing seizure disorders in patients may have a structural cause but that imaging studies in the past have not been sensitive enough to identify them.

Sleep Disorders

Alteration in sleep patterns may be a symptom of CNS neoplasm. Hypersomnolence is particularly striking in patients with hypothalamic tumors and in some patients with brainstem gliomas. In contrast, children who have difficulty sleeping may be experiencing nocturnal headaches. Although the older child will complain of awakening with headache, the infant can only respond to the pain with crying and irritability. Some children will develop disturbed sleep from undiagnosed nocturnal seizures associated with their brain tumor. Hence, change in sleep pattern should prompt neurologic evaluation.

Disorders of Eating

Disorders of eating may be the presenting symptom of a CNS neoplasm. The adolescent patient

diagnosed as having anorexia nervosa because of symptoms of weight loss, anorexia, and depression may actually harbor a tumor located in the hypothalamus or pituitary region. On examination, the patient may have deficits such as visual field abnormalities, papilledema, or optic atrophy. Failure to thrive in infancy is usually due to parental deprivation. Hence, many of these families may be referred for psychiatric care. However, failure to thrive is also the classic presenting symptom of the diencephalic syndrome in an infant with a hypothalamic tumor. In such cases, the child is alert and hungry but emaciated. Examination may reveal a large head with split sutures.

Weight gain may also be a symptom of either a mass located in the hypothalamic-pituitary axis or infiltration of the hypothalamus with malignant cells. In these cases, the patients develop a voracious appetite secondary to damage to the satiety center. This can be particularly difficult to diagnose in the child with leukemia. Although patients whose brain tumors are located in the hypothalamus usually have other clinical signs such as changes on funduscopic examination or endocrinopathies, infiltration of the hypothalamus by leukemic cells may be the first sign of central nervous system leukemia. Since this is an uncommon but well-reported complication of CNS leukemia, patients with this symptom should have a lumbar puncture for cytologic examination. Hyperphagia commonly occurs following surgery for craniopharyngiomas. In these cases, the excessive hunger is not due to psychic factors but rather damage to the satiety center.

Vomiting

Vomiting can be a symptom of bulimia. However, vomiting can also be due to increased intracranial pressure or can occur secondary to infiltration of the floor of 4th ventricle by tumor. If the vomiting is secondary to increased intracranial pressure, the clinical symptoms of headache and diplopia and the physical signs of papilledema and 6th nerve palsy are usually evident. However, when the lesion involves the floor of the 4th ventricle, it may be difficult to diagnose even on neuroimaging. Since patients with brain tumors often develop a variety of functional complaints, vomiting may often be dismissed as psychosomatic in origin. To complicate matters, we have seen several patients who develop persistent nausea following diagnosis of a brain tumor in whom there is no apparent organic etiology. It can be extremely difficult to determine how many of the child's problems are psychiatric and how many relate to organic pathology.

Declining School Performance

Declining school performance, depression, irritability, and apathy may be symptomatic of tumors located in the frontal or temporal lobes or may reflect increased intracranial pressure. Memory deficits and consequent decline in school performance may also occur in children with tumors located in the 3rd ventricle or hippocampus. Unsuspected seizures per se may be associated with poor performance in school. This may manifest as inattentiveness, short-term memory difficulties, and inconsistent schoolwork. Finally, the physician evaluating a patient with declining school performance must also be aware of treatment-induced dementia. Although many children with brain tumors do poorly in school because of emotional disturbances and depression, deteriorating school performance is usually due to organic etiology and should initiate further evaluation.

By-and-large, the psychiatrist who is evaluating a child with brain tumor-related psychiatric complaints will be seeing patients with supratentorial mass lesions. Most children with tumors of the brainstem and cerebellum have a host of neurologic deficits in addition to psychiatric symptoms. In contrast, children with supratentorial tumors, particularly those that are slow growing, may present with a paucity of neurologic signs and symptoms. Hence, the psychiatrist must be sensitive to alterations in school performance or seizure pattern, personality change, and disorders in sleep and eating, as they may be harbingers of serious structural pathology. Table 9.2 lists both psychiatric as well as neurologic signs and symptoms of the more common pediatric brain tumors. As noted, psychiatric symptoms do not generally occur in isolation. Therefore, a detailed neurologic history and physical should be performed in children whose signs and symptoms suggest organic etiology. The typical signs and symptoms of increased intracranial pressure as well as those relative to focal neurologic deficits usually accompany psychiatric manifestations. Neurologic consultation should be sought in any child with abnormalities on neurologic examination or symptoms that suggest organic pathology.

REFERENCES

Barlow CT. Headaches and brain tumor. Am J Dis Child 1982;136:99–100.

Bloom HJG, Glees, J, Bell J. The treatment and long-term prognosis of children with intracranial tumors: a study of 610 cases, 1950–1981. Int J Radiat Oncol Biol Phys 1990;18:745–773.

Clayton PE, Shalet SM, Price DA. Gonadal function after chemotherapy and irradiation for childhood malignancies. Horm Res 1988;30:104–110.

Cohen ME, Duffner PK. Brain tumors in children: principles of diagnosis and treatment. New York: Raven Press, 1984.

Cushing H. Experiences with the cerebellar astrocytomas. A critical review of seventy-six cases. Surg Gynecol Obstet 1931;52:129–191.

Duffner PK, Cohen ME, Myers MH, et al. Survival of children with brain tumors: SEER Program, 1973–1980. Neurology 1986;36:597–601.

Duffner PK, Cohen ME, Voorhess ML, et al. Long-term effects of cranial irradiation on endocrine function in children with brain tumors. A prospective study. Cancer 1985;56:2189–2193.

Ellenberg L, McComb JG, Siegel SE, Stowe S. Factors affecting intellectual outcome in pediatric brain tumor patients. Neurosurgery 1987;218:638–644.

Evans AE, Jenkin RDT, Sposto R, et al. The treatment of medulloblastoma. J Neurosurg 1990;72:572–582.

Freeman CR, Krischer J, Sanford RA, Burger PC, Cohen M, Norris D. Hyperfractionated radiotherapy in brainstem tumors: results of a Pediatric Oncology Group study. Int J Radiat Oncol Biol Phys 1988;15:311–318.

Honig PJ, Charney EB. Children with brain tumor headaches. Am J Dis Child 1982;136:121–124.

Hughes EN, Shillito J, Sallan SE, Loeffler JS, Cassady JR, Tarbell NJ. Medulloblastoma at the Joint Center for Radiation Therapy between 1968 and 1984. Cancer 1988;61:1992–1998.

Mulhern RK, Crisco JJ, Kun LE. Neuropsychological sequelae of childhood brain tumors: a review. J Clin Child Psychol 1983;12:66–73.

Packer RJ, Sutton LN, Atkins TE, et al. A prospective study of cognitive function in children receiving whole-brain radiotherapy and chemotherapy: 2-year results. J Neurosurg 1989;70:707–713.

Packer RJ, Zimmerman RA, Bilaniuk LT. Magnetic resonance imaging in the evaluation of treatment related central nervous system damage. Cancer 1986;58:635–640.

Page LK, Lombroso CT, Matson DD. Childhood epilepsy with late detection of cerebral glioma. J Neurosurg 1969;31:253–261.

Price RA, Birdwell DA. The central nervous system in childhood leukemia II. Subacute leukoencephalopathy. Cancer 1975;35:306–318.

Price RA, Birdwell DA. The central nervous system in childhood leukemia III. Mineralizing microangiopathy and dystrophic calcification. Cancer 1978;42:717–728.

Ron E, Modan B, Boice JD. Tumors of the brain and nervous system after radiotherapy in childhood. N Engl J Med 1988;319:1033–1039.

Segall HD, Batnitzky S, Zee CS. Computed tomography in the diagnosis of intracranial neoplasms in children. Cancer 1985;56:1748–1755.

Shalet SM, Gibson B, Swindell R, Pearson D. Effect of spinal irradiation on growth. Arch Dis Child 1987;62:461–464.

White PT, Ross AT. Inanition syndrome in infants with anterior hypothalamic neoplasms. Neurology 1963;13:974–981.

Chapter 10

Neuroradiologic Imaging in Children

Lisa M. Tartaglino, MD, and Jacqueline A. Bello, MD

NEURORADIOLOGIC IMAGING

Within the past decade, neuroradiologic imaging has made tremendous advances in the evaluation of neurologic and psychiatric disorders. This chapter addresses the imaging modalities available, with emphasis on computed tomography and magnetic resonance imaging of those neurologic disorders that may be encountered by the psychiatrist treating children and adolescents. Neurologic disorders presenting in the newborn and infant, as well as those predominantly affecting the spinal cord, are not considered except as they relate to other disease entities discussed.

Computed Tomography (CT)

CT scanning uses numerous ultrathin x-ray photons arranged in an arc or circle to obtain and reconstruct images in a single plane based on tissue density. Compared with conventional x-rays, CT scanning can separate not only bone from soft tissue but the various components in soft tissue, such as water, muscle, fat, and blood, due to their specific x-ray attenuation coefficients. Those substances that are more dense appear more "white", while less dense ones appear more "gray." Therefore, in descending order of density: bone or other calcification, hemorrhage, gray matter, white matter, cerebrospinal fluid (CSF), and fat appear progressively darker, and air appears completely black.

Contrast enhancement with various iodine-containing substances improves the detection and resolution of many abnormalities. It should be used whenever the possibility of an infection, tumor, or vascular anomaly is suspected. Contrast solutions normally reach the arterial and venous structures, but they are restricted to the intravascular compartment by an intact blood-brain barrier. With breakdown of the normal blood-brain barrier, which may occur with cerebral infarction, infection, active demyelination, hemorrhagic and neoplastic processes, parenchymal enhancement is seen. Often the pattern of enhancement is diagnostically useful.

Magnetic Resonance Imaging (MRI)

MRI has rapidly become the imaging modality of choice for many clinical problems. Information is extracted from molecules, particularly the protons in water as they align or realign in a magnetic field. The patient is placed in a uniform "background" magnetic field varying in strength from 0.3 to 1.5 Tesla. Protons inherent in the water molecules of various tissues become aligned within this magnetic field. A second magnetic field, called the radio frequency (RF) pulse, is then briefly applied. This pulse causes the protons to change their alignment. When the RF pulse is stopped, the protons realign to the "background" magnetic field, giving off a signal that is recorded by the RF coil. Images are then reconstructed by computer in various planes. Different images and information can be obtained by varying the interval between the RF pulses (TR) and the time at which the returning pulses (echo) are recorded (TE). These times, TR and TE, are expressed in milliseconds (msec).

The predominant technique used in brain imaging is the "spin echo" technique, which generates T1 weighted images using a short TR and short TE; T2 weighted images, using a long TR and long TE; and "balanced" or proton density weighted images, using a long TR and short TE pulse sequence. As in CT, information is presented on a gray scale. T1 weighted images are best at anatomic definition and take the shortest time to obtain. CSF appears dark or hypointense, gray matter appears gray, and white matter appears somewhat brighter or slightly hyperintense to gray matter. Fat is very bright on T1 pulse sequences.

T2 images show tissue with high water content to be brighter or hyperintense. CSF appears the most hyperintense, gray matter is slightly less intense, and white matter is more gray on T2 weighted images. Fat has a lower signal intensity than on T1 weighted images. Since most parenchymal lesions and/or associated edema results in increased water content, T2 weighted images are more sensitive in detecting pathology, even though the anatomic definition is less resolved compared with T1 images.

Balanced, or proton density, images also use a long TR pulse sequence. In general, structures follow the signal intensity of T2 images, although CSF is isointense or hypointense to adjacent brain parenchyma. Lesions adjacent to CSF spaces, such as periventricular plaques in multiple sclerosis, are therefore more easily visualized.

Flowing blood, cortical bone, dense calcification, and air appear as absent signal (black) on all pulse sequences. Paramagnetic contrast enhancement with Gadolinium (Gd-DTPA) is now often used, but it provides useful information only on T1 sequences.

MRI vs. CT

Considering imaging criteria alone, MRI is probably superior to CT, with a few exceptions (Brant-Zawadzki et al., 1984; Brant-Zawadzki et al., 1983; Johnson et al., 1983). As mentioned, compared with CT, MRI is more sensitive, particularly when using long TR pulse sequences for parenchymal abnormalities. There also is better visualization of the posterior fossa and brainstem, which is often suboptimal on CT due to beam-hardening artifacts and volume averaging (Brant-Zawadzki et al., 1984). MRI allows direct multiplanar imaging and superior anatomic definition, including gray-white differentiation, which is particularly useful for the evaluation of congenital anomalies, metabolic disorders, and white matter diseases (Brant-Zawadzki et al., 1983).

Unfortunately, there are several disadvantages to MRI. MR scans take considerably longer to obtain. Whereas a single CT image can be obtained in a few seconds, MRI can take up to 20 minutes per pulse sequence, and it is considerably more sensitive to patient motion. In children, this often requires sedation and monitoring. The availability of centers willing to sedate children with adequate MRI-compatible monitoring equipment is a limiting factor. Moreover, MRI availability and expense alone may preclude it as a practical option.

CT scanning will continue to be an important imaging tool. It is still the imaging modality of choice for the evaluation of most acute intracranial trauma. It is certainly more reliable for evaluation of fractures and intracranial calcified lesions (Atlas et al., 1988; Brant-Zawadzki et al., 1984). Because of the current problems with MRI, any unstable patients or those who are respirator dependent must still, in general, be done by CT. In many instances, although MRI may be slightly more sensitive, CT is often more than adequate to detect abnormalities (Naidich and Zimmerman, 1984). Patients with pacemakers, certain aneurysm clips, and some heart valves cannot enter the strong magnetic field of the MRI unit. Children who are claustrophobic often cannot tolerate the enclosed space of an MR scanner. Finally, while MRI does not use ionizing radiation, its long-term effects are not yet completely known.

INTRACRANIAL NEOPLASMS

If all ages are considered, pediatric brain tumors are more common in the posterior fossa, although supratentorial lesions dominate in the first 3 years (Farwell et al., 1977; Naidich and Zimmerman, 1984). As mentioned, MRI is superior to CT for the evaluation of intracranial neoplastic disease (Gentry et al., 1987; Pinto and Kricheff, 1984), especially in the posterior fossa. If CT is obtained initially, both noncontrast and contrast-enhanced images should be obtained. Gd-DTPA-enhanced MR images are not always necessary but often help to further characterize lesions and delineate tumor from edema (Elster and Rieser, 1989). The five most common histologic types, which account for

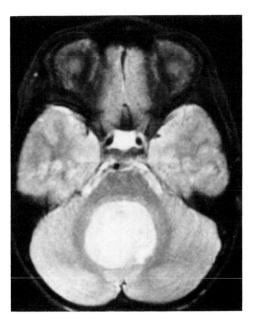

Figure 10.2.   Axial T2 of posterior fossa of same patient as in Fig. 10.1 showing mass now hyperintense to adjacent brain parenchyma. (Courtesy of T. Linda Chi, M.D., Montefiore Medical Center, Bronx, NY.)

80% of all intracranial tumors, are discussed (Farwell et al. 1977).

Posterior Fossa Neoplasms

MEDULLOBLASTOMA

Medulloblastoma (Figs. 10.1 and 10.2) is the most common posterior fossa neoplasm in children (Farwell et al., 1977; Naidich and Zimmerman, 1984). This is a highly malignant tumor affecting males three times as often as females. Seventy-five percent occur in children younger than age 10 (Barkovich and Edwards, 1990). They are usually midline lesions situated behind the fourth ventricle. Medulloblastomas appear hyperdense on noncontrast CT and enhance homogeneously after contrast infusion. There is mild to moderate vasogenic edema in the white matter surrounding the lesion, which appears hypodense on CT. These tumors often cause obstructive hydrocephalus, due to compres-

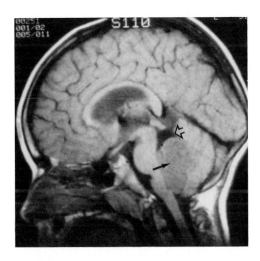

Figure 10.1.   Midline sagittal T1 showing slightly hypointense mass (*solid arrow*) inferior to the fourth ventricle (*open arrow*) with mass effect on the posterior brainstem in this patient with medulloblastoma. (Courtesy of T. Linda Chi, M.D., Montefiore Medical Center, Bronx, NY.)

sion of the fourth ventricle. Atypical features such as calcification, cysts, necrosis, or hemorrhage are occasionally seen (Barkovich and Edwards, 1990).

The MR appearance of medulloblastoma is more variable. These neoplasms are usually hypointense on T1 but hypo-, iso-, or hyperintense signal may be seen on T2 images. Surrounding edema is hyperintense on T2 sequences. There is a high incidence of CSF seeding, and gadolinium-enhanced T1 images are the most sensitive noninvasive imaging modality for detection of this complication (Barkovich and Edwards, 1990). Often a CT myelogram may be required to rule out intraspinal CSF seeding or drop metastases.

CEREBELLAR ASTROCYTOMAS

Cerebellar astrocytomas tend to be low-grade tumors (Murata et al., 1989) that affect the sexes equally. There is usually a cyst or necrotic component to the tumor, with less than 10% appearing completely solid. The cystic astrocytoma is most common in children younger than age 10. CT and MRI reveal a large, well-marginated cyst with an enhancing tumor nodule in its wall. The rim may also enhance. The fluid may be more dense than CSF on CT and of higher signal intensity than CSF on short TR MRI pulse sequences because of a high protein content (Segall et al. 1987). In older children, there may be more anaplastic change histologically and more solid components to the tumor (Murata et al., 1989). The solid portion is iso- or hypodense to brain parenchyma on CT, with irregular enhancement after contrast. MRI shows decreased signal on T1, with inhomogeneous enhancement after Gd-DTPA, and increased signal on T2. Cysts or necrotic components are typical. Calcification is infrequent, but hydrocephalus often occurs.

EPENDYMOMAS

Most ependymomas are solid, infiltrating-type tumors with a high recurrence rate. They have a propensity to grow from the ependyma of the fourth ventricle into the foramina of Luschka and subsequently into the cerebellopontine angle (CPA) cistern or foramen magnum. Calcification is present in 50% of lesions, while cysts are less common (Swartz et al., 1982). CT shows an iso- or hyperdense fourth ventricular mass with moderate inhomogeneous enhancement. The MR appearance is nonspecific, with decreased intensity on T1 and increased intensity on T2 (Barkovich and Edwards, 1990). Enhancement characteristics are similar to those in CT. Tumors extending into the CPA are highly suggestive of an ependymoma (Swartz et al., 1982). If seeding occurs, the tumor may be a malignant ependymoma or the more immature ependymoblastoma (Barkovich and Edwards, 1990).

BRAINSTEM ASTROCYTOMAS

Brainstem astrocytomas (Fig. 10.3) vary from low-grade to high-grade in malignancy. These tumors affect boys and girls equally and they are most common under the age of 10 (Naidich and Zimmerman, 1984). Whereas the three previously described neoplasms usually present with signs of cerebellar dysfunction and/or increased intracranial pressure, brainstem gliomas classically present with cranial nerve deficits. A large number may exhibit exophytic growth from the brainstem into the CPA (Barkovich and Edwards, 1990). Hemorrhage or cysts are present in 25% of cases (Lassiter et al., 1971).

CT exhibits a low-density expanded brainstem displacing the fourth ventricle posteriorly. Increased density may be seen secondary to blood or calcium. On MRI both T1 and T2 are prolonged, resulting in decreased signal on T1, with variable enhancement, and increased signal on T2. Both MRI and CT will show widening of the CPA cistern if exophytic growth occurs. The anatomic detail, multiplanar imaging capability, and absence of bone artifact on MRI make it the modality of choice for the brainstem glioma.

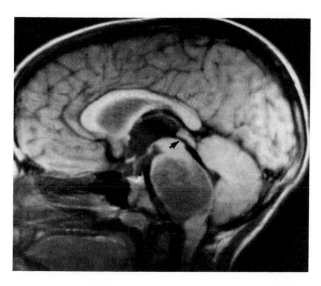

Figure 10.3.   Brainstem astrocytoma. Midline sagittal T1 revealing low intensity expansile mass in the pons. A dilated aqueduct (*arrow*) is seen. The obstruction is occurring inferior to the fourth ventricle.

Supratentorial Tumors

ASTROCYTOMAS

Astrocytomas are the most common supratentorial primary brain tumor in children (Fig. 10.4). In the cerebral parenchyma, the CT and MRI characteristics are similar to those described in the cerebellum. As astrocytomas become more aggressive and malignant, the amount of vasogenic white matter edema, enhancement, and incidence of hemorrhage all increase, and calcification becomes less common. Patients can present with signs of increased intracranial pressure, headache, or focal deficit. When the astrocytoma arises in the temporal lobe, the patient may present with seizures. These tumors also frequently occur in the region of the hypothalamus and optic chiasm. In this location, presenting symptoms may include visual field defects or endocrine abnormalities. Since it may not be possible to determine whether the tumor arises from the chiasm or the hypothalamus, findings suggesting von Recklinghausen's neurofibromatosis should be sought in support of a chiasmal lesion (see Chapter 1).

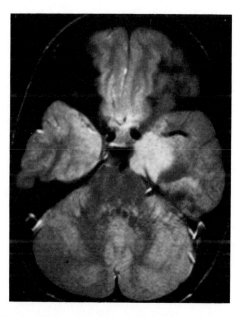

Figure 10.4.   This is an axial proton density MR image in a patient presenting with seizures. There is a hyperintense mass in the medial left temporal lobe with mild mass affect consistent with a low-grade astrocytoma.

EPENDYMOMAS AND EPENDYMOBLASTOMAS

When ependymomas occur supratentorially, the most common location is in the frontal lobe abutting the frontal horn of the lateral ventricle; a less common location is within the ventricle. The CT and MRI appearance has already been discussed under "Posterior Fossa Neoplasms."

CRANIOPHARYNGIOMA

In the suprasellar location, the craniopharyngioma is the most common tumor of childhood. The classic CT appearance is that of a cyst in the suprasellar region with "eggshell calcification" in its wall. Solid portions of the tumor enhance after contrast. Although the classic calcified cyst is not always seen, any tumor with solid, cystic, and calcified components in the suprasellar region is most likely a craniopharyngioma. MRI may show increased signal intensity within the cyst on short TR sequences, compatible with increased protein in the fluid. Approximately 25% of craniopharyngiomas extend into the posterior, middle, or anterior cranial fossa (Barkovich and Edwards, 1990). Symptoms may occur from: (1) impingement on the optic chiasm; (2) hydrocephalus from obstruction at the level of the third ventricle; or (3) endocrine abnormalities, such as diabetes insipidus from involvement of the hypothalamus.

PINEAL REGION TUMORS

Most tumors in the pineal region are germ cell tumors, including germinomas, teratomas, embryonal endodermal sinus tumors, and choriocarcinoma. Pineal cell tumors, such as pineocytomas and pineoblastomas, comprise the other major group of neoplasms. Symptoms usually result from local growth, obstruction at the aqueduct of Sylvius, and Parinaud's syndrome (paralysis of conjugate upward gaze) from compression on the tectum of the midbrain (Jooma and Kendall, 1983).

Germinomas account for more than half of all tumors in this location (Jooma and Kendall, 1983). Typically, presentation occurs in the teenage years, with a striking male preponderance. CT shows an iso- to hyperdense, well-defined mass in the region of the pineal gland, with uniform enhancement. Occasionally, germinomas may also occur in the suprasellar region. MRI may exhibit tumor isointensity or prolonged T1 and T2. Enhancement is similar to that on CT. These tumors seed the CSF, which is best detected with gadolinium-enhanced T1 MRI (Tien et al., 1990).

Teratomas, which are uncommon and rarely malignant (Jooma and Kendall, 1983), also occur in this location. Imaging studies may show evidence of fat, calcium, cysts, or solid components.

Pineocytomas are well-circumscribed, slow-growing tumors with an equal incidence in boys and girls. Compared with germinomas, they have a more lobulated appearance and frequently have calcification, cysts, or necrosis (Jooma and Kendall, 1983). Pineoblastomas may exhibit rapid growth and seeding of the CSF: otherwise they appear identical to their benign counterparts.

Other, less common tumors occurring in the pediatric population include primitive neuroectodermal tumors, choroid plexus papilloma, gangliogliomas, and ganglioneuromas.

THE PHAKOMATOSES

The phakomatoses are a group of congenital neurocutaneous disorders involving organs of ectodermal origin as well as the central and peripheral nervous systems. Often they present with seizures, mental retardation, or focal deficits. The most common phakomatoses are neurofibromatosis, tuberous sclerosis, and Sturge-Weber disease. They often have classic radiographic findings.

Neurofibromatosis

Neurofibromatosis has an autosomal-dominant pattern of inheritance with a high penetrance; however, approximately one-third of cases arise from spontaneous mutation (Holt, 1978). Although multiple forms have been described (Riccardi, 1987), two main types have been characterized by gene locus.

The most common form is neurofibromatosis I (NF I), which is also called von Recklinghausen's neurofibromatosis or peripheral neurofibromatosis. About 15% of patients have CNS lesions, including gliomas of the optic nerve, chiasm, and optic tracts, astrocytomas, hydrocephalus, vascular dysplasias, sphenoid wing and occipital bone dysplasias, plexiform neurofibromas, and benign hamartomas. The spinal axis may have nerve sheath tumors, scoliosis, and dural ectasia (Riccardi, 1987). MRI is the imaging modality of choice because of its overall increased sensitivity (Bognanno et al., 1988).

The most frequent lesion in NF I is the optic pathway glioma. On both CT and MRI, it is seen as a fusiform enlargement of the optic nerves and/or chiasm with variable contrast enhancement. Axial long TR sequences demonstrate increased signal and are best for evaluating whether the chiasm and posterior pathways are involved (Brown et al., 1987). Gliomas may also be seen

in the brainstem/tectum and cerebrum. As with most parenchymal tumors, gliomas are low density on CT precontrast and enhance variably in proportion to their aggressiveness on postcontrast studies. CT is more sensitive than MRI for detecting calcium, but the absence of bone artifact in the posterior fossa as well as the increased sensitivity of long TR pulse sequences give MRI a considerable advantage. Both CT and MRI show minimal to moderate surrounding edema (Barkovich, 1990D; Bognanno et al., 1988).

Hydrocephalus results from obstruction at the aqueduct from brainstem gilomas or benign aqueductal stenosis (Bognanno et al., 1988). Plexiform neurofibromas (Fig. 10.5) occur most commonly near the orbital apex or superior orbital fissure. They arise from small, unnamed nerves and grow into the intracranial space or orbit. Enhancement is variable on CT, although MRI may show heterogeneous enhancement (Barkovich, 1990D).

Benign hamartomas are commonly seen in the pons, cerebellar white matter, and globus pallidus. Long TR images visualize them best as

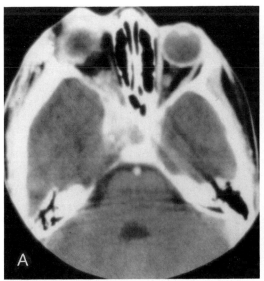 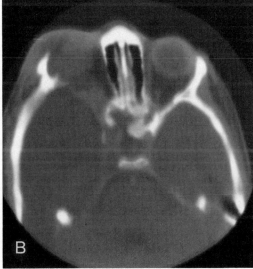

Figure 10.5.   A and B, Contrast-enhanced CT of the brain with bone windows showing enhancing mass in right cavernous sinus extending into the orbit consistent with a plexiform neurofibroma. The sphenoid wing is absent.

hyperintense foci. Unlike astrocytomas, they do not enhance, have little mass effect, and do not grow (Bognanno et al., 1988; Mirowitz et al. 1989). Vascular dysplasias (e.g. vessel occlusions with moyamoya collaterals) affect the internal carotid and the proximal anterior and middle cerebral arteries. Stenosis may also occur secondary to radiation arteritis. MRI and CT may show large vessels in the basal ganglia and thalamus secondary to the enlarged lenticulostriate collaterals (moyamoya), but detailed analysis of the intracranial vessels is best seen via cerebral arteriography (Barkovich, 1990D).

Neurofibromatosis II (NF II), or central neurofibromatosis, which is the less common variety, is associated with bilateral acoustic neuromas. There is also an increased incidence of multiple meningiomas, gliomas, and other cranial nerve neuromas, as well as paraspinal neurofibromas, spinal cord ependymomas, and spinal meningiomas (Riccardi, 1987). Skin changes, skeletal dysplasias, optic gliomas, and vascular dysplasias are uncommon.

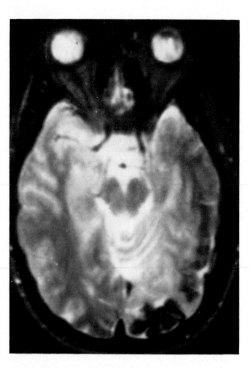

Figure 10.7. Sturge-Weber syndrome. Axial T2 MRI shows markedly decreased signal in a gyral pattern corresponding to tram track calcification.

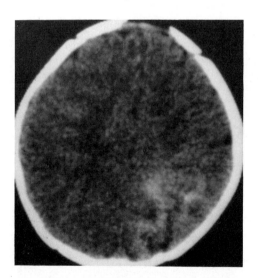

Figure 10.6. Noncontrast CT of the brain revealing early calcification in the left parietal occipital lobe in a patient with Sturge-Weber syndrome.

Sturge-Weber (encephalotrigeminal angiomatosis)

Sturge-Weber syndrome (Figs. 10.6 and 10.7) is a diffuse, usually unilateral angiomatosis involving the face, choroid plexus, and leptomeninges. The facial angioma, or port-wine stain, is in the distribution of the fifth nerve, most commonly in the ophthalmic division (V_1). It is associated with ipsilateral intracranial pial and choroid angiomatosis with hemiatrophy. Children present with seizures, mental retardation, and hemiparesis. Most cases are sporadic, but familial cases have been described (Gean and Taveras, 1989). The predominant intracranial finding is "tram track" calcification in the subcortical region of the parietal and occipital lobes. Enhancement of the adjacent meninges and enlarged choroid plexus may also be seen

(Fernandez et al., 1990). The globe may be enlarged with congenital glaucoma (buphthalmos) secondary to glaucoma that results from angiomatosis's affecting the ciliary body, and retinal detachment may occur due to involvement of the choroid in the globe (Barkovich, 1990D).

CT is more sensitive than MRI in detecting calcification that can be seen as early as 1 year of age. Enhancement of the meninges and choroid plexus as well as hemiatrophy can be seen on both CT and MRI (Wasenko et al., 1990). Increased signal in the choroid on long TR pulse sequences has been described (Stimac et al., 1986) possibly secondary to slow-flowing thrombosed, or increased blood in the deep venous system. An enlarged deep venous system may be due to shunting, since superficial veins in the region of the pial angiomatosis are absent (Wasenko et al, 1990).

Tuberous Sclerosis

The characteristic lesion in tuberous sclerosis is a hamartoma involving multiple organ systems. Most cases are thought to represent a spontaneous mutation, although an autosomal-dominant pattern of inheritance is present (Hanno and Beck, 1987). The classic clinical triad consists of seizures, mental retardation, and adenoma sebaceum.

Intracranially, hamartomas, or tubers, are present in the subependymal region of the ventricles and the cortical gyri (Fig. 10.8). Hamartomas appear as hypodense nodules along the surface of the ventricles. On long TR sequences, there may be increased signal in the cortical tubers. If enough calcification is present, a hypointense signal within the hyperintense nodule may be seen on long TR sequences (Altman et al., 1988; Iwasaki et al., 1990). Enhancement is rare. About 5 to 10% have malignant degeneration of a subependymal hamartoma due to a subependymal giant cell astrocytoma (Barkovich, 1990D). These malignancies usually occur near the foramen of Monro, where they can cause

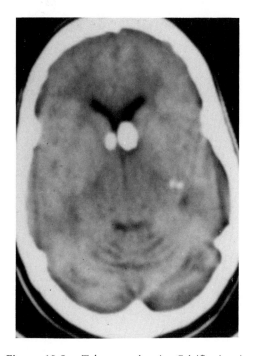

Figure 10.8. Tuberous sclerosis. Calcification is seen in the region of the foramen of Monro bilaterally and in left periatrial area consistent with calcified subependymal tubers.

obstructive hydrocephalus. Both CT and MRI will demonstrate an enlarging mass near the foramen of Monro that enhances postcontrast (Fig. 10.9).

CNS INFECTION

The most common form of CNS infection is meningitis. Patients may present with fever, headache, nausea, vomiting, stiff neck, altered mental status, visual disturbances, and cranial nerve deficits. The most common source is an adjacent otitis media or sinusitis. CT and MRI are often normal even when contrast is administered. An exception to this is tuberculous (TB) meningitis (Fig. 10.10) in which intense meningeal enhancement can be seen on both CT and MRI (Chang et al., 1990). As expected, Gd-DTPA-enhanced MRI is superior since meningeal enhancement is more readily seen without

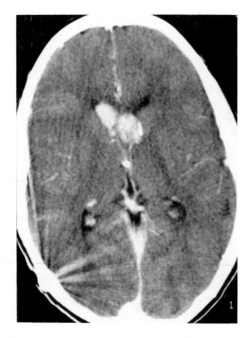

Figure 10.9. Contrast-enhanced CT of brain showing subependymal tuber that has undergone degeneration to a subependymal giant cell astrocytoma. Note the isodense mass that enhances postcontrast in the region of the foramen of Monro.

the resorption of CSF by the arachnoid villi over the convexity. If the fourth ventricle remains small compared with the lateral and third ventricles, then the hydrocephalus is termed noncommunicating or obstructive and is often secondary to debris or adhesions occurring at the aqueduct of Sylvius. Both forms may show transependymal resorption of CSF around the ventricles. MRI is most sensitive for detecting this abnormal fluid as increased signal immediately around the ventricles on proton density and T2 weighted images.

Sinus thrombosis can be visualized on both CT and MRI. Children are more likely to have this complication when they become dehydrated. On noncontrast CT the sagittal sinus may appear dense. On postcontrast studies, the superior sagittal sinus exhibits a triangular filling defect within the sinus called the "empty delta sign" (Rao et al., 1981). MRI can sometimes be difficult to evaluate. One should clearly see the

the beam-hardening or volume-averaging artifacts of CT (Chang et al. 1990).

Although it is not always necessary to obtain an imaging study when meningitis is suspected (Gold, 1989), it is advisable if the diagnosis is unclear, if the patient develops a focal deficit, or if there is further deterioration. Regardless of whether CT or MRI is performed, the examination usually should include both pre- and postcontrast studies.

Complications of meningitis include communicating and noncommunicating hydrocephalus, venous thrombosis, arterial infarctions, subdural effusions and empyemas, cerebritis, and ventriculitis (Figs. 10.11 and 10.12), all of which may be seen on neuroimaging studies.

Hydrocephalus will appear as enlarged ventricles. If all four ventricles are enlarged, then the hydrocephalus is most likely communicating and resulting from the meningitis's impeding

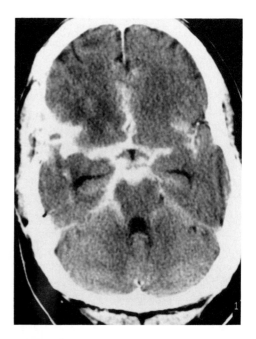

Figure 10.10. TB meningitis. Contrast-enhanced CT of the brain through the suprasellar cistern. Diffuse enhancement of the suprasellar cistern and right sylvian fissure greater than left.

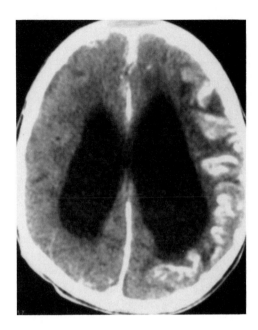

Figure 10.11. Contrast-enhanced CT of brain 3 weeks after presenting with meningitis. There is massive enlargement of the lateral ventricles consistent with hydrocephalus. There is prominent gyral enhancement in the middle cerebral artery territory consistent with a subacute left MCA infarct.

sequences (Weingarten et al., 1989). Often, simple effusions are bilateral. In addition, the subdural empyemas can involve the epidural space or be associated with adjacent cerebritis. Enhancement may be absent early on but increases as a capsule develops (Weingarten et al., 1989).

While cerebritis may occur secondary to meningitis it often follows hematogenous dissemination of infection or a penetrating wound (Barkovich, 1990B). It is the earliest stage of a focal parenchymal infection. If untreated, the brain will liquify. The development of a surrounding capsule of granulation tissue and collagen results in a cerebral abscess. It can be difficult to determine whether there is true abscess formation in the intermediate stages. Again, this determination is important because a frank abscess often requires surgical intervention. Cerebritis apears as an ill-defined hypodensity on CT with irregular enhancement, mild-to-moderate mass effect, and vasogenic

absence of flow on several pulse sequences and in several planes. In addition, clot changes characteristics with age but should be confirmed on several projections to differentiate it from various flow artifacts (Rippe et al. 1990; Sze et al., 1988). Secondary venous infarcts with small petechial or subcortical hemorrhages can be seen in 25% of cases (Rao et al., 1981). Arterial infarcts secondary to a periarteritis can also be seen in a territorial or lacunar-like pattern (Chang et al., 1990) (please see the discussion later in this chapter of infarcts in the vascular section for the CT and MR appearance).

Subdural effusions are particularly common in children with *Haemophilus influenzae* infections. It can be very difficult to differentiate a subdural effusion from an empyema, especially by CT. The distinction is important since an empyema is a surgical lesion. On MRI there may be slight difference from CSF intensity on various pulse

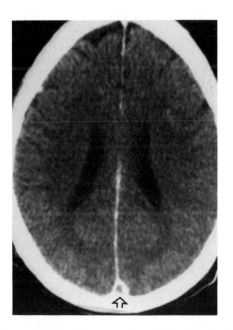

Figure 10.12. Contrast-enhanced CT of the brain exhibiting triangular filling defect in the sagittal sinus consistent with "empty delta sign" (*arrow*).

edema. Both T1 and T2 are prolonged on MRI studies. As an abscess evolves its center liquifies. CT shows a ring-enhancing lesion with a well-defined, smooth, thin wall and a center of near-CSF density (Fig. 10.13). This is most commonly seen at the gray-white junction. The medial wall is usually thinner and there is considerable vasogenic edema and mass effect. On MRI, the wall may be hypointense on long TR pulse sequences. The center is slightly hypointense on short TR and hyperintense on long TR sequences (Hamies et al., 1989). It usually does not look like CSF on all pulse sequences because of the high protein content of the purulent center.

Viral encephalitis is a more diffuse, though often nonspecific, process. Most viral encephalitides result in neuronal degeneration and inflammation. A nonspecific increase in water content is seen on MRI and CT in the affected area. Herpes simplex encephalitis, a common

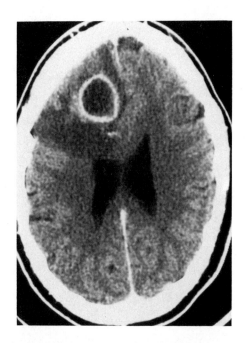

Figure 10.13. Contrast-enhanced CT shows a ring-enhancing mass with extensive surrounding edema and mass effect compatible with a right frontal cerebral abscess.

infection in children, affects the anteromedial temporal lobe, insular cortex, and gyrus rectus. Petechial hemorrhage and occasionally, gyral enhancement may be seen (Barkovich, 1990B). Findings are often bilateral but asymmetric. MRI is often very helpful especially when correlated with electroencephalogram (EEG) and possibly scans. CT is notoriously negative in the early stages.

Subacute sclerosing panencephalitis (SSPE) can present as a progressive onset of behavior changes and mental retardation followed by myoclonic seizures. Both CT and MRI are nonspecific, showing diffuse atrophy and multifocal patchy periventricular and subcortical white matter involvement without enhancement.

Lyme disease is a spirochetal infection affecting the CNS in 10 to 15% of cases. Multiple abnormalities have been reported, including periventricular white matter lesions, thalamic and basal ganglia abnormalities, meningeal enhancement, and hydrocephalus. It can mimic multiple sclerosis or vasculitis (Fernandez et al., 1990).

Acquired immune deficiency syndrome (AIDS) can present with a myriad of symptoms, including cognitive impairment, developmental delay, dementia, or focal neurologic deficit (Chapter 17). The most common findings on imaging studies include diffuse atrophy, ventricular dilation, and calcification in the basal ganglia. The cause of the latter is not clear, although it may be secondary to a vasculitis (Bradford et al., 1988). White matter degeneration and destruction may also be seen with diffuse hypodensity in the white matter on CT and prolonged T1 and T2 on MRI (Bradford et al., 1988). When only a few patchy lesions are seen, progressive multifocal leukoencephalopathy (PML) or vasculitis should be considered. Although PML, toxoplasmosis, and cryptococcosis are considerably less common in children than in adults, when they do occur in children, MRI is considerably more sensitive in detecting lesions, especially when Gd-DTPA is administered (Post et al., 1988).

Metabolic and White Matter Disorders

WHITE MATTER DISEASES

White matter disease may be classified as *dysmyelinating*, in which myelin never forms properly, versus *demyelinating*, in which myelin breaks down after it has been formed. Imaging alone usually cannot differentiate the two. However, MRI is superior to CT in detecting the number and extent of white matter abnormalities (Nowell et al., 1988).

Those diseases predominantly dysmyelinating in origin include Alexander's disease, Canavan's disease, Krabbe's disease, and metachromatic leukodystrophy. Adrenoleukodystrophy exhibits characteristics of both. All of these conditions show diffuse confluent bilateral white matter changes with decreased attenuation on CT, decreased signal on T1, and increased signal on T2. Alexander's disease (Fig. 10.14) classically

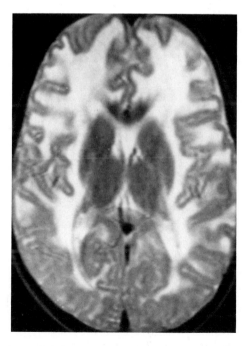

Figure 10.14. Axial T2 weighted image in patient with Alexander's disease. Note extensive increased signal throughout the white matter but more prominent anteriorly.

begins in the frontal lobes and spreads posteriorly. There may be enhancement near the frontal horns (Shah and Ross, 1990). Adrenoleukodystrophy more commonly begins in the occipital white matter and progresses anteriorly. Involvement of the splenium of the corpus callosum, cerebellar white matter, and cerebral peduncles is typical. The leading edge may also show enhancement secondary to breakdown of the blood-brain barrier and active inflammation with demyelination (Knaap and Valk, 1989). Krabbe's disease, in addition to diffuse white matter abnormalities, exhibits increased density in the thalami and caudate nuclei on CT (Barkovich, 1990C). Further differentiation can be made in conjunction with age of onset and clinical symptoms.

Multiple sclerosis (MS) is predominantly a demyelinating disease of adults that can be seen in adolescents. In the adolescent, there is a more striking female predominance and more severe disease characteristics, and infratentorial structures are more frequently involved (Ebner et al., 1990; Osborn et al., 1990). MRI is more sensitive in detecting lesions, particularly on balanced (long TR, short TE) sequences. The classic MS plaques are seen in the periventricular white matter. In children, there is also an increased number of lesions in the deep cerebellar white matter, brainstem, and spinal cord. Acute plaques may enhance with gadolinium and on contrast-enhanced CT. On initial presentation, MS plaques may mimic tumors, acute disseminated encephalomyelitis, progressive multifocal leukoencephalopathy, and CNS lymphoma (Ebner et al., 1990). When the diagnosis is in doubt, sequential MR studies will reveal changes in size and configuration of the lesions.

Acute disseminated encephalomyelitis (ADEM) usually develops late in the course of a viral illness. Clinical presentations include seizures and focal neurologic signs. Resolution is the rule, although 10 to 20% may have permanent damage. CT and MRI reveal moderate-to-large areas of demyelination in the subcortical white matter that do not enhance (Barkovich, 1990C).

METABOLIC DISORDERS

Most metabolic disorders are evident early in life. CT and MRI may help in evaluating response to therapy and whether the disease is progressing.

Phenylketonuria (PKU), if not treated at birth, can present as mental retardation, autism, seizures, hyperactive behavior, and hyperreflexia (Pearsen et al., 1990). Evidence of decreased myelination is present on CT and MRI. On long TR pulse sequences there is symmetric increased signal in the periventricular white matter, most prominently in the posterior cerebral hemispheres (Pearsen et al., 1990).

The mucopolysaccharidoses I, II, III, and VII often have a predominant neurologic component in their presentation, usually manifested as developmental delay. CT and MRI show varying amounts of atrophy, hydrocephalus, and mul-

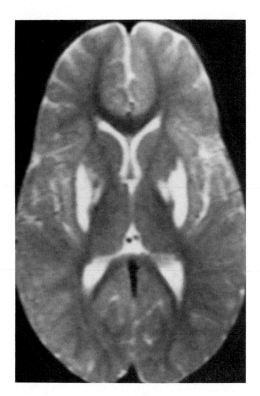

Figure 10.16.   T2 sequence demonstrating increased signal predominantly in the putamen in patient with Leigh's disease. (Courtesy of T. Linda Chi, MD, Montefiore Medical Center, Bronx, NY.)

tiple discrete white matter foci (Fig. 10.15). As the disease progresses, these foci may also represent demyelination or lacunar infarct.

Leigh's disease, Wilson's disease, and mitochondrial encephalomyopathies all have in common lesions that affect the basal ganglia. On CT, all show symmetric hypodensity within the basal ganglia, while MRI shows prolonged T1 and T2. Leigh's disease (Fig. 10.16) primarily affects the putamen, but the globus pallidus, caudate nuclei, and periaqueductal gray matter may also be involved (Medina et al., 1990). Wilson's disease targets the basal ganglia, the thalamus, and, occasionally, the white matter. The mitochondrial encephalomyopathies include atrophy and white matter lesions and also affect the basal ganglia (Barkovich, 1990C).

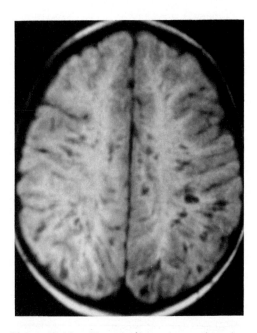

Figure 10.15.   Hunter's disease (mucopolysaccharidosis type II). Multiple diffuse lesions with prolonged T1 in the white matter, most likely representing cavitation and pitting around blood vessels. (Courtesy of I. Rapin, MD, Albert Einstein Hospital, Bronx, NY.)

TRAUMA

Most authors agree that CT scanning is the procedure of choice in *acute* trauma because skull fractures, subarachnoid hemorrhage, and often, parenchymal hemorrhages are more reliably detected (Gentry et al., 1980; Kelly et al., 1988). In addition, MRI is often not a practical choice because of its relatively long scan times, the inability to sedate unstable patients, and the need for monitoring and life support equipment. However, when a patient's clinical signs and symptoms are unexplained by CT, MRI often yields important findings. In the subacute and chronic stages of hematoma, MRI is superior to CT because of its greater sensitivity to hemorrhage in these stages and overall sensitivity for parenchymal lesions on long TR sequences (Fobben et al., 1989; Gentry et al., 1990; Kelly et al., 1988).

The appearance of hemorrhage on MRI is affected by many factors, including age, field strength, scan parameters, CSF properties, and location. Acute hemorrhage reflects deoxyhemoglobin and appears isointense to hypointense on T1 and markedly hypointense on T2 weighted imaging. Subacute hemorrhage begins as hyperintense signal seen at the periphery on T1 weighted imaging. This reflects conversion from deoxyhemoglobin to intracellular methemoglobin. As methemoglobin becomes extracellular, both T1 and T2 will appear hyperintense in the late subacute stage. During the chronic phase, the long TR images demonstrate a markedly hypointense ring representing hemosiderin and ferritin. This appearance may persist for years (Gammal et al., 1987).

Any discussion of head trauma in children should include the possibility of child abuse. Nonaccidental trauma is a significant cause of head injury, with 10 to 44% of abused children having intracranial abnormalities (Sato et al., 1989). It should be suspected when: (*1*) the visualized injury does not correspond with the reported mechanism of injury; (*2*) there is evidence of separate injuries of different ages; (*3*) shear injuries are seen; and (*4*) an interhemispheric subdural hematoma is seen. The latter two findings often occur as a result of shaking injuries. However, all of the entities discussed below can be seen. MRI is particularly helpful in identifying hemorrhage of various ages. It is the study of choice when screening in the subacute or chronic stages (Sato et al., 1989).

Cerebral contusions are essentially bruises to the cerebral cortex and variable amounts of underlying white matter. In the acute stage there is usually associated petechial or patchy hemorrhage that appears dense relative to normal brain on CT. In several days, the hemorrhage becomes more isodense relative to brain, and reactive surrounding edema may become severe. After about 1 week, enhancement may be seen. As the hemorrhage and edema resolve, focal hypodensity and atrophy are seen at the site (Zimmerman, 1987A). Patients may persist with focal deficits, behavioral abnormalities or seizures.

Coup injuries result from an object's impacting the stationary brain; the frontal and temporal lobes are most commonly affected. Contrecoup injuries occur when the brain is in motion relative to the calvaria. In this case the anterior temporal lobes, inferior frontal lobes, or temporal lobe opposite the side of impact are most affected. There is also a high association of subdural hematoma (Zimmerman, 1987A).

Shearing injury is an injury that occurs with rapid acceleration and deceleration of the cerebral hemispheres. "Shearing" of the axons and small blood vessels occurs notably at the gray-white junctions, corpus callosum, internal capsule, basal ganglia, and upper brainstem (Zimmerman, 1987A; Kelly et al., 1988). On CT, the clinical state often seems out of proportion to the abnormalities on the scan. Diffuse cerebral edema with loss of sulci and basal cisterns is seen, with variable numbers of punctate hemorrhages in the above locations. MRI can also detect those lesions unaccompanied by hemorrhage, especially on T2-weighted sequences (Zimmerman 1987B, Gentry et al., 1980). Patients may have severe, permanent brain damage, and long-term follow-up often shows considerable atrophy.

Subdural hematomas (Fig. 10.17) occur in a potential space between the dura and leptomeninges secondary to tearing of small bridging veins. Often there is associated underlying brain injury. Classically, a peripheral crescentic dense collection between the skull and parenchyma is visualized on CT. It may extend into the interhemispheric fissure or along the tentorium. During the subacute phase of 1 to 3 weeks, the hematoma may appear isodense to brain parenchyma. There is still mass effect, with compression of the ventricle and displacement of the gray-white junction medially. Contrast often enhances the inner membrane, rendering it more visible. In the chronic stage, the hematoma becomes hypodense compared with adjacent gray matter. The MRI appearance of subdural hematoma follows the same progression through acute, subacute, and chronic stages as does parenchymal blood; however, in the chronic stage there is iso- or slightly hypointense signal relative to gray matter on short TR sequences, and on long TR sequences the hemosiderin and ferritin ring is rarely visualized (Fobben et al., 1989).

Epidural hematomas (Fig. 10.18) occur in the potential space between the cranial periosteum and bone, secondary to laceration of a branch of the middle meningeal artery or vein, or to tearing of one of the dural venous sinuses. As opposed to subdurals, epidurals are limited by the cranial sutures and have a biconcave or lens-shaped appearance. Ninety percent are associated with skull fractures, although children have an increased occurrence unassociated with fractures (Scatliff, 1987). There is usually no underlying brain injury; however, epidurals can grow rapidly, causing herniation and death if not detected early. CT density and MRI signal characteristics are similar to those discussed for subdural hematomas.

Subarachnoid hemorrhage from any cause appears as increased density in the sulci and basal cisterns on CT. It tends to be most extensive when it is due to a ruptured aneurysm. CT is considerably more sensitive to subarachnoid hemorrhage than is MRI, especially in the acute stage (Zimmerman 1987B; Gentry et al., 1980). Often there are other associated injuries such as contusion or subdural hematoma.

Congenital Anomalies

The congenital cerebral anomalies represent abnormal or arrested growth in utero. Common presenting symptoms are developmental delay, mental retardation, and seizures. Most of the other entities described in this chapter manifest lesions of abnormal density or signal intensity on CT and MRI, respectively. The congenital anomalies are recognized by distortions in the anatomy, usually with normal signal intensity. Although late-generation CT scanners have markedly improved anatomic definition and gray-white matter differentiation, MRI has un-

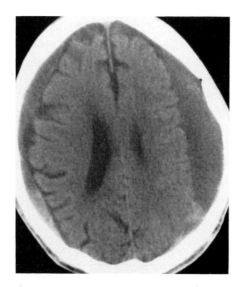

Figure 10.17. Noncontrast CT of the brain demonstrates bilateral isodense to hypodense subdural hematomas greater on the left. There is a slightly more acute component posteriorly.

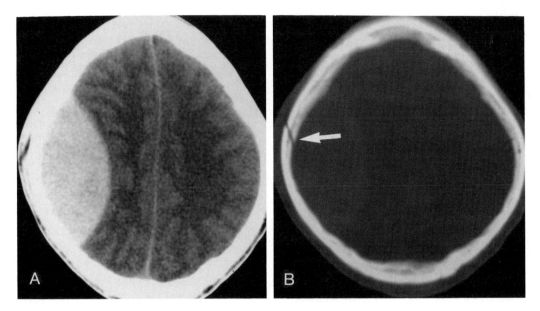

Figure 10.18.   A, Noncontrast CT acute trauma. Note lens-shaped density of right parietal convexity buckling both gray and white matter, consistent with acute epidural hematoma. **B,** Bone window reveals associated parietal skull fracture (*arrow*).

questionably become the imaging modality of choice. The ability to image in essentially any plane as well as the superior gray-white differentiation and anatomic definition are just some of the reasons why (Barkovich et al., 1987; Barkovich, 1990A; Knaap and Valk, 1988; Wolpert et al., 1987).

There are three types of holoprosencephaly: alobar, semilobar, and lobar in decreasing order of severity. Holoprosencephaly represents an incomplete division of the cerebral hemispheres, ventricles, and thalami. In the most severe form there is a single common ventricle, fused thalami, and absence of the third ventricle, falx, septum pellucidum, and corpus callosum (Barkovich, 1990). There is a high association with midline facial anomalies, cyclops, and cleft palate and lip. The semilobar and lobar types are more commonly encountered. With these entities there is progressive separation of occipital and temporal horns as well as hemispheres. There may still be partial fusion of the thalami. In all cases, the septum pellucidum is absent. The mildest forms may be confused with septooptic dysplasia. This entity consists of absence of the septum pellucidum in addition to hypoplasia of the optic chiasm, nerves, and pituitary gland. Patients often present with hypothalamic pituitary dysfunction (Barkovich, 1990A).

Dyke-Davidoff-Masson syndrome results in hemiatrophy of one cerebral hemisphere. Any prenatal or perinatal insult such as ischemia, infection, or trauma can be the underlying cause. CT and MRI reveal asymmetric cerebral hemispheres (Fig. 10.19). One the atrophic side, the skull may exhibit increased pneumatization of the paranasal sinuses, elevation of the petrous ridge, or thickening of the calvaria.

Gray-white differentiation is very important in the evaluation of neuronal migration anomalies. Often these patients may present in late childhood or adolescence with seizures, mental retardation, or abnormal motor skills (Barkovich et al., 1987).

Lissencephaly refers to a cerebral cortex that is agyric (without gyri) or agyric with pachygyric

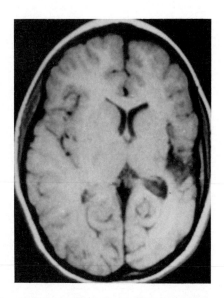

Figure 10.19. Dyke-Davidoff-Masson syndrome. Axial T1 of the brain showing asymmetry of the brain and marked atrophy of the left hemisphere. (Courtesy of G. Solomon, MD, Cornell Medical Center.)

areas (few broad, thick gyri). The gray matter is markedly thickened and the shape of the cerebral mantle is that of an oval or hourglass (Byrd et al., 1988). There may be abnormal venous drainage.

Heterotopia refers to abnormal areas of gray matter within the white matter. It is associated with schizencephaly (see below), Chiari II malformation, polymicrogyria, and other congenital anomalies (Barkovich et al., 1987). As with all the migrational anomalies, the gray and white matter maintain normal signal intensity and density but are in an abnormal location or shape.

The hallmarks of schizencephaly (Fig. 10.20) are holochemispheric clefts extending from the cortical surface to the ventricles throughout the thickness of the hemisphere. In contrast to porencephaly, these clefts are lined with gray matter. The differentiation is important, especially since genetic counseling is warranted with migrational anomalies (Barkovich et al., 1987). Heterotopia and polymicrogyria are often found.

Polymicrogyria may appear very similar to pachgyria on CT and MRI, with increased thick-

ness of the cortex and excessive small convolutions that may be hard to detect (Barkovich et al., 1987; Wolpert et al., 1987). It is most common in the insular cortex and again may be seen in association with other congenital anomalies.

Agenesis of the corpus callosum is a relatively commonly anomaly. Patients may have normal brain function or may present with seizures, intellectual impairment, or neurologic deficits. Often the symptoms are a result of the associated anomalies. Sagittal T1 MRI is ideal in visualizing the entire corpus callosum. With agenesis of the corpus callosum, axial and coronal MRI and CT show the lateral ventricles to be relatively parallel in orientation, and the third ventricle approximates the interhemispheric fissures. It is associated with many other congenital anomalies including Dandy-Walker syndrome, Chiari malformation, lipoma of the corpus callosum, interhemispheric cysts, and heterotopias (Barkovich, 1990A; Scatliff, 1987).

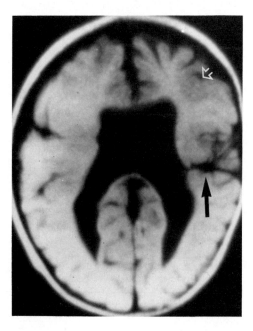

Figure 10.20. Schizencephaly. T1 axial image demonstrating pachgyria (*open arrow*) and holohemispheric fissure lined by gray matter (*closed arrow*).

DANDY-WALKER SYNDROME

The Dandy-Walker syndrome (Fig. 10.21) includes vermian hypoplasia (at least inferiorly), cystic enlargement of the fourth ventricle, and a large posterior fossa. Sagittal T1 MR images ideally show the relationship of the fourth ventricle, cyst, tentorium, and vermis. Hydrocephalus may or may not be present. There is an increased incidence of agenesis of the corpus callosum and holoprosencephaly. When there is partial vermian agenesis with or without a cyst and a small posterior fossa, this is termed a *Dandy-Walker variant*. It is possible that Dandy-Walker syndrome, variant, and giant cisterna magna are all entities within the same spectrum (Barkovich, 1990A).

The Chiari I malformation is a disorder in which there is caudal extension of the cerebellar tonsils below the foramen magnum into the cervical canal. Twenty-five percent of cases are associated with hydrocephalus and syringomyelia

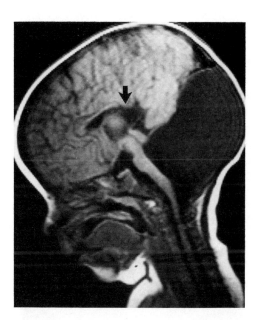

Figure 10.21. Sagittal T1 of brain in severe Dandy-Walker syndrome. Note markedly enlarged posterior fossa secondary to cyst. There is no recognizable residual cerebellum and a small brainstem. Associated partial agenesis of the corpus callosum posteriorly (*arrow*) is present.

of the cervical cord. C1–2 anomalies and Klippel-Feil anomalies also occur with an increased incidence. Clinical symptoms usually can be referred to the cervicomedullary junction, syrinx, or hydrocephalus.

CHIARI II MALFORMATION

The Chiari II malformation is a group of findings that includes an elongated, small cerebellum and brainstem with inferior displacement through the foramen magnum into the cervical canal. Virtually all cases are associated with a myelomeningocele of the spine that is evident at birth. Associated findings visualized on MRI and sometimes on CT include: (1) beaking of the tectum from fused colliculi; (2) aqueductal stenosis, either primary or secondary to compression; (3) hydrocephalus; (4) erosion and scalloping of the clivus and petrous bones; (5) falx deficits with interdigitation of the hemispheres: (6) agenesis or partial agensis of the corpus callosum; (7) protrusion of the cerebellum through the tentorium; and (8) polymicrogyria (Gammal, et al., 1987). Most patients are intellectually normal. Morbidity is associated primarily with the associated myelomeningocele or compression of the brainstem. MIR in the sagittal plane is informative for evaluation and surgical planning (Gammal et al., 1987).

VASCULAR OCCLUSIVE DISEASE

In comparing vascular occlusive disease in the adult and pediatric populations, several differences must be stressed. Although the most common etiologies for cerebral infarction in adults include atherosclerosis and hypertension, the major cause of arterial occlusion in children is congenital cyanotic heart disease. Therefore, intracranial arterial occlusion occurs more often in children, while extracranial arterial occlusion occurs more often in adults. Stroke occurs much less frequently in children, with an incidence of 2.5 per 100,000, compared with up to 50 per 100,000 in adults. In children the incidence of stroke is 50% that of primary brain tumors. The male-to-female incidence ratio is equal for stroke affecting infants, children, and adolescents. In adults older than age 45, the incidence of stroke doubles each decade, and it is higher in males than in females. Following ischemic insult in children, there is generally greater improvement (75% recovery rate) and a lower recurrence rate (10-fold) than in adults (Gold, 1989).

Due to these differences in pathophysiology and prognosis, the radiologic investigation of pediatric and adult stroke differs. However, CT and MRI appearances are similar in both populations. On CT, the acute stroke usually appears as an area of hypodensity conforming to a vascular distribution that has subtle mass effect with sulcal and/or ventricular effacement. The white-gray differentiation may be obscured by edema in the affected area. The hypodensity of infarction typically extends through the cortex. By contrast, the hypodensity from the reactive edema in infection and neoplasm is confined to the white matter.

Acutely, MRI is more sensitive than CT in detecting hemorrhagic infarction. This appears as low signal on T2 weighted images and is usually isointense to gray matter in T1 weighted images.

In the subacute phase of infarction (i.e., from 4 to 7 days through 3 weeks), enhancement occurs with the administration of iodinated contrast on CT and of Gd-DTPA on T1 weighted MR images. The mechanism for enhancement, as previously discussed, is breakdown of the blood-brain barrier (Imakita et al., 1988).

Chronic infarction appears as porencephaly with focal atrophy. Altered parenchymal signal at this stage typically "tracks" or follows the CSF signal (i.e., hypointensity on T1 and hyperintensity on T2 pulse sequences). These general imaging characteristics apply for strokes of all etiologies.

The particular vascular distribution affected, as well as the associated findings, may suggest the etiology of a given stroke. Cyanotic congen-

ital heart disease may cause cortical branch occlusions, typically the middle cerebral artery (MCA), or may result in infarctions of the watershed territories, which are the border zones between major vascular distributions. These vulnerable regions occur between the anterior and middle cerebral arteries, between the middle and posterior cerebral arteries, and at the distal convexity subcortical white matter, which is the part of the brain farthest from the heart.

Although usually cardiogenic in origin, emboli in children may result from arrhythmias, rheumatic valvular disease, coagulopathy, umbilical vein and cardiac catheterization, or cardiac surgery (Fig. 10.22). Septic emboli, which may result from bacterial endocarditis, cause branch occlusions, abscess formation, or mycotic aneurysms. Tumor emboli may fragment from left atrial myxomas; fat emboli may arise from long bone fractures; and air emboli may occur iatrogenically. Regardless of their etiology, emboli typically result in cortical branch occlusions,

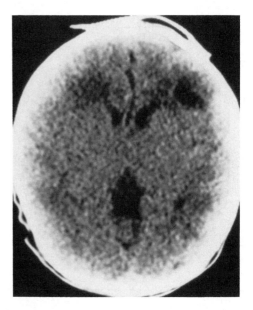

Figure 10.22. Axial noncontrast CT of the brain demonstrates low attenuation and focal atrophy due to a left frontal cortical and subcortical infarct in an infant with tetralogy of Fallot.

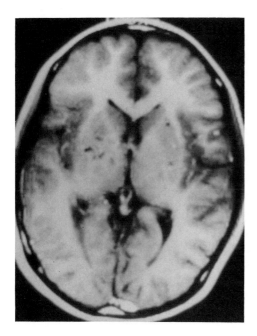

Figure 10.23. Axial T1 weighted MRI demonstrates signal void within the basal ganglia due to flow within lenticulostriate collaterals in this patient with moyamoya disease.

and an infarction ensues if arterial collateral supply is inadequate. Arteritis in children may accompany infections of the ears, nose, and throat; an inflammatory response within the vascular wall may be incited by the "reactive CSF" which surrounds the cerebral vessels within the basal cisterns. Resultant vascular occlusions are usually transient; focal deficits resolve to near or complete recovery, and the self-limited event rarely recurs. The angiographic counterpart of this clinical entity is basal occlusive disease without telangiectasia. Narrowing of the supraclinoid internal carotid artery is apparent, typically unilateral, and without collaterals from the lenticulostriate vessels.

Moyamoya disease refers to a pattern of collateral supply attempted by lenticulostriate telangiectasia, which usually occurs in the setting of bilateral supraclinoid internal carotid occlusion past the origin of the ophthalmic artery. Although such occlusion may result from an idi-

opathic immunologic arteritis; moyamoya collaterals may also be seen with proximal vascular occlusions in neurofibromatosis, certain collagen vascular diseases, including Kawasaki's disease, polyarteritis, radiation therapy, and sickle cell disease (Suzuki, 1983).

The prominent collateral supply via lenticulostriate telangiectasia has an angiographic appearance likened to a "puff of smoke," described in Japanese as moyamoya (Suzuki, 1983) (Fig. 10.23). On all MRI pulse sequences, these collateral vessels are visualized within the basal ganglia as serpiginous structures devoid of signal due to flow within them (Fig. 10.24). They may proliferate to such an extent that they bleed, resulting in parenchymal hemorrhage. Blood dyscrasias predisposing to stroke in the pediatric population include sickle cell disease, leukemia, and thrombotic thrombocytopenia.

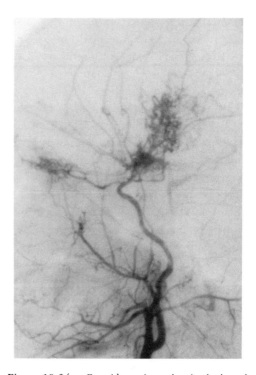

Figure 10.24. Carotid arteriography, in the lateral projection, demonstrates the prominent lenticulostriate collaterals as a result of supraclinoid occlusion of the internal carotid in another patient with moyamoya disease.

Cerebrovascular complications occur in 6 to 25% of patients with sickle cell disease, most often with hemoglobin SS, less commonly with sickle C, and rarely with sickle trait. The incidence of recurrent infarction in untreated children is 67% (Gold, 1989). Proposed mechanisms include small vessel occlusion due to sickling, vascular occlusions due to endothelial proliferation, and underlying arteriopathy.

Although rare in children, arteritis may accompany connective tissue disorders, such as scleroderma, polyarteritis, rheumatoid arthritis, and lupus. Circulating anticardiolipin antibody, which is often, but not exclusively found in association with lupus, predisposes to embolic phenomena.

Illicit drugs, including heroin, LSD, and especially methamphetamines, may cause a necrotizing vasculitis. Cocaine abuse may result in spontaneous subarachnoid hemorrhage.

Vascular trauma, most often resulting in arterial dissection, accounts for 5% of ischemic strokes in children. Internal carotid artery occlusion in the neck may result from blunt trauma. Arterial dissection results in stroke in children less commonly than in adults because of the greater collateral potential of children. Hematomas within the vessel well beneath the intimal flap are easily detected noninvasively by MRI. Their appearance follows that expected for hemorrhage in its various stages.

Cortical venous and dural sinus thrombosis likewise follow the expected course of hemorrhage degradation on MRI. The CT and MRI appearances have been discussed previously. Bilateral, often symmetric subcortical venous infarctions, which are frequently hemorrhagic, may ensue. Predisposing factors include dehydration, sepsis, disseminated intravascular coagulopathy, polycythemia, sickle cell disease, paroxysmal nocturnal hemoglobinuria, and platelet disorders.

Metabolic dysfunction marked by distinct biochemical abnormalities may result in clinical "stroke." A well-documented example is the MELAS syndrome (Mitochondrial myopathy, Encephalopathy, Lactic Acidosis, and Strokelike episodes; (Pavlakis et al., 1984) (see Chapter 14). Neuropathologically, this and similar syndromes result in spongy degeneration of the brain. Atrophy is apparent on imaging studies. Affected areas may demonstrate hypodensity on CT, correlating with abnormal high signal on T2 weighted MRI. Alteration in regional cerebral blood flow has been shown by SPECT studies in these patients (Suzuki et al., 1990). These CT and MR imaging findings do not necessarily correspond to a vascular distribution, and they may be transient (Abe et al., 1990). Furthermore, cerebral angiography may be unrevealing. This suggests that transient capillary endothelial dysfunction rather than finite arterial occlusions might be the underlying cause of the clinical syndrome, and that the neuropathologic findings at postmortem examination represent the end result of repeated and/or irreversible ischemia.

Homocystinuria, another metabolic disorder caused by cystathionine synthase deficiency, can involve the intima and media of large and medium-sized vessels, resulting in thromboembolism of arteries and veins. Arterial and venous infarcts as well as dural sinus thrombosis can occur (Swarman, 1990).

VASCULAR MALFORMATIONS

Children with cerebral vascular malformations may present with headache, seizures, or hemorrhage and a focal neurologic deficit. Vascular malformations may be categorized into four major types: arteriovenous malformations (AVMs), cavernous malformations, venous angiomas, and capillary telangiectasia (Wilson and Stein, 1984). Of these, AVMs carry the greatest risk of hemorrhage with neurologic sequelae. AVMs represent abnormal shunts between arteries and veins without an intervening capillary bed. They are more common supratentorially than in the posterior fossa. Contrast-enhanced CT demonstrates serpiginous enhancement due to the abnormal vessels. With hemorrhage, CT shows a density due to hemorrhage and mass effect due to edema. On MRI, the abnormal vessels are seen as signal void structures due to blood flow within them (Fig. 10.25). Hemorrhage has characteristic T1 and T2 appearances, depending on its stage. Angiography is necessary to define the arterial supply, vascular nidus, and venous drainage. It is crucial to treatment planning. Arterial aneurysms, which are otherwise uncommon in children, may arise in the arterial supply to the AVM.

Cavernous malformations are low-flow malformations consisting of vascular sinusoids without intervening normal brain parenchyma. Subclinical repeated bleeds typically occur and account for the pathognomonic MRI appearance of these lesions, which have mixed signal intensity due to hemorrhage degradation products on T1 and T2 images. They may or may not be seen on contrast CT studies as faintly enhancing lesions. Common locations include the temporal

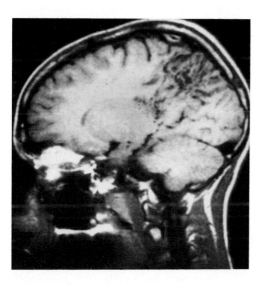

Figure 10.25. Sagittal T1 MRI of the brain showing multiple areas of signal void consistent with AVM. (Courtesy of G. Solomon, MD, Cornell Medical Center.)

lobes and brainstem. Angiography is notably normal, which explains the reference to these lesions as "cryptic" malformations.

Venous angiomas are comprised of abnormal medullary veins with intervening normal white matter that drain into a single prominent vein. The typical appearance on angiography is likened to a "caput medusae." Common locations include the frontal lobes and posterior fossa. Since hemorrhage rarely occurs, treatment is not usually indicated. The cluster of medullary veins is not seen on CT and MRI; however, on CT the single prominent draining vein may appear as linear enhancement, whereas on MRI, depending on the relative rate of blood flow, it may appear as a linear structure that may or may not contain signal.

Capillary telangiectasias consist of abnormally dilated capillaries between normal arteries and veins. These lesions typically occur in the brainstem, and do not bleed.

Mesial Temporal Sclerosis

A frequent cause of intractable temporal lobe partial complex seizures is mesial temporal sclerosis. Although the cause is unknown, pathologically one sees neuronal necrosis and a decreased number of glial cells in the medial temporal lobe (Brooks et al., 1990). Occasionally, MRI may demonstrate increased signal in the medial temporal lobe with ipsilateral enlargement of the temporal horn secondary to atrophy. If atrophy is not present, differentiation from a low-grade astrocytoma may be difficult.

CT and MRI have provided remarkable structural detail of the intracranial anatomy. Technologic advances, such as MR angiography, may further decrease the need for invasive procedures such as angiography. MR spectroscopy is in its infancy but has considerable potential for evaluation of metabolic function. Needless to say, both CT and MR are, and will continue to be, invaluable tools of the clinician in the evaluation of pediatric neurologic disorders.

REFERENCES

Abe K, Inui T, Hirono N, Mezaki T, Kobayashi Y, Kameyama M. Fluctuating MR images with mitochondrial encephalopathy, lactic acidosis, stroke-like syndrome (MELAS). AJNR 1990;32:77.

Altman NR, Purser RK, Post MJD. Tuberous sclerosis: characteristics at CT and MR imaging. Radiology 1988;167:527–532.

Atlas SW, Grossman RI, Hackney DB, et al. Calcified intracranial lesions: detection with gradient-echo-acquisition rapid MR imaging. AJNR 1988;9:253–259.

Barkovich AJ. Congenital malformations of the brain. In: Pediatric neuroimaging. New York: Raven Press, 1990A:77–121.

Barkovich AJ. Infections of the nervous system. In: Normal D, ed. Pediatric neuroimaging. New York: Raven Press, 1990B:293–325.

Barkovich AJ. Metabolic and destructive brain disorder. In: Norman D, ed. Pediatric neuroimagining. New York: Raven Press, 1990C:35–75.

Barkovich AJ. Phakomatosis. In: Norman D, ed. Pediatric neuroimaging. New York: Raven Press, 1990D:123–147.

Barkovich AJ, Chuang SH, Norman D. MR of neuronal migration anomalies. AJNR 1987;8:1009–1017.

Barkovich AT, Edwards MSB. Brain tumors of childhood. In: Norman D, ed. Pediatric neuroimaging. New York: Raven Press, 1990:149–204.

Bognanno JR, Edwards MK, Lee TA, Dunn DW, Roos KL, Klatte EC. Cranial MR imaging in neurofibromatosis. AJNR 1988;9:461–468.

Bradford BF, Adbenour GE, Frank JL, Scott GB, Beerman R. Usual and unusual radiologic manifestations of acquired immunodeficiency virus (HIV) infection in children. Radiol Clin 1988;26 (2):341–353.

Brant-Zawadzki M, Badami P, Mills CM, Norman D, Newton H. Primary intracranial tumor imaging: a comparison of magnetic resonance and CT. Radiology 1984;150:435–440.

Brant-Zawadzki MR, Davis PL, Crooks LE, et al., NMR demonstration of cerebral abnormalities: comparison with CT. AJNR 1983;4:117–124.

Brooks BK, King DW, El Gammal T, et al. MR imaging in patients with intractable complex partial epileptic seizures AJNR 1990;11:93–99.

Brown EW, Riccardi VM, Mawad M, Handel S, Goldman A, Bryan RN. MR imaging of optic pathways in patients with neurofibromatosis. AJNR 1987;8:1031–1036.

Byrd SE, Bohan TP, Osborn RE, Naidich TP. The CT and MR evaluation of lissencephaly. AJNR 1988;9:923–927.

Chang KH, Han MH, Roh JK, Kim IO, Han MC, Kim CW. Gd-DTPA-enhanced MR imaging of the brain in patients with meningitis: comparison with CT. AJNR 1990;11:69–76.

DeVries LS, Regev R, Connell JA, et al. Localized cerebral infarction in the premature infant: an ultrasound diagnosis correlated with computed tomography and magnetic resonance imaging. Pediatrics 1988;81:36–40.

Dunn DW, Daum RS, Weisberg L, Vargas R. Ischemic cerebrovascular complications of *Haemophilus influenzae* meningitis. The value of computed tomography. Arch Neurol 1982;39:650–652.

Dunn DW, Weisberg LA. Computed tomography of the brain in asphyxiated infants. Radiology 1987;11 (3):147–150.

Ebner F, Milner MM, Justich E. Multiple sclerosis in children: value of serial MR studies to monitor patients. AJNR 1990;11:1023–1027

Elster AD, Rieser GD. Gd-DTPA-enhanced cranial MR imaging in children: initial clinical experience and recommendations for its use. AJNR 1989;10:1027–1030.

Farwell JR, Dohrmann GJ, Flannery JT. Central nervous system tumors in children. Cancer 1977;40:3123–3132.

Fernandez RE, Rothberg M, Ferencz G, Wujack D. Lyme disease of the CNS: MR imaging findings in 14 cases. AJNR 1990;11:479–481.

Fobben ES, Grossman RI, Atlas SW, et al. MR characteristics of subdural hematomas and hygromas at 1.5T. AJNR 1989;10:687–693.

Gammal TE, Mark EK, Brooks BS. MR imaging of Chiari II malformation. AJNR 1987;8:1037–1044.

Gean AD, Taveras JM. The phakomatoses In: Taveras JM, ed. Radiology, vol. 3: Neuroradiology and radiology of the head and neck. Philadelphia: JB Lippincott, 1989:ch. 35, pp. 1–18.

Gentry LR, Godersky JC, Thompson B. MR imaging of head trauma: review of the distribution and radiopathologic features of traumatic lesions. AJNR 1980;9:101–110.

Gentry LR, Jacoby CG, Turski PA, et al. Cerebellopontine angle-petromastoid mass lesions: comparative study of diagnosis with MR imaging and CT. Radiology 1987;162:513–520.

Gold AP. Stroke in children. In: Rowland LP, ed. Merritt's textbook of neurology (ch. 34) Philadelphia: Lea & Febiger, 1989:219–225.

Hamies AB, Zimmerman RD, Morgello S, et al. MR imaging of brain abscesses. AJNR 1989;10:279–291.

Hanno R, Beck R. Tuberous sclerosis. Neurol Clin 1987;5:351–360.

Holt JF. Neurofibromatosis in children. AJNR 1978; 130:615–639.

Imakita S, Nishimura T, Yamada N, et al. Magnetic resonance imaging of cerebral infarction: time course of Gd-DTPA enhancement and CT comparison. Neuroradiology 1988;30:372–378.

Iwasaki S, Nakagawa H, Kichikawa K, et al. MR and CT of tuberous sclerosis: linear abnormalities in the cerebral white matter. AJNR 1990;11:1029–1034.

Johnson MA, Pennock JM, Bydder GM, et al., clinical NMR imaging of the brain in children: normal and neurologic disease. AJNR 1983;4:1013–1026.

Jooma R, Kendall BE. Diagnosis and management of pineal tumors. J Neurosurg 1983;58:654–665.

Kelly AB, Zimmerman RD, Snow RB, Gandy SE, Heier

LA, Deck MDF. Head trauma: comparison of MR and CT-experience in 100 patients AJNR 1988;9:699–708.

Knapp MSV, Valk J. MR of adrenoleukodystrophy: histopathologic correlations. AJNR 1989;10:512–514.

Knapp MSVD, Valk J. Classification of congenital abnormalities of the CNS. AJNR 1988;9:315–326.

Kolawofe TM, Patel PJ, Mahdi AH. Computed tomographic changes in juvenile hemiplegia. Radiology 1987; 11(3):125–130.

Lassiter KRL, Alexander E, Courtland H, Davis CH, Kelly DL. Surgical treatment of brain stem gliomas. J Neurosurg 1971;34:719–725.

Weese-Mayer DE, Brouiellette RT, Naidich TP, et al. Magnetic resonance imaging and computerized tomography in central hypoventilation. Am Rev Respir Dis 1988; 137:393–398.

Medina L, Chi TL, DeVivo DC, Hilal SK. MR findings in patients with subacute necrotizing encephalomyelopathy (Leigh syndrome): correlation with biochemical defect. AJNR 1990;11:379–384.

Mirowitz SA, Sartor K, Gado M. High-intensity basal ganglia lesions on T1-weighted MR images in neurofibromatosis. AJNR 1989;10:1159–1163.

Murata R, Nakajima S, Tanaka A, et al. MR imaging of the brain in patients with mucopolysaccharidosis. AJNR 1989;10:1165–1170.

Naidich TP, Zimmerman RA. Primary brain tumors in children. Semin Roentgenol 1984;19(2):100–114.

Nowell MA, Grossman RI, Hackney DB, Zimmerman RA, Goldberg HI, Bilaniuk LT. MR imaging of white matter disease in children. AJNR 1988;9:503–509.

Osborn AG, Harnsberger HR, Smoker WRK, Boyer RS. Multiple sclerosis in adolescents: CT and MR findings. AJNR 1990;11:489–494.

Pavlakis SG, Phillips PC, DiMauro S, DeVivo DC, Rowland LP. Mitochondrial myopathy, encephalopathy, lactic acidosis, and strokelike episodes: a distinctive clinical syndrome. Ann Neurol 1984;16(4):481–488.

Pearsen KD, Marton ADG, Levy HL, Davis KR. Phenylketonuria: MR imaging of the brain with clinical correlation. Radiology 1990;177:437–440.

Pinto RS, Kricheff II. Neuroradiology of intracranial neuromas. Semin Roentgenol 1984;14:44–52.

Post MJD, Berger JR, Hensley GT. The radiology of central nervous system disease in acquired immunodeficiency syndrome. In: Tavaras JM, ed. Radiology, vol. 3: Neurodiology and radiology of the head and neck (ch 38a). Philadelphia: JB Lippincott, 1988:1–26.

Rao KCVG, Knipp HC, Wagner EJ. Computed tomographic findings in cerebral sinus and venous thrombosis. Radiology 1981;140:391–398.

Riccardi VM. Neurofibromatosis. Neurol Clin 1987;5:337–349.

Rippe DJ, Boyko OB, Spritzer CE, et al. Demonstration of dural sinus occlusion by the use of MR angiography. AJNR 1990;11:199–201.

Satho S, Shibuya H, Matsushima Y, Suzuki S. Analysis of the angiographic findings in cases of childhood moyamoya disease. AJNR 1988;30:111–119.

Sato Y, Yuh WTC, Smith WL, Alexander RC, Kao SCS, Ellerbroek CJ. Head injury in child abuse: evaluation with MR imaging. Radiology 1989;173:653–657.

Scatliff JH. Supratentorial congenital abnormalities. In: Taveras JM, ed. Radiology, vol. 3: Neuroradiology and radiology of the head and neck (ch 34). Philadelphia: JB Lippincott, 1987:1–18.

Segall HP, Zee C, Alimadi J, Becker TS. Posterior fossa neoplasms in children. In: Taveras Jm, ed. Radiology, vol. 3: Neuroradiology and radiology of the head and neck (ch 74). Philadelphia: JB Lippincott, 1987:1–7.

Shah M, Ross JS. Infantile Alexander disease: MR appearance of a biopsy-proved case. AJNR 1990;11:1105–1106.

Stimac GK, Solomon MA, Newton TH. CT and MR of angiomatous malformations of the choroid plexus in patients with Sturge-Weber disease. AJNR 1986;7:623–627.

Suzuki J. Moyomoya disease. New York: Springer-Verlag, 1983.

Suzuki T, Koizumi J, Shiraishi H, et al. Mitochondrial encephalomyopathy (MELAS) with mental disorder—CT, MRI and SPECT findings. AJNR 1990;32:74–76.

Swarman KF. Inborn metabolic errors affecting the nervous system. In: Joynt RJ, ed. Clinical neurology, vol. 4. Philadelphia: JB Lippincott, 1990: ch. 56, pp. 67–70.

Swartz JD, Zimmerman RA, Bilaniuk LT. Computed tomography of intracranial ependymomas. Radiology 1982;143:97–101.

Sze G, Simmons B, Krol G, et al. Dural sinus thrombosis: verification with spin echo techniques. AJNR 1988; 9:679–686.

Tien RD, Barkovich AJ, Edwards MSB. MR imaging of pineal tumors. AJNR 1990;11:557–565.

Wasenko JJ, Rosenbloom SA, Duchesneau PM, Lanzieri CF, Weinstein MA. The Sturge-Weber syndrome: comparison of MR and CT characteristics. AJNR 1990;11:131–134.

Weingarten K, Zimmerman RD, Becker RD, Heier LA, Haimes AB, Deck MDF. Subdural and epidural empyemas: MR imaging. AJNR 1989;10:81–87.

Wiklund LM, Uverbrant P, Flodmark O. Morphology of cerebral lesions in children with congenital hemiplegia. AJNR 1990;32:179–186.

Wilms G, Marchal G, Van Frayenhoven L, et al. Unilateral moya-moya disease: MRI findings. AJNR 1989;31:442.

Wilson C, Stein B. Intracranial arteriovenous malformations. Baltimore: Williams & Wilkins, 1984.

Wolpert SM, Anderson M, Scott RM, Kwan ESK, Runge VM. Chiari II malformation: MR imaging evaluation. AJNR 1987;8:783–792.

Zimmerman RA. Evaluation of head injury: supratentorial. In: Taveras JM, ed. Radiology, vol. 3: Neuroradiology and radiology of the head and neck (ch 37). Philadelphia: JB Lippincott, 1987A:1–18.

Zimmerman RA. Magnetic resonance of head injury. In: Taveras JM, ed. Radiology, vol. 3: Neuroradiology and radiology of the head and neck (ch 37). Philadelphia: JB Lippincott, 1987B:1–12.

Chapter 11

HEADACHES IN CHILDREN*

Shlomo Shinnar, MD, PhD

INTRODUCTION

Headaches are among the most common complaints in children. By age 7, almost 40% of children will have experienced headaches. By age 15 the figure rises to 75%. Many of these headaches are infrequent, intermittent, and nonrecurrent. Of more concern to parents and physicians is the sizable group of children with frequent recurrent headaches. This group includes 2 to 5% of 7-year-olds and as many as 15% of 15-year-olds (Bille, 1962). Chronic headache constitutes one of the most common reasons for referral to a pediatric neurology practice.

The majority of childhood headaches are not associated with intracranial structural lesions. Diagnosis can usually be made by means of careful history and physical examination; extensive laboratory investigations are rarely required. Most children can be managed with reassurance, simple analgesics, and mild sedation. For more severe cases, particularly of migraine, effective pharmacologic agents are available.

This chapter reviews those aspects of the diagnosis and treatment of childhood headache of most concern to the child psychiatrist.

TYPES OF HEADACHE

There are many causes of headache in children (Table 11.1). An accurate diagnosis can usually be made on the basis of the history and physical examination (Shinnar and D'Souza, 1982A). Different headache syndromes in children are described below.

Migraine

Migraine, a vascular disorder characterized by paroxysmal attacks of vasoconstriction and/or vasodilation, occurs in all age groups, including young children. Notably, it is the most common headache type in children younger than 7 years of age, accounting for more than two-thirds of recurrent headaches in this age group. There is an equal sex incidence prior to puberty, but in adolescents migraine occurs more frequently in females. In 70 to 80% of affected children a first- or second-degree relative also has migraine.

There are no uniformly accepted diagnostic criteria for childhood migraine. Vahlquist (1985) has proposed criteria that include paroxysmal headache separated by pain-free intervals and at least two of the following: unilateral pain, nausea, aura, and positive family history. A high incidence of associated sleep disturbances such as nightmares, somnambulism, and bed-wetting has also been reported. However, there is little evidence to support the concept of a "migraine

*Portions of this chapter are adapted from a review article by Shinnar S and D'Souza B, The diagnosis and management of headaches in childhood, Pediatr Clin North Am 1982;29:79-94.

Table 11.1.
Classification of Childhood Headaches

Migraine:	Muscle contraction headaches
Classic migraine	Posttraumatic headaches
Common migraine	Psychogenic headaches:
Complicated migraine	Depression
Hemiplegic	School avoidance
Ophthalmoplegic	Malingering
Basilar artery	Traction headaches:
Acute confusional state	Tumor
Alice in Wonderland syndrome	Hematoma
Migraine variants	Abscess
Cyclic vomiting	Postlumbar puncture
Cluster headache	Pseudotumor cerebri
Nonmigrainous vascular headaches:	Headaches with cranial inflammation
Systemic infection with fever	Headaches due to diseases of other head or neck structures:
Convulsive states	Eyes
Hypoxia	Sinuses
Miscellaneous	Temporomandibular joint

personality." Migraine headaches are typically unilateral, throbbing, and associated with nausea and vomiting. They occur at any time of day, last from 30 minutes to 2 to 3 days, and are often relieved by vomiting or sleep. Precipitating factors include stress, fatigue, exertion, head trauma, illness, or dietary factors (Cooper et al., 1987; Shinnar and D'Souza, 1982B). Migraine is closely related to certain other periodic disorders of childhood such as cyclic vomiting and benign paroxysmal vertigo (Barlow, 1984; Congdon and Forsythe, 1979; Prensky, 1979; Shinnar and D'Souza, 1982B).

Classic Migraine. The best known form of migraine, classic migraine, is far less frequent than common migraine. It accounts for less than one-third of cases of migraines in childhood. Classic migraine is a biphasic illness in which the initial phase is characterized by an aura that is usually a visual aberration. Visual disturbances, which may be dramatic, include blurred vision, scotomata, flashing lights, and hemianopsia. Sometimes children can draw pictures of the aura better than they can describe it. Although the aura may be an isolated phenomenon, it is usually followed by a throbbing hemicranial headache that can be incapacitating.

Common Migraine. This is the most fre-

quent form of migraine in childhood. Although there is no well-defined aura, the child may complain of generalized malaise, dizziness, or nausea prior to the onset of the headache. The listlessness may be misinterpreted as abnormal behavior. Headaches may be generalized, bifrontal, or bitemporal in location. Nausea, vomiting, pallor, and other autonomic findings are prominent features and may be more pronounced than the pain. The headache often ends with the child's falling asleep.

Complicated Migraine (Barlow, 1984; Dalessio, 1972; Shinnar and D'Souza, 1982B). Complicated migraine is the association of migraine with transient neurologic deficits or alterations in state of consciousness. The deficits are presumably due to prolonged vasoconstriction and ischemia to the affected cerebral areas. The onset of the deficit usually precedes the headache. The symptoms are extremely diverse and depend on the vascular territory involved. The natural course of complex migraine is usually benign, and most patients later go on to develop typical migraine. It is important to differentiate migraine syndromes from more serious intracranial pathology. In general, children with complex migraine should be referred to a child neurologist for evaluation. The more common complex migraine syndromes are listed in Table 11.1.

Abdominal Migraine, or Cyclic Vomiting. This migraine variant may not be recognized in children before the more characteristic features of migraine develop. In very young children these periodic attacks consist of abdominal pain, nausea, and vomiting lasting for hours to days (Brown, 1977; Prensky, 1979; Shinnar and D'Souza, 1982A; Shinnar and D'Souza, 1982B). Irritability, listlessness, and other behavioral disturbances may also occur. A family history of migraine may be present.

Cluster Headache. Although cluster headache is sometimes included among the migraine syndromes, it is a distinct entity. Patients do not have a family history of migraine, nor do they progress to typical migraine. Cluster attacks are characterized by intense, nonthrobbing periorbital pain that may then generalize to the entire hemicranium. The headaches are often associated with unilateral conjunctival injection, lacrimation, and rhinorrhea. The attacks are brief, not preceded by an aura, last 30 minutes to 1 hour, and occur in groups of one to three daily for a period of 6 to 12 weeks. The cluster of headaches is followed by prolonged periods of remission lasting months to years (Dalessio, 1972). Cluster headaches are rarely seen in children less than 10 years of age. Cluster headaches are usuall refractory to simple analgesic therapy and should be referred to a neurologist.

Nonmigrainous Vascular Headaches

Convulsive States. Headache may occur as a postictal symptom but is rarely the sole manifestation of a seizure (Swaiman and Frank, 1978). On occasion, patients with nocturnal seizures may afterward awaken with a postictal vascular headache. Although the incidence of electroencephalographic abnormalities and seizures is higher in migraine patients than in the general population, migraine and epilepsy are distinct syndromes that can usually be differentiated on clinical grounds (Andermann and

Lugaresi, 1987; Shinnar and D'Souza, 1982A). However, some cases of complex migraine that may involve altered states of consciousness and transient neurologic deficits may be difficult to distinguish from seizures.

Muscle Contraction Headaches

Muscle contraction headache, which results from sustained contraction of the muscles of the neck and scalp, is the most common form of headache in adolescents and adults. Adolescents with these headaches typically describe a sensation of tightness or pressure in a band-like distribution around the head. Physical examination may reveal tenderness or tightness of the muscles in the occipital scalp or posterior cervical region. These headaches are often quite frequent and may last all day if untreated. They usually do not interrupt regular daily activities and often respond well to mild analgesics such as acetaminophen or ibuprofen. Muscle contraction headaches are also known as "tension headaches." They differ from migraine headaches in the absence of vomiting and associated autonomic symptoms and in the ability of patients to continue their daily activities during the attack.

Posttraumatic Headaches

Although the existence of this entity is controversial, in this author's experience it is a real entity that occurs even when litigation is not an issue. The headaches are often self-limited and usually resolve after a few weeks. However, they can persist for months to years, even after relatively minor trauma. Other symptoms of the posttraumatic syndrome, such as sleep disturbances and behavior changes, are often present (Levin et al., 1989). The headaches may be vascular or muscle contraction in character.

Headaches and Childhood Depression

A serious cause of chronic headache is childhood depression (Ling et al., 1970). The child usually complains of a dull, constant headache that may be generalized or localized to the occipital region. Other symptoms of childhood depression can often be elicited (e.g., significant mood changes, withdrawal, increasingly poor school performance, school problems, sleep disturbances, aggressive behavior, lack of energy, weight loss, anorexia, and other somatic complaints). Appropriate treatment depends on recognition of the underlying depression.

Headaches as a primary manifestation of childhood depression are relatively uncommon and must be distinguished from muscle contraction or migraine headaches, whose frequency and severity have been increased by stress (Cooper et al., 1987). Commonly, children with a past history of headaches have more frequent headaches in the context of family or school stress.

Traction Headaches

As the name implies, a traction headache is caused by traction on the intracranial pain-sensitive structures. The traction may be exerted by a mass lesion such as a brain tumor, abscess, or subdural hematoma, by the weight of the brain after removal of cerebrospinal fluid by lumbar puncture, or by distortion of intracranial structures from increased intracranial pressure, as in hydrocephalus or pseudotumor cerebri. Although a relatively uncommon form of headache, it is often associated with serious intracranial pathology.

Tumor Headaches. Although headache can be the first sympton of a brain tumor, brain tumors are an infrequent cause of headache in childhood. Several characteristics help to distinguish brain tumor headaches from more benign varieties. Headaches associated with brain tumors are usually chronic and progressive, present in the morning on first arising, and exacerbated by changes in position, coughing, or a Valsalva maneuver. Unlike a child with a migraine or muscle contraction headache, the child with a brain tumor headache often does not seem to be his or her usual self, even between attacks. The

patient's response to analgesics is also not a reliable diagnostic clue, since simple analgesics may temporarily relieve a brain tumor headache and provide a false sense of security. Localization of the headache is also of limited value because a mass lesion may cause distortion of distant pain-sensitive structures.

Headaches are rarely the only symptom of a progressing brain tumor. Associated symptoms such as vomiting, diplopia, weakness, ataxia, and personality changes are usually present within a few weeks of the onset of headache (Honig and Charney, 1982). The physical examination often reveals papilledema, nuchal rigidity, irritability, focal neurologic deficits such as a field cut, or a hemiperesis. As a general rule, the child with headaches of more than 6 months' duration who still has a normal neurologic exam is exceedingly unlikely to have a brain tumor.

Pseudotumor Cerebri. The syndrome is characterized by the clinical manifestations of increased intracranial pressure in the absence of hydrocephalus or a mass lesion. It occurs most frequently in obese young women but is not uncommon in children. In children, there is no clear sex predilection and obesity is often not present (Weisberg and Chutorian, 1977). Headache is the most common presenting complaint and is frequently associated with nausea and vomiting. Visual symptoms such as diplopia are not uncommon and are usually present even between headaches. Imaging studies are typically normal. However, on examination, papilledema is almost invariably present. Children with headaches and papilledema should be referred immediately to a child neurologist for further evaluation and treatment, which are beyond the scope of this chapter. Prompt treatment is necessary to prevent visual loss.

Headache Associated with Other Head or Neck Structures

Refractive errors and eye muscle imbalance are common in children but only rarely cause frank headaches. Instead, they may cause dull pain localized to the periorbital or frontal area that is clearly related to prolonged eye strain. Correction of the visual deficit leads to prompt resolution of the headache. Headache from ear disease is usually associated with acute otitis externa, acute otitis media, or serous otitis media. The associated ear pain and the physical examination should make the diagnosis clear. Dental disease can also cause headache in association with severe local pain. However, in the absence of local pain, temporomandibular joint (TMJ) dysfuntion is very rarely a cause of headaches.

Headaches from sinus disease are rare in young children, since the frontal sinuses are not fully developed prior to age 12. In adolescents, however, sinus disease can cause a chronic headache, with pain and tenderness to percussion over the forehead and maxillary regions A history of chronic sinus disease or recurrent upper respiratory tract infection is usually present.

HISTORY

In most children with headaches, the diagnosis rests almost exclusively on the history. A history should be obtained from both patient and parent, including information regarding the characer of the headache, its frequency and severity, and associated symptoms. A change in the pattern of the child's headaches requires reevaluation. Unlike other features of the headache, the severity of pain is not a reflection of the gravity of the underlying process: it is best assessed by the degree of interference with the child's activity level. For example, a child still willing to play or watch television while complaining of a headache does not have a severe headache. In contrast, the child with a migraine attack often wants to lie down and sleep in a quiet dark room and is unwilling to participate even in favorite activities.

A detailed investigation of the triggering events and the events surrounding the first attack may provide a clue not only to the diagnosis but also to treatment. The duration and frequency of the headache might indicate whether the problem requires urgent attention or an outpatient evaluation. In contrast to recurrent morning headaches with vomiting, a daily constant headache is most likely psychogenic in origin. An aura may point to the diagnosis of migraine or temporal lobe seizures. Associated deficits between headaches, such as weakness, ataxia, personality change, and visual disturbances, should make one suspicious of a mass lesion. Weight loss, fatigue, and irritability can be seen in childhood depression.

Because headaches are often familial conditions, a family history of tension headache, migraine, seizures, and brain tumors should be elicited. Migraine, in particular, is a familial disorder, with a positive family history obtainable from 70 to 90% of patients. A family history of affective disorders, chronic abdominal pain, renal disease, collagen vascular disease, and hypertension may also be significant.

The type and number of medications used in the past is an indication of the perceived magnitude of the problem. Prolonged use of multiple medications should alert the physician to the potential for drug dependence or abuse. A therapeutic response to a previously used agent may be of diagnostic as well as therapeutic significance. At the end of the interview (Table 11.2), the physician should have a good idea as to the type of headache present.

PHYSICAL EXAMINATION

Although often normal in children and adults with headache, a complete general and neurologic examination is essential to rule out organic disease. In the general examination, blood pressure should be determined. Disturbances in growth parameters, including head circumference, height, and weight, may indicate hydrocephalus, chronic disease, or the presence of a pituitary tumor. Particular attention should be given to the structure of the head and neck. A

Table 11.2.
Sample Questions in the Headache Interview

Age of onset	Triggering events:
Events surrounding onset	Stress (school, family, etc.)
Prodrome	Exertion/fatigue
Characteristics of attacks:	Food intake
Frequency	Medications
Duration	Irregular habits (meals, sleep, etc.)
Severity	Behavior between headaches:
Localization	Personality change
Type of pain	Clumsiness or change in gait
Time of day	Irritability
Associated autonomic symptoms	Change in school performance
Associated neurologic deficits:	Change in appetite or weight
Type	Change in sleep patterns
Temporal relation to headache	Frequent urination
Duration	What makes headache better
Whether localization of deficit corresponds	What makes headache worse
to site of headache	Medications for headache:
Postictal state	Currently used
Family history:	Previously used
Headaches	Whether they help
Seizures	What patient currently does when
Psychiatric disorders	he/she gets a headache
Previous laboratory evaluations	Number of days of school missed
Previous consultations for headaches	How significantly headaches are interfering with normal life
Prior history of abdominal pain	

physician should palpate for scalp defects and for tenderness over the posterior cervical and occipital scalp area, percuss the sinuses, and auscultate for cranial bruits. Nuchal rigidity should always be excluded. Inspection of the skin may reveal evidence of a neurocutaneous disorder such as neurofibromatosis, tuberous sclerosis, or Sturge-Weber syndrome.

In the neurologic examination, a thorough fundoscopic examination, visual acuity, visual fields, and assessment of extraocular movements, including smooth pursuit and saccades, are essential. Abnormalities of other cranial nerve or cerebellar functions may indicate a posterior fossa mass. Gait disturbances and asymmetric motor findings also point to possible structural abnormalities. When a properly performed general and neurologic examination fails to reveal any significant abnormalities and the history is reassuring, the physician can usually rule out an intracranial structural lesion and make a clinical diagnosis without laboratory testing.

LABORATORY STUDIES

Illingworth (1975) reports that of all children referred for the evaluation of headache, laboratory tests were helpful in only 5% or fewer. In these 5%, the underlying abnormality can usually be suspected on the basis of a careful history and physical examination. Rarely does a laboratory test reveal significant organic disease in the presence of a normal history and examination. Hence, in the majority of children with chronic headache, no laboratory studies are needed. When indicated, blood counts, sedimentation rate, urinalysis, Lyme titer, lead level, and sinus films may be of value. When intracranial pathology is suspected, neurodiagnostic procedures are indicated.

MRI and CT Scans. Both magnetic resonance imaging (MRI) and computed tomographic (CT) scanning of the head offer relatively safe, sensitive imaging for detecting a variety of structural lesions of the central nervous system, including brain tumors, hematomas, hydrocephalus, and hemorrhages. In the select group of children in whom a mass lesion is suspected or a persistent neurologic deficit is present, one of these imaging studies is mandatory. However, they are overused in the evaluation of patients with headache. They are not indicated in the child with no other symptom or sign of intracranial pathology. Minor abnormalities on CT scan have been reported in a few patients with migraine, but their significance is unclear. Imaging studies are often indicated in children with complex migraine and in children in whom the headaches are consistently lateralized exclusively to one side. For such cases, referral to a child neurologist is usually appropriate. In general, the MRI has become the imaging study of choice due to its superior abilities to detect arteriovenous malformations and low-grade tumors as well as to avoid the risks of intravenous contrast injection.

Electroencephalography. The electroencephalogram (EEG) is of minimal usefulness in the evaluation of headaches because of problems with both sensitivity and specificity. The EEG may be abnormal in a large number of otherwise normal children with headache, particularly migraine. It may also be completely normal in children with well-documented epilepsy. Even if the electroencephalogram is abnormal, the physician should always treat the patient and not the EEG. The EEG remains an important diagnostic test in children for whom the differential diagnosis includes both migraine and seizures.

Skull X-ray. Skull x-rays can be abnormal in a wide variety of conditions. However, the abnormalities are usually nonspecific except for fractures and are often normal in the presence of serious intracranial pathology such as a brain tumor. Skull x-rays have been replaced by the MRI and CT scans and no longer have a role in the evaluation of chronic headaches.

WHEN TO REFER TO THE CHILD NEUROLOGIST

In the majority of cases, a referral to the child neurologist is not necessary. Referral to the child neurologist is indicated when the diagnosis is uncertain or when the headaches are refractory to routine treatment. It is also indicated whenever there is a history of an associated neurologic deficit or an abnormality in the examination. Guidelines for referral to the neurologist are listed in Table 11.3. It should be emphasized that these guidelines are meant as screens that

Table 11.3.
Indications for Referral to the Child Neurologist

Evaluation of headaches with unusual or worrisome features:
    Complicated migraine
    Consistently unilateral headaches
    Any neurologic abnormality (transient or persistent)
    Headaches that awaken the child at night
    Morning headaches
    Persistent vomiting
    Sudden unexplained change in character or frequency of headaches
Differentiating headaches from other conditions:
    Headaches vs. seizures
    Brain tumor
    Arteriovenous malformation
    Headache vs. childhood depression
Headaches in children at risk for serious neurologic disorders:
    Children younger than 5 years of age
    Children with a neurocutaneous syndrome
    Children with macrocephaly
    Children with growth abnormalities
    Children with diabetes insipidus
    Children with any chronic systemic or neurologic disorder
Management of headaches:
    Headaches refractory to standard therapy
    Headaches requiring treatment with medications that are:
        Unusually large in quantity
        Associated with serious side effects
        Narcotics

should identify the vast majority of children with potentially serious pathology. Most children who meet one of the criteria in Table 11.3 do not have structural brain abnormalities.

TREATMENT

In treating recurrent childhood headaches, the emphasis should be placed on reassurance, removal of precipitating factors, and simple analgesics. Aggressive pharmacologic therapy should be avoided. The parent and child are often more concerned about the possibility of a serious systemic illness or intracranial pathology than about the headache itself. Understanding that the child has migraine or tension headaches, with reassurance of the benign nature and good prognosis of these disorders, relieves most of the anxiety. A small number of children with chronic headache nevertheless require pharmacologic therapy. The approach to these children is discussed below.

Nonpharmacologic Therapy

A large number of external and constitutional factors play a role in triggering and exacerbating both migraine and tension headaches in children. Although these factors often cannot be completely eliminated, their identification and reduction reduce the frequency and severity of the child's symptoms. Foremost among precipitating factors are the emotional stresses of school, peer relations, and family tensions. In adolescents, the stresses of maturation, puberty, and the struggle to become independent are additional factors. For each child, there is usually a particularly prominent area of tension that can be addressed.

The irregular lifestyle of many adolescents contributes to their headaches, particularly in those with migraine. Fasting or missing meals, sleeping late, or lack of sleep have all be implicated in triggering headache attacks. Other triggering factors include bright and flashing lights, such as those in discos, and heavy exertion. Contrary to popular belief, dietary factors have not been conclusively implicated in studies of large numbers of migraineurs. However, in selected patients, where there is a clear history of headaches following the ingestion of specific foods, dietary manipulation may be beneficial. In adolescent females, both migraine and tension headaches are often associated with menstruation. Oral contraceptives may exacerbate headaches in some women.

Biofeedback and relaxation techniques are relatively new nonpharmacologic tools that are playing an increasingly accepted role in the management of chronic headaches. They are particularly effective in muscle contraction headaches but are also proving effective in the management of migraine (Adler and Adler, 1976; Diamond, 1979). Studies to date have been done mainly in adults, but at least one group reports successfully using the technique on headache patients as young as 9 years of age (Diamond, 1979). The safety of these techniques and their avoidance of the potential pitfalls of drug dependency and abuse make them very attractive for use in adolescents with chronic headaches of all causes. Biofeedback and relaxation techniques work best when provided in the context of a comprehensive stress management approach.

Acute Pharmacologic Treatment

In a large number of children with chronic headaches, both migrainous and tension, therapy with a mild analgesic, such as acetaminophen, combined with rest in a quiet room offers adequate relief. Migraine attacks in children are generally shorter in duration than in adults, and reassurance and sedation, especially in the younger child, often are enough to get the child through the attack. However, drugs such as Fiorinal and its various congeners, which combine an analgesic with a short-acting barbiturate, should be used with restraint. Although effective in treating muscle contraction headaches, they are not very useful in the treatment of migraine except that they may help the child fall asleep. If used frequently, they may be habit-forming.

They are appropriate for the child or responsible adolescent with an occasional severe headache that is not frequent enough to warrant prophylactic therapy.

Ergotamine. In adults with classic migraine, ergot compounds, usually given in combination with caffeine, are the mainstay of therapy (Dalessio, 1972). However, the use of ergotamine in younger children is very difficult. Most children do not have an aura. When an aura does occur, it is briefer than in adults and does not provide adequate warning. Because the medicine must be taken at the onset of symptoms, the child must carry it along at all times, including school and play, and be responsible for taking it. In general, ergotamine should be avoided in children younger than 10 years of age but can be used in responsible adolescents with classic migraine. The usual dose is 1 to 2 mg p.o. at the onset of the aura and an additional 1 mg 30 to 60 minutes later if necessary. A maximum of 12 mg per week may be used. Ergotamine is contraindicated in patients with complicated migraine, as the drug may theoretically prolong the ischemic phase.

Migraine Prophylaxis

In the great majority of pediatric patients with migraine, prophylactic therapy is neither necessary nor desirable. Given the choice of taking simple analgesics when the attack occurs or taking daily medications, all of which have potential side effects, most families either reject prophylactic therapy or become noncompliant after a short time. However, for the child with severe and frequent migraine attacks and for the child with complex migraine, several effective agents are available.

Propranolol. Propranolol is an excellent agent for migraine prophylaxis and has been studied in children as well as adults (Bille et al., 1977; Ludvigsson, 1974). It is well-tolerated by most children. The most common side effects include nausea and easy fatigability on exertion. Since it is a beta-blocker, it is contraindicated in patients with bronchial asthma, sinus bra-

dycardia, and congestive heart failure. It is relatively contraindicated in children with major affective disorders because it can exacerbate them. Rarely, it can cause nightmares. Propranolol's effectiveness in classic, common, and complex migraine in all age groups and the low incidence of side effects in children make it, in the author's opinion, the drug of choice for migraine prophylaxis. However, propranolol is not effective in muscle contraction headaches and is only rarely effective in cluster headaches. The starting dose in children younger than 12 is 20 to 40 mg orally daily. In older teenagers, 40 to 80 mg daily is an appropriate starting dose. These doses may need to be increased. Adolescents often need a full adult dose.

Amitriptyline. Amitriptyline is an effective and well-tolerated agent in the prophylactic treatment of adult migraines and chronic muscle contraction headaches. The migraine prophylaxis effect is independent of its antidepressant activity (Couch and Hassanein, 1979). Although no studies on its efficacy in children are available and it is not approved for children under 12 years of age, amitriptyline has been widely used in treating children with migraine, particularly those in whom propranolol is contraindicated. The author considers it the drug of choice for children and adolescents with a combination of migraine and muscle contraction headaches, severe and frequent muscle contraction headaches, and posttraumatic headaches, particularly if other features of the posttraumatic syndrome are present.

The dosages of amitriptyline for headaches are relatively small. Hence, the medicine is well-tolerated and relatively free of the disabling side effects associated with higher doses. In children 6 to 12 years old, the starting dose is approximately 10 mg q.h.s., which can be gradually increased if needed to a dose of 30 to 50 mg q.h.s. In adolescents, a starting dose of 25 mg q.h.s. is often effective and can be increased, if needed, to 50 to 75 mg q.h.s. Therapy must be instituted gradually, and a therapeutic effect may require several weeks. Although other antidepressants may also have analgesic properties, there is little experience with them in the treatment of headaches. As child psychiatrists gain more experience with the newer antidepressants, data will accumulate on their relative safety and efficacy in treating headaches.

Calcium Channel Blockers. Calcium channel blockers such as verapramil are effective in the prophylaxis of migraine headaches. They can be used in asthmatic children, in whom beta-blockers, such as propranolol, are contraindicated. The author has found them to be poorly tolerated in children because these drugs have a high incidence of GI side effects. In general, calcium channel blockers should be reserved for children with migraines refractory to beta-blockers and amitriptyline.

Anticonvulsants. Although phenobarbital and phenytoin are not considered effective in the treatment of migraine in adults, they were reported to be very effective in the treatment of childhood migraine in two large but uncontrolled studies in which they were taken in therapeutic anticonvulsant doses (Millichap, 1978). The effectiveness of anticonvulsants in treating childhood headaches is reportedly unrelated to the presence or degree of EEG abnormalities. Due to their unfavorable side effect profile and the lack of controlled trials demonstrating efficacy, the use of anticonvulsants should be reserved for intractable cases that do not respond to conventional agents.

Cyproheptadine. Cyproheptadine (Periactin), an antihistamine with antiserotonergic effects, has been reported to be effective in childhood migraine (Bille et al., 1977). Some authors have advocated it as the drug of choice in childhood migraine. The author has found it to be of limited benefit, particularly due to the common side effects of sedation and weight gain.

Methysergide. Methysergide, a potent antiserotonergic medication, was one of the first agents used in migraine prophylaxis (Dalessio, 1972). It is effective in adults and probably also in children. However, it carries a high incidence of side effects. The most common are nausea,

vomiting, and overstimulation or sedation. Less common, but more serious, is the development of retroperitoneal fibrosis. The drug should not be used in children except in rare cases, and then only with careful monitoring under the supervision of an experienced neurologist.

Long-Term Management

Children older than 10 years of age who are placed on medication should, in general, also be treated with biofeedback and stress management techniques. Although medications may be needed initially, nonpharmacologic techniques alone may be sufficient at a later time or at least may reduce the need for chronic medications. Children who are on long-term prophylactic management for migraine should have periodic attempts at medication withdrawal, since there is a high rate of spontaneous remission. A convenient time is after the end of the school year. Even if complete remission has not occurred, the symptoms may have improved sufficiently to warrant discontinuation of daily medication.

Since many children with chronic headaches, particularly adolescents, may have headaches for many years, the potential for drug dependence in later life is high. One of the major problems faced in the treatment of adults with chronic headaches is trying to wean them from the veritable pharmacy of potent drugs that they are often taking. The physician caring for the child with headache has a major influence on how that child will cope with headache and stress when he or she becomes an adult. Emphasis on nonpharmacologic techniques and on prophylaxis of headaches rather than seeking acute pharmacologic relief for each symptom will help prevent some of the excesses commonly found in the treatment of chronic headaches.

PROGNOSIS

The prognosis of chronic headache in childhood is generally favorable. Approximately two-thirds of all children with migraine will be improved or asymptomatic in long-term follow-up. There appears to be little correlation between type of migraine, severity of symptoms, and frequency of attacks, and the ultimate prognosis. In Bille's study (1962), the patients with severe migraine did almost as well as the unselected migraine group. The type of therapy employed, whether simple analgesics, ergotamine, or prophylactic medications, also had little effect on outcome (Bille, 1962; Congdon and Forsythe, 1979; Prensky and Sommer, 1979). In contrast, age of onset was a significant prognostic factor. Patients with onset of migraine after puberty tend to have continuing symptoms, and they have a prognosis similar to that of adult-onset migraine. Congdon and Forsythe (1979), who report a spontaneous remission of 3 to 14% per annum between the ages of 7 and 17 years, believe that remission is unlikely to occur after 18 years of age. Relapses in patients who have spontaneous remission for more than 2 years do occur but are relatively uncommon.

In a 6-year follow-up of 52 children with non-migrainous headaches, Bille found 88% to be improved or asymptomatic (Bille, 1962). These data are similar to those in children with migraine. Once again age was a significant prognostic variable, with onset in adolescence carrying a somewhat poorer prognosis. Not surprisingly, a large number of adults with chronic headaches report the onset of these symptoms in adolescence.

Long-term follow-up of a large number of children with chronic headache in whom the initial work-up was negative shows that only a tiny fraction (less than 1%) go on to develop significant intracranial pathology in later years. In almost all these cases, a change in the headache pattern or the appearance of neurologic deficits and signs of systemic illness give a clue to the development of new pathology. Physicians should be alert to a change in headache pattern in a patient with chronic headache. However, chronic headache in itself does not carry a significantly increased risk for development of serious intracranial pathology.

REFERENCES

Adler CS, Adler SM. Biofeedback psychotherapy for the treatment of headaches: a 5-year follow-up. *Headache* 1976;16:189–191.

Andermann F, Lugaresi E, eds. *Migraine and epilepsy.* Boston: Butterworths, 1987.

Barlow CF. *Headaches and migraine in childhood.* Clinics in developmental medicine no. 91. London: Spastics International Medical Publications, 1984.

Bille B. Migraine in school children. *Acta Paediatr Scand* 1962;51 (suppl 136):1–151.

Bille B, Ludvigsson J, Sanner G. Prophylaxis of migraine in children. *Headache* 1977;17:61–63.

Brown JK. Migraine and migraine equivalents in children. *Dev Med Child Neurol* 1977;19:683–692.

Congdon PJ, Forsythe WI. Migraine in childhood: a study of 300 children. *Dev Med Child Neurol* 1979;21:209–216.

Cooper PJ, Bowden HN, Camfield PR, Camfield CS. Anxiety and life events in childhood migraine. *Pediatrics* 1987;79:999–1004.

Couch JR, Hassanein RS. Amitriptyline in migraine prophylaxis. *Arch Neurol* 1979;36:695–699.

Dalessio DJ. *Wolff's headache and other head pain.* 4th ed. Oxford and New York, Oxford University Press, 1980.

Diamond S. Biofeedback and headache. *Headache* 1979; 19:180–184.

Honig PJ, Charney EB. Children with brain tumor headaches: distinguishing features. *Am J Dis Child* 1982; 136:121–124.

Illingworth RS. *Common symptoms of disease in children.* 5th ed. Oxford, UK: Blackwell Scientific Publications, 1975:98.

Lapkin ML, Golden GS. Basilar artery migraine: a review of 30 cases. *Am J Dis Child* 1978;132:278–281.

Levin HS, Eisenberg HM, Benton AL, eds. *Mild head injury.* New York: Oxford University Press, 1989.

Ling W, Oftedal G, Weinberg W. Depressive illness in childhood presenting as severe headache. *Am J Dis Child* 1970;120:122–124.

Ludvigsson J. Propranolol used in prophylaxis of migraine in children. *Acta Neurol Scand* 1974;50:109–115.

Millichap JC. Recurrent headaches in 100 children: electroencephalographic abnormalities and response to phenytoin (Dilantin). *Child's Brain* 1978;4:95–105.

Prensky AL. Migraine and migrainous variants in pediatric patients. *Pediatr Clin North Am* 1979;23:461–471.

Prensky AL, Sommer D. Diagnosis and treatment of migraine in children. *Neurology* 1979;29:506–510.

Shinnar S, D'Souza BJ. The diagnosis and management of headaches in childhood. *Pediatr Clin North Am* 1982A; 29:79–94.

Shinnar S, D'Souza BJ. Migraine in children and adolescents. *Pediatr Rev* 1982B;3:257–262.

Swaiman KF, Frank Y. Seizure headaches in children. *Dev Med Child Neurol* 1978;20:580–585.

Vahlquist BO. Migraine in children. *Int Arch Allergy* 1955; 7:348–355.

Weisberg LA, Chutorian AM. Pseudotumor cerebri of childhood. *Am J Dis Child* 1977;131:1243–1248.

Chapter 12

Child and Adolescent Sleep Disorders

Ronald E. Dahl, MD

INTRODUCTION

By early school age, the average child has spent nearly half of his or her life asleep. Despite the ubiquity of this state in young children, the basic function of sleep and its relationship to development remain a mystery. The absence of an identified function becomes even more intriguing when one considers sleep as an *active* process. Research has shown that sleep is not a uniform state of rest but an active cycling of different states. These states appear to create categoric changes in awareness and responsiveness to the environment and altered regulation in many physiologic systems such as muscle tone and temperature regulation.

In clinical practice, sleep problems face clinicians and parents on a daily basis. Sleep-related complaints are raised by families in an estimated 5% of all visits to pediatricians and 10% of visits to child psychiatrists. More comprehensive assessments of sleep in these populations (with semistructured interviews) indicate that sleep-related problems occur in up to 30% of children seeking health care services. A wide range of behavioral, psychiatric, and medical disorders can disturb sleep in children. In turn, sleep disturbances can influence many behaviors and physiologic systems. These interactions complicate the evaluation and treatment of sleep disorders in children. Some understanding of sleep physiology and the normal development of sleep patterns in children is an essential component of the clinical evaluation and treatment of these problems.

PHYSIOLOGY AND NORMAL DEVELOPMENT

Sleep is traditionally described in terms of stages based on measures of electroencephalogram (EEG), muscle tone (EMG), and eye movements (EOG). The three broad categories of state (see Table 12.1) consist of awake, rapid eye movement (REM) sleep, and non-REM sleep. Non-REM sleep is further subdivided into stages 1, 2, 3, and 4. Stage 1 is light sleep or drowsiness. Stage 2 is the most commonly occurring stage of sleep; it is of medium depth and characteristically has features of spindles and K-complexes in the EEG. Stages 3 and 4 are also given the name *slow-wave sleep* or *delta sleep* because of the low-frequency and high-amplitude waves in the delta frequency band (0.5 to 2 Hz) in EEG terminology.

From a physiologic perspective, a contrast between REM and delta sleep (as shown in Table 12.2) is most illustrative. REM sleep is also called "paradoxical sleep" because it has some aspects of being a deep sleep stage and some aspects of a light sleep. During

Table 12.1.
Sleep Stages

Awake
Rapid eye movement (REM) sleep
Non-REM sleep:
    Non-REM Stage 1—(drowsiness or light sleep)
    Non-REM Stage 2—(spindle sleep)
    Non-REM Stage 3 ⎫
                 ⎬(delta or slow wave sleep)
    Non-REM Stage 4 ⎭

REM sleep the tone of most voluntary muscles drops dramatically, the result of active postsynaptic inhibition emanating from a small region in the pons of the brain. This relative muscle paralysis may, according to one hypothesis, prevent body movements from occurring with activation of motor cortex during dreams. The regulation of temperature, blood pressure, heart rate, and respiration appears to have greater variability and less precise control during REM sleep. In contrast, cerebral metabolic activity and total brain oxygen consumption are relatively high during REM sleep. The timing of REM sleep is linked to the circadian cycle of body temperature regulation, with the majority of REM usually occurring at 4 to 6 o'clock a.m. (near the body temperature nadir). When one is awakened from REM sleep, the return of alertness is relatively rapid and frequently is followed by descriptions of dream activity.

In contrast to REM sleep, delta (or slow-wave) sleep is a very deep stage of sleep resistant to arousal. If one is awakened from delta sleep, there is usually a state of being disoriented or in a "fog" that requires a few minutes' transition before being completely alert. Most delta sleep occurs early in the night within 1 to 3 hours of going to sleep. The amount and intensity of delta sleep are strongly influenced by the amount of prior wakefulness. Individuals who get by on very little sleep have relatively high percentages of delta sleep. Children show large amounts of deep delta sleep. During this intense delta sleep, children are very resistant to being awakened. One study examining the threshold of arousal in children showed that 123-dB tones delivered through earphones failed to result in any behavioral or EEG arousal in most children during delta sleep. When a tired child falls into delta sleep during a car ride or in the living room, parents can often pick up the child, change him into his pajamas, and place him in bed without any sign of the child's waking up.

Sleep stages can be further understood by examining the patterning of these stages in a typical child. Figure 12.1 shows an example of a sleep histogram from a 10-year-old child studied in our laboratory. The vertical axis is labeled with "awake" at the top, with stages 1, 2, 3, and 4 at progressively

Table 12.2.
Physiology of REM and Delta Sleep

REM	Delta (Stages 3 and 4)
Heart rate, respiratory rate, and BP variable	Heart rate and respiration rate slow; BP low but stable
Muscle tone absent	Muscle tone lower than when awake
Occurs primarily in the 2nd half of sleep	Occurs primarily in first third of night
Arousal from REM occurs easily with rapid return to an alert state, often with the description of a detailed dream	Very difficult to arouse from delta; afterward one is often in a confused "fog"
Amount and duration of REM is related to the core temperature cycle	Amount and duration of delta related to the length of previous wakefulness
EEG shows desynchronized, fast activity	EEG shows large, synchronized slow waves

SLEEP PATTERN IN AN EARLY SCHOOL-AGE CHILD

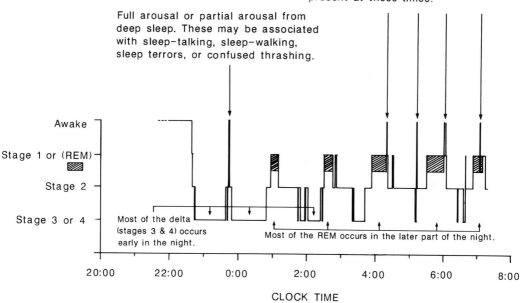

Brief wakings from stage 2 and REM; difficulties going back to sleep can present at these times.

Full arousal or partial arousal from deep sleep. These may be associated with sleep-talking, sleep-walking, sleep terrors, or confused thrashing.

Awake

Stage 1 or (REM)

Stage 2

Stage 3 or 4

Most of the delta (stages 3 & 4) occurs early in the night.

Most of the REM occurs in the later part of the night.

20:00   22:00   0:00   2:00   4:00   6:00   8:00

CLOCK TIME

Figure 12.1.   Sleep Pattern in an Early School-Age Child.

lower levels. "REM" is shown at the same level as stage 1, but with striped boxes, indicating its paradoxic relationship to sleep depth. After falling briefly into stage 1, this child quickly descended into stage 2 and after a few minutes proceeded into stages 3 and 4 (or delta sleep). The first delta period lasted approximately 60 minutes, then after a return to stage 2 (and a brief arousal), a second delta period occurred, lasting approximately another hour. In an older adolescent or an adult, the first REM period may have occurred 90 minutes into sleep (where stage 2 and a brief arousal occurred in this child). Children often skip this first REM period opportunity and go back to deep sleep, possibly because of their increased depth of sleep and increased sleep needs. As the night progressed, the child's sleep returned to lighter stage 2 followed by the first REM period.

REM periods are interspersed approximately every 60 to 90 minutes for the rest of the night with increased length of REM periods toward early morning.

Three important points are illustrated by this typical pattern of sleep and are relevant to our later discussion of specific sleep disorders. (1) Most of the delta sleep occurs within the first 1 to 3 hours after sleep onset. Hence, most of the disorders related to delta sleep (sleep terrors, sleepwalking, confused arousals) occur at this time of night. (2) Most of the REM sleep occurs in the second half of the night. Hence, most REM-related disorders (such as nightmares) are more frequent in the early morning hours. (3) Short periods of wakefulness typically occur five to seven times a night in normal sleep. During most of these arousals, the child quickly returns to sleep after a brief adjustment in sleeping position, covers, pillows, etc., with no memory of the event in the morning. Difficulties going back to sleep following these normal arousals can often present to the parents as if something is recurrently waking the child.

Age-Related Changes in Sleep

Among the factors that influence sleep, age appears to exert the greatest effect. The total amount of sleep, the patterning of stages, and the rate of cycling all change significantly across ages. The most dramatic alterations occur through infancy. Newborns spend more than 16 of 24 hours asleep. They begin their sleep cycle with REM sleep (this is called "active sleep" in newborns) and cycle from REM to non-REM every 50 to 60 minutes. The short sleep bouts of infants (equally distributed between night and daytime) gradually give way to longer periods of wakefulness predominating (the parents hope) during daylight hours. By age 1, the average child sleeps 11 hours at night and obtains another 2½ hours of sleep from two daytime naps. By age 3, the average child sleeps 10½ hours at night with one 1½ hour nap. The average American child ceases to nap by age 4 or 5 years. There is a gradual decrease in total amount of sleep from age 5 (approximately 10.5 hours) to adult levels (of approximately 8 hours a night) at age 18. There is a great deal of individual variation in total requirements. There is also considerable social influence on sleep and napping behavior; for example, daytime naps continue through adulthood in some cultures.

In addition to changes in the total amount of sleep, increasing age is also accompanied by significant changes in certain sleep stages. There is a gradual drop of REM sleep, and a very significant decrease in delta sleep. Both the amount of delta sleep and wave amplitude of delta EEG waves decrease from age 4 to adolescence. Between the ages of 10 and 20, although there are small changes in the total

amount of nocturnal sleep, delta sleep decreases by nearly 40%. One hypothesis suggests that this age-related decline in delta sleep parallels loss of cortical synaptic density.

Age also influences sleep efficiency. Young children have very short intervals of arousal during the night. Almost all of the time from going to bed to waking up in the morning is spent in stages 2, 3, 4 and REM sleep, resulting in very high sleep efficiency. With increasing age, this sleep efficiency goes down, with more frequent wakefulness and stage 1 interspersed through the nocturnal period.

Symptoms of daytime sleepiness also change with age. Daytime sleepiness is determined objectively in sleep laboratories with tests such as the Multiple Sleep Latency Test (MSLT). The MSLT measures the ability to fall asleep during specific daytime nap opportunities. Young children, ages 6 to 12 (who are such efficient sleepers at night), are remarkably alert and nonsleepy on these tests during the daytime. The daytime sleepiness increases significantly with the onset of adolescence. Although some of the adolescent sleepiness may be the result of inadequate nighttime sleep, evidence also suggests that physiologic changes in sleep regulation (occurring with puberty) may account for part of this increase in sleepiness.

In addition to any physiologic increase in sleepiness during adolescence, there is also substantial evidence that many adolescents in our society are relatively sleep-deprived. Research in this area indicates that early morning school schedules combined with late-night social schedules frequently contribute to inadequate sleep in this age group. Although some high school students can get by on 6 to 7 hours of sleep during the school week, their sleep behaviors on weekends and vacations support the idea that their true sleep needs are greater. At least one study indicates that many of these adolescents show significant sleepiness in the classroom. The effects of this relative sleep deprivation are not well-understood at this time. From a clinical standpoint, many adolescents evidently develop problems with sleep scheduling because of increasingly later schedules, erratic napping, and dramatically altered sleep on the weekends. Many adolescents develop such disturbed sleep/wake schedules that they are unable to awaken consistently for school even when they are highly motivated.

PEDIATRIC SLEEP DISORDERS

Some understanding of sleep disorders is essential for child psychiatrists because: (1) Sleep disorders can be mistaken for psychiatric disorders; (2) psychiatric disorders can cause sleep disturbances; and (3) both the primary sleep disorders and sleep complaints secondary to psychiatric disorders can present for psychiatric evaluation.

There are a number of classification systems for sleep disorders, including those developed by the American Sleep Disorders Association and the DSM III-R diagnoses in the psychiatric literature. These classification systems were developed primarily for adult sleep disorders, and some of the details of these classification systems are not applicable to the younger age groups. (At the time of this writing, a new International Classification of Sleep Disorders (ICSD) system is being developed.) For this discussion a very simple classification of problems is used, dividing the disorders into three general categories. The first is problems of insomnia or the sleepless child. The second includes sleepiness/hypersomnolence in children and adolescents. Under the category of hypersomnolence the topics of sleep-disordered breathing, narcolepsy, and scheduling disorders are addressed. The third category consists of the parasomnias or abnormal

behaviors associated with sleep (sleep-related problems), including night terrors, sleepwalking, nightmares, headbanging, enuresis, and sleep-related seizures.

Assessment/Interview

The initial assessment of the child or adolescent with sleep complaints involves a thorough interview of the patient and family members to obtain a wide range of sleep-related information. This should include usual sleep/wake habits, bedtime routines, descriptions of middle-of-the-night behaviors (including parental responses to these arousals), wake-up times, morning routines, and symptoms of daytime sleepiness or irritability. The interview should assess the duration, frequency, and patterns of symptoms, including timing, changes with weekends and vacations, and changes with stresses or special events. Past medical history, medications (especially stimulants, asthma medications, antiseizure drugs, and sedatives), and family history of sleep problems can also be important. A 2-week *prospective* sleep log or diary can be an excellent source of more detailed and accurate information. Parents and/or the patient should record the details of bedtime, estimated time to fall asleep, wake-up times, and the details of symptoms. Additional aspects of the interview and assessment are addressed within discussions of specific sleep complaints and disorders.

INSOMNIA/SLEEPLESS CHILD

Resistance to going to bed or to sleep is a very frequent complaint of parents of younger children. Bedtime and middle-of-the-night struggles are often a source of considerable stress to both parents and children and often contribute to inadequate sleep for many family members. Studies suggest that approximately 30% of 1- and 2-year-olds have frequent nighttime arousals that disturb their parents. There is further evidence that nighttime awakenings continue to be a problem in as many as 30% of children up to school age. Although medical problems (such as pain from an ear infection, allergy to cow's milk, colic, or the itching of atopic dermatitis) can contribute significantly to this problem in some children, the majority of cases result from behavioral and learned factors. Sleep-onset associations and learned self-comforting behaviors are crucial factors in children's learning to sleep through the night. The focus of this chapter is school-aged and adolescent problems, so this topic is not discussed in detail here; preschool-aged sleep problems have been well reviewed elsewhere (Ferber, 1987B).

In school-aged children and adolescents, additional issues must be considered in conjunction with symptoms of insomnia. Anxieties and worries can contribute to difficulties falling asleep in a manner similar to that in adults. For many active children, lying down to go to sleep is a time when they begin to reflect on conflicts from the day and sources of anxiety. In some children, this becomes a habit that interferes with going to sleep. Periods of anxiety and tension can become associated with bedtime to the point of severe insomnia. There is a wide range of individual patterns to this problem. Some children lie quietly in bed, making no noise, and the parents are unaware of the insomnia. Other children are disruptive, repeatedly get out of bed, or require parental intervention for a long time every night. Identifying the sources of anxiety and worry, encouraging the child to express these in appropriate ways during waking hours, and using relaxation exercises can all be important aspects to treating this problem. Helping the child learn to focus on positive images (which bring on relaxation) at bedtime can be essential. Consistent limit-setting by the parents, helping the child maintain a regular schedule, and helping the child establish new positive associations with bedtime can also be important factors. Although hypnotic medications such as diphenhydramine (Benedryl) are commonly used by many clinicians, these drugs often result in very limited, short-termed improvement and development of tolerance to the drug, with little long-term benefit. Short-term use of hypnotics can be combined with behavioral programs to help break the cycle of bad habits and negative associations with bedtime.

When insomnia is persistent it is important to also consider sleep/schedule or circadian disorders, or the possibility of psychiatric disorders such as depression and separation anxiety. These topics are addressed in later sections.

THE SLEEPY CHILD AND ADOLESCENT

Complaints of excessive sleepiness and/or increased needs for sleep occur occasionally in the older child and frequently in adolescents. A thorough and detailed history is an essential part of the evaluation of these complaints. It is important to characterize the nature of the sleepiness (that is, drifting off to sleep during boring activities versus sleep attacks), the frequency and duration of symptoms, and whether the symptoms are occurring at particular times of day or only during certain situations. A family history of increased sleep needs and sleepiness can be important in the consideration of narcolepsy and idiopathic central nervous system hypersomnolence. It is also essential to be aware of the wide individual variations in sleep needs. One perfectly normal child may require 2 more hours of sleep per night than does a same-aged peer or sibling.

The approach to the sleepy child or adolescent (see Table 12.3) consists of considering four basic categories of problems (see Table 12.4): (1) inadequate amounts of sleep; (2) disturbed nocturnal sleep; (3) increased sleep requirements despite adequate nocturnal sleep and (4) circadian and scheduling disorders. The history and evaluation should be directed at characterizing the problem with respect to these categories.

Inadequate Amounts of Sleep

The most common cause of mild-to-moderate sleepiness in adolescents is an inadequate number of hours in bed. A combination of social schedules leading to late nights with early-morning school requirements can significantly compress the number of hours of sleep. Part-time jobs, sports activities, hobbies, and active social lives can exacerbate this problem. The catch-up sleep of naps, weekends, and holidays can further contribute to the problem by leading to erratic schedules and even later nights. In taking a sleep history, it is important to ask specific questions concerning schedules. Many families will say the adolescent "usually" goes to bed at a certain time, but when asked for an exact time covering the previous few nights, a much later hour is reported. When assessing the amount of sleep, it is important to obtain details of bedtime (with lights out and the child or adolescent attempting to fall asleep), estimates of sleep latency, nighttime arousals, time of getting up in the morning, difficulty getting up, and the frequency, timing, and duration of daytime naps. It is also essential to get details of sleep/wake schedules on weekends as well as during the school week. When this type of specific information is obtained (either by interview or by having the family maintain a sleep diary), evidence of inadequate sleep is often evident. A prospective detailed sleep diary seems to provide the most reliable information.

When inadequate sleep is identified, recommendations that the adolescents go to bed earlier are unlikely to lead to significant changes in behavior for most adolescents. Often the primary role of the clinician is to help the entire family understand (and acknowledge the consequences resulting from) the inadequate sleep. Sleep deprivation frequently contributes to many factors that the family identifies as problems, including falling asleep in school, oversleeping in the morning, fatigue, and irritability. With respect to sleep (as in many areas of health), strategies of prevention and maintaining healthy habits make great common sense but have little salience in the decision-making processes of many adolescents until problems become severe. In cases in which the adolescent's school or social functioning is significantly impaired by the sleep problem, a strict behavioral contract (agreed upon by the family) can be essential. The contract should specify hours in bed (with only *small* deviations on the weekends) and target the specific behaviors contributing to bad sleep habits, such as specific late-night activities, erratic napping, oversleeping for school, etc. The choice of rewards for successes and negative consequences for failures as well as an accurate method of assessing compliance are essential components of the contract. (Also, see "Circadian and Scheduling Disorders;" these can lead to inadequate sleep.)

Disturbed Nocturnal Sleep

When symptoms of sleepiness occur despite an adequate schedule of hours in bed, disruptions of sleep should be considered. Disturbances within sleep can be more difficult to assess by history alone. Although some families may describe that the child or adolescent is waking frequently, in other cases the family may be unaware of subtle disruptions of sleep leading to daytime sleepiness. The use of drugs or alcohol is an important consideration in these cases. In addition to the obvious effects of late-night stimulants such as cocaine, there are also more complex drug/sleep interactions. Alcohol, for example, can facilitate sleep onset but can lead to decreased delta and REM sleep. Further, the

Table 12.3.
Approach to the Sleepy Adolescent

Carefully collect information on hours in bed, hours asleep, patterns of symptoms, napping, drugs/alcohol/medications, etc.

Adequate number of hours in bed?

— **YES** → Adequate number of hours asleep?

    YES

1. Symptoms of narcolepsy? Refer for sleep studies.
2. Symptoms of disrupted sleep? (snoring, restless sleep, frequent arousals) Evaluation and treatment; may require sleep studies
3. Symptoms of depression? Evaluation and treatment
4. Symptoms of Kleine-Levin syndrome? Evaluation and treatment
5. Evidence of drugs/alcohol? Evaluation and treatment
6. Evidence of objective sleepiness despite adequate night sleep? Consider idiopathic hypersomnolence; may require sleep studies

    NO

1. Evidence of delayed sleep phase insomnia? Consider chronotherapy
2. Evidence of depression? Evaluation and treatment
3. Evidence of drugs or alcohol? Evaluation and treatment
4. Evidence of conditioned insomnia? Consider behavioral therapy

— **NO** → Does the sleepiness significantly impact function or mood?

    YES

What are the specific causes of late night/early morning schedule? Problem-solve with family around specific late-night activities, early rising schedules, erratic sleep/wake hours, etc.

    NO

Recommend increased sleep, good sleep habits

Table 12.4.
Sources of Sleepiness in the Adolescent

Inadequate amounts of sleep:
  Light-night and erratic schedules
  Difficulty falling asleep
  Early morning awakening
Disturbed nocturnal sleep
  Sleep apnea syndrome
  Frequent nocturnal arousals
  Medical problems disturbing sleep
  Use of drugs and/or alcohol
  Withdrawal from drugs/alcohol
Increased sleep requirements:
  Narcolepsy
  Idiopathic CNS hypersomnolence
  Some cases of depression
  Kleine-Levin syndrome
Circadian and scheduling disorders:
  Delayed sleep phase syndrome

withdrawal from stimulants, alcohol, and marijuana can produce transient but severe sleep disruptions. Caffeine is also a commonly used substance in the adolescent population in the form of caffeinated sodas, coffee, and tea. Elimination of caffeine can be an important step in treating symptoms of difficulty falling asleep, which can lead to daytime sleepiness. Prescription medications such as beta-adrenergic agonists for asthma or stimulants for attention deficit disorder can also result in significant sleep disruptions.

A few *specific* sources of daytime sleepiness should be considered in this age group (sleep-disordered breathing, narcolepsy, and sleep/wake schedule disorders) and are discussed in greater detail.

Sleep Disordered Breathing. During sleep, and particularly in REM sleep, there is a considerable drop in muscle tone. This decreased tone affects the musculature maintaining the airway and the muscles assisting in respiration. In susceptible individuals, these physiologic changes can lead to obstructive sleep apnea syndrome (OSAS). In adults the clinical picture of OSAS is typically an obese, hypersomnolent, lethargic in-

dividual. In children the clinical appearance is quite different. The most common cause of OSAS in children is hypertrophy of adenoids and tonsils. Many of these children have little difficulty breathing when awake; however, with decreased muscle tone during sleep, the airway becomes smaller, airway resistance increases, and the work of breathing increases. An analogy can be made of breathing through a small, flimsy straw with the straw occasionally collapsing and obstructing air flow. In its severe form, these apneic episodes result in nocturnal hypoxemia and bradycardia and can lead to pulmonary hypertension with cor pulmonale. More commonly in children, however, they result in frequent brief arousals from sleep. Many of the short apneas (lasting only a few to 10 seconds) cause a brief arousal that increases the muscle tone to the neck and pharyngeal muscles, opens the airway, and allows the child to resume breathing. In some cases without actual obstruction or apnea, the increased work of breathing through a very small airway can significantly disturb sleep in children (Guilleminault, 1982). Although the actual number of minutes of arousal during the night may be small, the repeated, chronic, but brief disruptions in sleep can lead to significant daytime symptoms in children. (A comparable image would be answering a wrong number on the telephone 15 to 30 times a night.) It is important to note that the child is usually unaware of waking up, and the parent often describes very restless sleep but usually does not describe the child's waking up completely. The most frequent symptoms reported by families include loud chronic snoring (or noisy breathing), restless sleep with unusual sleeping positions (attempts by the child to move and open the airway), a history of problems with tonsils, adenoids, and/or ear infections, and *signs of inadequate nighttime sleep.* Although OSAS is being discussed under the heading of excessive sleepiness, it is important to note that preadolescent children often express inadequate sleep through a wide range of behavioral disturbances. Irritability, difficulty concentrating, decreased school performance, and oppositional behavior are often frequent components of sleepiness in younger children. Many of these children appear hyperactive (particularly in situations such as school) as a result of inadequate nighttime sleep. Previous researchers have noted the frequency of "hyperactivity" in children with obstructive sleep apnea (Guilleminault, 1982). Within the group of children diagnosed with OSAS in our center, 40% had previously been diagnosed with attention deficit disorder and were receiving psychostimulant medication. In many of these cases, the medication had improved symptoms of irritability and inattention. In some of these cases, the stimulants were primarily treating the symptoms of inadequate sleep.

The diagnosis of OSAS can often be made clinically. Many pediatric otolaryngologists are experienced in assessing children with signs of snoring and disturbed sleep for evidence of adenoidal hypertrophy. It is important to understand that even moderate-sized adenoids and tonsils (which cause no problems in the awake exam by the otolaryngologist) may produce obstructive symptoms during sleep. In questionable cases, or if there are reasons why tonsillectomy/ adenoidectomy are being discouraged, polysomnographic studies can aid in the diagnosis. However, it should be noted that sleep studies in children with this syndrome can be difficult to interpret. There are few normative studies in this age group that include nighttime pulmonary monitoring. Even more importantly, some children show such brief apneas that they do not meet published criteria for obstructive sleep apneas. Nonetheless, some of these children are working

so hard to breathe during their sleep that during weeks to months, they show significant signs of disturbed sleep. Laboratories that primarily study adults with sleep apnea or pulmonary laboratories that do not carefully assess the quality of the child's sleep can have difficulties diagnosing some of these cases. We have seen a number of children with relatively low apnea/hypopnea indices (which would fail to meet any criteria for OSAS) with convincing evidence of chronically disrupted sleep secondary to sleep-disordered breathing difficulties. Although the initial study may be borderline "normal", these children show significant improvements in sleep following tonsillectomy/ adenoidectomy. We recently reported a case of a 13-year-old boy whose sleep studies did not have sufficient apnea to meet any criteria for OSAS but whose sleep patterns were very suggestive of sleep-disordered breathing. He was referred to the pediatric otolaryngology center, where (although he had small tonsils) an adenoidectomy was scheduled because of the sleep study results. At surgery, a large polyp was discovered almost completely obstructing his airway. Following removal of the polyp, this boy had a significant improvement in his sleep and decrease in daytime symptoms of irritability and sleepiness.

The treatment of sleep-disordered breathing is most frequently the treatment of adenotonsillar hypertrophy. Referral to an otolaryngologist experienced with these problems is usually indicated. Certain categories of children are at high risk for sleep apnea, including those with maxofacial abnormalities, micrognathia, a history of cleft palates (particularly with pharyngeal flap repairs), and Down's syndrome.

Disorders of Increased Sleep Needs

Narcolepsy in Children.   Narcolepsy is a chronic disorder characterized by excessive daytime sleepiness and other abnormally timed elements of REM physiology such as muscle paralysis (cataplexy and sleep paralysis) and dream imagery (hypnogogic and hypnopopic hallucinations). It is not a rare disorder, affecting approximately 1 of 10,000 people in this country (a prevalence approximately that of multiple sclerosis). Narcolepsy appears to be a neurologic disorder with a strong genetic predisposition. Nearly all identified cases of narcolepsy have HLA-DR2 antigen. Family history of narcolepsy and/or excessive sleepiness can be helpful, though it is negative in many cases. Although traditionally the onset of narcolepsy is thought to be late adolescence and adulthood, there is increasing evidence that symptoms often begin in childhood.

The classic tetrad of symptoms in narcolepsy includes: (1) sleep attacks; (2) cataplexy (the sudden loss of muscle tone without change of consciousness); (3) sleep paralysis (inability to move after waking up); and (4) hypnogogic hallucinations (dream-like imagery before falling asleep). These symptoms do not all occur together or consistently in many cases of narcolepsy. Particularly in younger patients, signs of sleepiness may be the only initial symptom. Cataplexy is typically provoked by laughter, anger, or sudden emotional changes. It may be as subtle as a slight weakness in the legs, or as dramatic as a patient's falling to the floor limp and unable to move. If cataplectic attacks last long enough, full sleep can occur. In two of the childhood narcolepsy cases in our sleep center, mild symptoms of cataplexy were clearly evident only in retrospect following the diagnosis. In one case, the family indicated only after the sleep studies that for the previous year the girl had become "like Jello" whenever she laughed, but the family had not related this state to the questions that physicians had asked about paralysis or weakness. In another case a boy with cataplexy

had been frightened by the episodes and would not talk about them with anyone. Although a few events had occurred during school, the rapid recovery from the events and their strange quality had led people to believe that he was "faking it." Likewise, hypnogogic hallucinations can be difficult to elicit from a child's history. To further complicate matters, these symptoms often wax and wane in individuals with narcolepsy.

The diagnosis of narcolepsy requires evaluation in a sleep laboratory. Narcoleptics show early REM periods near sleep onset, fragmented nighttime sleep, excessive daytime sleepiness in objective nap studies during the day, and sleep-onset REM periods in naps. In prepubertal children, this diagnosis can be very difficult to establish (Kotagal et al., 1990). Repeat studies may be necessary before reaching a final diagnosis. One case recently diagnosed in our center occurred in a 13-year-old boy who had been hospitalized for 1 month with a diagnosis of "psychotic depression" before the diagnosis of narcolepsy was considered and established. This boy had withdrawn from school and social activities, was spending most of his time alone in his room (sleeping), and was having hallucinations that he would not discuss. In this case, the boy was so frightened by the hypnogogic hallucinations that he was fighting going to bed and going to sleep. He became sleep deprived, which further exacerbated his symptoms. His state of functioning deteriorated so severely that it led to the initial impression of psychosis and severe depression. The lack of response to psychotropics and observed episodes of cataplexy in the hospital eventually led to a sleep evaluation and the correct diagnosis of narcolepsy.

Treatment of narcolepsy is generally focused on (1) education and counseling of the patient and family, (2) adherence to a regular schedule to obtain optimal sleep with good sleep habits (often including scheduled naps), (3) use of short-acting stimulant medication for treatment of daytime sleepiness (with drug holidays to avoid build-up of tolerance), and (4) use of REM-suppressant medications (such as protriptyline) when symptoms of cataplexy are problematic.

Idiopathic Hypersomnolence. Some patients have signficantly increased sleep needs without evidence of the REM abnormalities seen in narcolepsy. This condition has been called *idiopathic hypersomnolence.* There is often a familial history of excessive sleep needs, and these individuals show clear objective sleepiness in nap studies despite having obtained what appears to be adequate amounts of nighttime sleep. These disorders are also frequently treated with stimulant medication when the diagnosis is definitively established and daytime functioning is impaired.

Kleine-Levin Syndrome. Symptoms of excessive somnolence, hypersexuality, and compulsive overeating were first described in adolescent boys by Kleine (1925) and Levin (1929). Mental disturbances (irritability, confusion, and occasional auditory or visual hallucinations) have also been reported in these cases.

This syndrome (with more than 100 published cases) occurs more frequently in males (3 : 1). Typically, symptoms being during adolescence either gradually or abruptly, and in about half the cases the onset follows a flu-like illness or injury with loss of consciousness. Frequently, there is an episodic nature to the symptoms, with cycles lasting from 1 to 30 days. The syndrome usually disappears spontaneously during late adolescence or early adulthood.

Laboratory tests, imaging studies, EEGs, and endocrine measures do not appear to be helpful in making the specific diagnosis of Kleine-Levin syndrome. It is important to rule out other organic causes of similar symptoms such as a hypothalamic tumor, localized CNS infection, or vascular accident. The presence of neurologic signs, evidence of increased CNS pressure, abnormalities in temperature regulation, abnormalities in water regulation, or other endocrine abnormalities point to an organically based abnormality. A family history of bipolar illness or other signs suggesting an early-onset bipolar illness should also be considered in the differential.

Although stimulant medication or use of lithium carbonate has been reported to be helpful in individual cases, there is no clear consensus on treatment.

CIRCADIAN AND SCHEDULING DISORDERS

Our understanding of normal circadian physiology has advanced considerably during the past 10 years. The presence of a biologic clock in the suprachiasmatic nucleus of the hypothalamus and our understanding of how the clock must be reset daily has contributed significantly to our understanding of jet lag, difficulties with shift work, and sleep disturbances resulting from altered circadian regulation. Circadian physiologists have elucidated a number of principles relevant to discussions dealing with sleep/schedule problems: (1) Without the input of external time cues, the human clock runs on a 25-hour period. Hence, in situations with weak time cues or low schedule demands, we tend to drift to later bedtimes and wake-up times (as often occurs on weekends). (2) There are individual components to this rhythmic system, including temperature rhythm, hormone rhythms, and sleep/wake rhythms. (3) Different components in the system have altered capacities for shifts and different adjustment rates following perturbation of the system. Hence, although the sleep/wake rhythm may adjust quickly to a new schedule, the circadian temperature rhythm may not realign for 5 to 7 days. (4) There are intervals of time (roughly corresponding to subjective dawn and dusk) when the circadian system seems to be much more sensitive to time cue information such as light, social interactions, and activity. (5) During certain phases of the circadian system, such as when the body temperature cycle is peaking, it is very difficult to go to sleep despite being tired and motivated by the knowledge that one needs to go to sleep.

These five principles are important in evaluating and treating disorders of the circadian system. (For a good review and discussion of circadian physiology see Moore-Ede, 1985.) The most common specific problem with this system, relevant to adolescents, is delayed sleep phase syndrome (DSPS). DSPS often begins with a tendency to stay up late at night, sleeping late, and/or taking a late afternoon nap. This process often begins on weekends, holidays, or summer vacations. Problems become apparent when school schedules result in morning wake-up battles and difficulties getting to school. Often these adolescents cope by taking afternoon naps and getting catch-up sleep on the weekends. Although some of these behaviors occur in many normal adolescents, in extreme cases the circadian system can become set to such a late time that even highly motivated adolescents can have difficulty shifting their sleep back to an earlier time. In some instances, the adolescents' (and their families') attempts to correct the problem go against circadian principles. For example, an adolescent who has been going to bed at 3 a.m. and getting up at noon during vacation tries to go to bed at 10 p.m. the Sunday night before the first day back at school and finds that her physiology is quite resistant to sleep. For a few days she manages to get up for school by overriding the system (despite inadequate sleep) but then takes a long nap

after school. Despite numerous nights of trying to go to bed at 10 p.m. she is unable to consistently shift her temperature cycle and circadian system back to an earlier phase.

The treatment of delayed sleep phase syndrome consists of two parts. The first is to *gradually* align the sleep system to the desirable schedule. The second is to maintain that alignment. The process of alignment consists of gradual, small, *consistent* advances in bedtime and wake-up time (15 minutes a day). It is often best to begin from the time the adolescent usually goes to sleep without difficulty. It is important during this process to avoid any naps and to be consistent across weekends and holidays. In severe cases, some adolescents on very late schedules respond more favorably to going around the clock with successive *delays* in bedtime. This process has been described as phase delay "chronotherapy." Since the biologic clock tends to run on a 25-hour cycle, it accommodates phase delays more easily than phase advances. Hence, the schedule changes can proceed with larger (2 to 3 hour) delays per day. An example is described for an adolescent who has been falling asleep at 3 a.m. and getting up at noon. On day 1 he stays up until 6 a.m. then sleeps until 3:00 p.m. On day 2 he goes to bed at 9 a.m. and sleeps until 6 p.m. On day 3 he sleeps from noon until 9 p.m.; day 4, from 3 p.m. until midnight; day 5, from 6 p.m. until 3 a.m.; day 6, from 9 p.m. until 6 a.m.; and day 7, from 10 p.m. until 7 a.m. He then strictly maintains the 10 p.m. to 7 a.m. sleep schedule. It is important that during the chronotherapy the adolescent take no naps. Upon waking up he should get some activity and, if possible, bright light exposure such as walking outdoors. Although many adolescents do very well with this type of phase delay chronotherapy, the first weekend or vacation of returning to old habits can undo a lot of hard work. Particularly in the first 2 to 3 weeks following chronotherapy, rigid requirements should be set about wake-up time 7 *days a week*. Later, if the adolescent wants to stay up late on an occasional weekend night, he may be able to do so but should not be permitted to sleep more than 1 or 2 hours later than his usual wake-up time for school. Strict behavioral contracts (worked out with the parents), with specific rewards for success and serious consequences for failures, are essential in this type of intervention.

At least two other disorders can mimic a delayed sleep phase syndrome. One disorder involves adolescents who appear to have trouble following an early schedule but are not particularly troubled by their late schedule. These adolescents are not motivated to correct the problem, are not particularly troubled by their recurrent experiences of being late for or missing school, and do not show great motivation to change their late-night habits. These adolescents are essentially *choosing* a late night schedule. Unless the clinician is able to alter the larger realm of priorities and motivators, these adolescents are very unlikely to respond to any treatment of a sleep/schedule problem.

A second group of adolescents, who initially appear to have delayed sleep phase syndrome, reveals a history of requiring very long periods of time to fall asleep, no matter how late they go to bed. In these adolescents, a conditioned insomnia (as described in "Insomnia/Sleepless Child") is a larger component of the problem than the schedule itself. For an overview of the clinical approach to the adolescent with sleep delay symptoms, see Figure 12.2.

Occasionally, one encounters a child or adolescent who appears to have a totally chaotic sleep schedule. Sleep appears to be scattered across night and day in a random fashion, with no clear pattern. One of the most helpful assessment tools for such a problem is a well-documented sleep diary or sleep chart.

Details of individual sleep bouts collected prospectively can then be plotted on a chart, which can indicate patterns not evident by taking the history alone. An example of one such child is shown in Figure 12.3 in what is termed a "double-plot." Sleep is shown in black and awake in white, with 48 hours of data on each line. The history of this child was that his sleep was completely erratic. He was described as staying up all day and all night followed by interspersed long sleep, then short naps, etc. The chart shows that between the dates of 8/19 and 9/7, his sleep was following a periodicity of 25.6 hours. This was despite the fact that he was going to school from 8 a.m. to 3 p.m. This child had a free-running circadian system, with his sleep following that cycle. This boy had some features of autism, and we believe his free-running rhythm was related to his pattern of social interactions. As shown in the diagram, following intervention with a structured behavioral program to eliminate naps and enforce a strict sleep and social schedule, his sleep lined up in a 24-hour rhythm. It was interesting to us that following the intervention he no longer showed evidence of inadequate sleep, and the family reported significant improvements in irritability and behavioral problems. Although this is a very unusual case in many ways, it points out the value of obtaining specific sleep schedule information in a way that permits visual evaluation of the pattern of sleep.

PARASOMNIAS

Parasomnia is the term given to one of a group of unusual behaviors emerging from sleep. These include sleepwalking, night terrors, confused partial arousals, enuresis, and nightmares. Headbanging and nocturnal seizures are also addressed under this topic as other unusual sleep-related events in children.

Partial Arousals

Sleepwalking, sleeptalking, and sleep terrors are all variations of partial arousals from deep (usually stages 3 and 4) sleep. As discussed earlier, most children have a very deep period of slow-wave sleep during the first 1 to 3 hours after sleep onset. At the end of this very deep sleep period, the transition to lighter sleep, REM sleep, or a brief arousal is often accompanied by unusual transition behaviors. If observed closely (as in a sleep lab), many children are seen to mumble, grimace, or demonstrate some awkward movements during this transition. Sometimes these transition episodes consist of talking, calm sleepwalking, agitated sleepwalking, confused partial arousals, and, at times, what appears to be a panic-like event. During these episodes, the child remains essentially asleep and has no memory of the event in the morning. The episodes can last from seconds to 30 minutes, with most events lasting 2 to 10 minutes. Because many parents think the child is having a nightmare or dream, they often attempt to wake and reassure the child. This can result in a very disorienting process for the parent, since the child often stares blankly, does not recognize the parents, and can appear incoherent. Sometimes children thrash wildly, let out blood-curdling screams, and bolt away from parents. The event usually terminates spontaneously with the child's returning to deep sleep. Attempts at waking the child are usually unsuccessful. The child is often completely unaware of the event (occasionally there is a vague image or fragmented memory, but nothing like the detailed imagery related to dreaming or nightmares).

The cause of these events is unknown. It appears as if some fragmentation of the normal transition from deep sleep to light sleep results in part of the child's system's being in a very high arousal state while part of the system is still in a very deep sleep. The individual characteristics of these partial arousals (whether they are intense, associated with fear, etc.) may be related to the level and location of the areas involved in the arousal. The intensity of deep delta sleep appears to have an important relationship to the occurrence of these events. The frequency of these events is highest in the age groups with the highest amount of delta sleep. These events also occur more often in families with higher amounts of deep delta sleep and with increased sleep needs. In addition, conditions that lead to increased delta sleep within an individual, such as sleep loss or being overly tired, are associated with increased partial arousals. As the pressure for delta sleep goes up, the transition out of delta sleep appears to be more difficult. The history of children with frequent night terrors or partial arousals often indicates that these events occur in conjunction with chaotic sleep schedules, on the nights of recovery sleep following sleep loss, in conjunction with a change in schedule (such as beginning earlier mornings for school or daycare), or following periods of stress.

There has also been considerable discussion about the role of psychologic characteristics in these events. Previous authors have written about the association of anxiety with night terrors, describing the role of unexpressed anxieties, fears, and conflicts in contributing to the occurrence of partial arousals at night. Clinical experience from our sleep center supports these impressions. We have observed many children with frequent night terrors as anxious, tense children whose parents describe them as extremely well-behaved. Although there appears to be some convergence of clinical impressions, at this time there is little empiric evidence to support these observations.

Some partial arousals are quite common in younger children. Sleepwalking episodes occur in approximately 10% of children aged

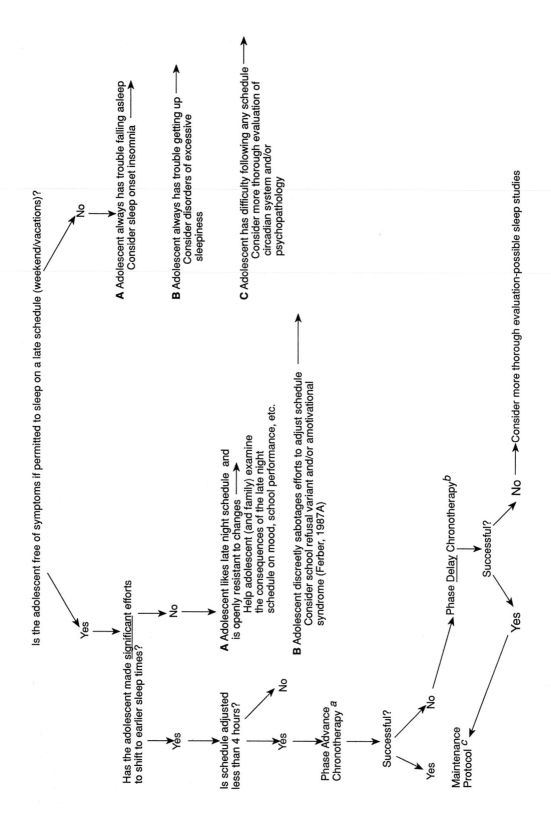

3 to 12 years. Other estimates indicate that approximately 5% of the children in this age group sleepwalk regularly and that as many as 20% have had at least one episode of sleepwalking. Sleep terrors appear to be less frequent, with estimates ranging from 1 to 6% in this age group. There are some discrepancies among reported rates of partial arousals. One source of variance may be the difficulty in measuring the occurrence of these events, which the children do not remember and the parents may not observe. Surveys are more likely to measure the rates at which these problems affect the parents rather than their true incidence. Clearly, however, as delta sleep drops off in adolescence, the frequency of all of these delta-related events drops off dramatically. Adult sleep clinicians have expressed the opinion

that the persistence of these partial arousals into adulthood is often associated with psychopathology or organic disorders.

There are a number of considerations in the clinical evaluation and treatment of these problems. The first is to identify clearly that the episode is in fact a partial arousal. A contrast between night terrors and nightmares is given in Table 12.5. Occurrence during the first third of the night, a state of confusion and partial arousal, the duration of the event, lack of memory of the event in the morning, a quick return to deep sleep following the event, and an increase in the frequency of events following sleep loss (or being overly tired) all strongly support the diagnosis of partial arousals. Once the problem is identified, it is important to explain to the parents and the rest of the family what

---

Figure 12.2.   Approach to the adolescent with delayed sleep phase symptoms (difficulty going to sleep until very late hours and great difficulties getting up in the morning until late hours). *ᵃPhase advance chronotherapy*. (*1*) Shift bedtime and wake-up time gradually (15 min/day) to earlier time, beginning at adolescent's "desired" schedule. (*2*) Encourage bright light exposure and moderate activity within 30 to 60 minutes of wake-up time (ideally, a 5 to 10 minute walk outside). (*3*) During the phase advance, absolutely no: (a) naps; (b) deviations in the schedule for weekends, vacations; (c) caffeine, alcohol, drugs. (*4*) Behavioral contract signed by family specifying each night's bedtime (with lights out, no TV, radio, phone, etc.) and wake-up time (awake, standing, with lights on) with contingent rewards for success and loss of privileges for failures. (*5*) After schedule has aligned to desired time, adolescent is to follow the schedule rigidly for 2 weeks (including weekends) before beginning maintenance protocol. *ᵇPhase delay chronotherapy*. (*1*) Delay bedtime and wake-up time by 3 hours each night, beginning at adolescent's usual time of falling asleep. (*2*) During phase delay process, adolescent is to take no naps and no caffeine or alcohol. (*3*) At "bedtime" lights are out, no TV, phone, music; at wake-up time, adolescent is to be awake, standing, with lights on. (*4*) A behavioral contract signed by family members should be made specifying rewards for success and loss of privileges for failures to follow the schedule and rules. (*5*) When bedtime and wake-up align to desired time (e.g., 10:30 p.m. to 6:30 a.m.), that schedule should be followed rigidly for 2 weeks (including weekends), again with a behavioral contract specifying bedtimes, wake-up times, and absence of naps, caffeine, etc., before beginning maintenance protocol. *ᶜMaintenance protocol*. Following successful chronotherapy and 2 weeks of rigid scheduling, the adolescent must understand that he/she is vulnerable to slipping back to the old schedule and problems. To prevent recurrence, the following steps should be followed: (*1*) On weekends/vacations, the schedule should not deviate by more than 2 hours, trying to stay as close as possible to the usual weekday schedule. (*2*) If the adolescent stays up very late one night for a special event, he/she is still to get up within 2 hours of the usual school wake-up time and avoid naps. (*3*) Follow rules of good sleep hygiene: (a) Bed should be used only for sleeping. (b) Regular prebedtime ritual followed by lights out at a specific time. (c) Focus on positive, relaxing images while trying to fall asleep. (d) Brisk wake-up and get-up routine with bright light exposure and moderate activity within 30 to 60 minutes. (e) Avoid daytime naps, and avoid caffeine after 12:00 noon. (*4*) A behavioral contract should be made specifying the exact rules with contingent rewards/loss of privileges for continuing the maintenance protocol. (Adapted from Ferber R. Circadian and schedule disturbances. In: Guilleminault C, ed. Sleep and its disorders in children. New York: Raven Press, 1987A.)

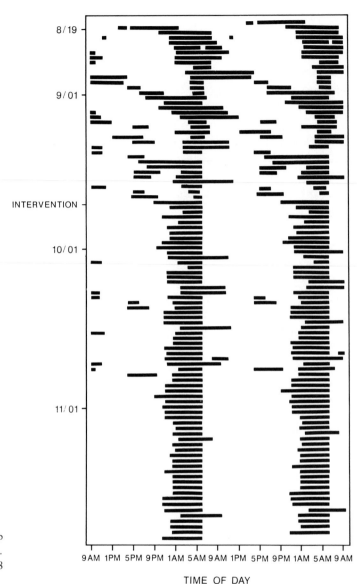

Figure 12.3. Double plot of sleep in a boy with a free-running rhythm. Sleep is shown in black bars with 48 hours of data on each line.

the event is and what it is not. Reassurance of the family is one of the most important roles of the clinician. The next step should be to address the adequacy of the child's sleep and schedule. Increasing the amount of sleep and introducing more consistency into the schedule of the child can result in a dramatic decrease in the frequency of events. In ad-

dition, it is important to identify the child with an occult insomnia. Some children go quietly to bed and lie awake 1 to 2 hours (without disturbing their parents) before going to sleep. Also, disturbances in the quality of sleep (such as sleep-disordered breathing or frequent middle-of-the-night awakenings) also result in a relative sleep def-

Table 12.5.
Contrast Between Night Terrors and Nightmares

Night Terrors	Nightmares
Occur during stage 4 sleep	Occur during REM sleep
Usually occur in first third of night	Usually occur in last half of night
Child appears confused, half asleep, or extremely agitated	Child often describes detailed dream
Child often does not recognize parents, is difficult to reassure	Child usually wants parental reassurance
Event usually lasts 2 to 10 minutes and terminates abruptly with return to deep sleep	Child often has difficulty going back to sleep, may want to stay with parents, talk, leave lights on, etc.
Can be accompanied by extreme autonomic arousal (dilated pupils, tachycardia) as well as piercing screams	Child can appear frightened and typically calms in response to reassurance

icit, increased intensity of delta, and more frequent partial arousals. In addition to identifying and treating the causes of disturbances in the amount and quality of sleep, at least one author has shown evidence that in some cases, helping the child to express feelings and emotions during the day has decreased the frequency of night terrors (Klackenberg, 1987).

Medications such as a bedtime dose of diazepam or imipramine significantly decrease delta sleep and temporarily improve the situation in the child with frequent night terrors. Often when the medication is stopped, however, there are rebound delta and rebound partial arousals. In some cases when night terrors or partial arousals are extremely frequent, occur repeatedly within a single night, or are severely disruptive to the family, medications can be an important temporary adjunct to treatment. In these situations, often so much tension and fear are associated with going to bed and going to sleep that it is important to "break the cycle" of sleep deprivation, disturbed sleep, increased pressure for delta, and frequent night terrors. Short-term use of medication (such as 25 to 75 mg of imipramine at bedtime) in this situation can help create a window for more lasting intervention.

Ensuring physical safety for the child with partial arousals is essential. In this state, children can fall down stairs, walk through windows, or fall from upper bunks. Altering the sleep environment to minimize the risk of serious injuries is an essential aspect of dealing with these problems.

Nightmares

Nightmares, in contrast ot night terrors, are REM-related events. These are quite common in children, occurring occasionally in most youngsters. However, frequent and recurrent nightmares are not common. One of the first steps in assessing frequent nightmares is distinguishing them from night terrors. Since nightmares occur more frequently during REM, they are much more likely to happen in the second half of the night. The child is not awake during the nightmare: they awake *following* the nightmare. When a parent encounters the child awakening from a nightmare, the child is alert and often describes detailed scenes of frightening images. The child typically has difficulty going back to sleep and often wants to remain with the parents. (With night terrors, in contrast, the child often does not recognize the parent and returns quickly to a very deep sleep.) Another important distinction is that in the morning, children frequently continue to remember and talk about their nightmares, whereas children with night terrors usually have no memory or only the vaguest image of the night terror. Although these distinctions are relatively easy to make in the older child, they can be difficult in a younger child with limited verbal abilities.

Frequent and recurrent nightmares do occur in children. Frightening television programs, movies, and threatening events during the day are often important factors contributing to these events. Often, parents are unaware of their children's access to material on cable television and video cassette recorder that can be extremely disturbing to children and adolescents. In addition, traumatic events can lead to recurrent nightmares. Common-sense approaches to addressing the sources of a child's fears and anxieties are sufficient in many cases. However, there is a wide range of clinical opinions (particularly in the psychoanalytic literature) on issues of dream content and nightmares.

Enuresis

Nocturnal enuresis is an extremely common sleep-related problem that has been the focus of writings by many psychologists, psychiatrists, pediatricians, urologists, endocrinologists, and other health care workers. It is likely that a variety of etiologic factors are relevant in different cases of nocturnal enuresis. There is an increasing understanding of small functional bladder capacity, variance in the strength of the child's urethral sphincter, and variance in the neurologic connections sensing and responding to bladder contractions and sphincter tone. One additional factor in many cases of enuresis is the subset of children for whom very deep sleep is an important component of their nocturnal enuresis. In some of these children enuresis occurs in the first third of the night. It is hard to imagine that bladder capacity or inadequate amounts of a hormone to concentrate urine are important factors in children who wet the bed an hour after going to sleep. A large number of children with enuresis show a good response to any of the traditional treatments: imipramine, nocturnal alarm, reinforcement techniques, or combinations of these. However, there is a subgroup of children who do not respond to these treatments. In these children, enuresis may be a variant of a partial arousal as described previously. It is important to note that the same factors contributing to sleep loss and partial arousals (sleep loss, obstructive sleep apnea syndrome, being over-tired) are also associated with enuresis. In some of these cases, identifying and treating the cause of inadequate or disturbed sleep can significantly improve the enuresis. In other children, enuresis occurring during deep sleep seems to be related to genetic or constitutional factors.

The approach at our center with these difficult cases is to use a treatment program that addresses multiple components of the system. Specifically, bladder and sphincter training exercises are combined with self-awakening exercises and a behavioral program. When necessary, a battery-operated underwear wetness alarm is added. The children are on a program in which they delay urination as long as possible with the goal of increasing the volume of the void. They then void into a measured container, trying to break their previous mark on the container. The child is also instructed, when he is in the state of having a very full bladder, to go into his bedroom, get into bed under the covers, turn out the lights, and, as much as possible, simulate the state of being asleep. Then while imagining that he is asleep, he is to focus on the sensation of the full bladder. He is then to get up from bed and void into his container and try to break his record. Before going to sleep at night, he is to review the entire scene and tell himself that when he has that familiar sensation he will wake up on his own and go to the bathroom. The use of the alarm can be an adjunct to this program if the child is not able to wake up sufficiently to complete the rest of the program. The motivation of the child, the co-operation of the family, and "star" charts with appropriate rewards for the child's successes are also central parts of the program. A good description of this type of program for parents is also available (Ferber, 1985).

Recently there has been considerable interest in the use of intranasal vasopressin (DDAVP) in the treatment of enuresis. DDAVP is a synthetic version of the endogenous peptide vasopressin, which is involved in concentrating urine. There is a theory that abnormal circadian fluctuations in vasopressin contribute to enuresis in some children. In short-term trials, DDAVP clearly increases urine concentration, decreases urine volume, and decreases problems with enuresis. For situations such as overnight stays with friends or going to camp, DDAVP can be extremely helpful. In general, we have found medications to be unnecessary if the child and family are able to carry out the bladder training and behavioral programs.

Headbanging and Variants—Rocking, etc.

Headbanging (jactatio capitas nocturna) is the stereotypic, rhythmic movement of the head and upper body during sleep, drowsiness, or rest. This occurs frequently in young infants, with estimates that 3 to 15% of normal, healthy children evidence some headbanging in the first year of life. The behavior usually disappears by age 4 but can persist through adolescence and into adulthood. Persistence beyond 10 years of age is reported to be associated with mental retardation or psychopathology.

Most headbanging occurs at the onset of sleep, beginning during the drowsiness prior to sleep onset. Many children have recurrence of headbanging in the middle of the night during sleep stage transitions back to wakefulness; that is, these children also seem to headbang in order to go back to sleep after waking up during the night. Some studies have shown that many children continue headbanging into stage 2 sleep. Some children seem to use headbanging as a self-comforting behavior even when they are awake during times of rest. Episodes typically last 5 to 15 minutes; however, many last as long as 1½ to 4 hours. The activity is often more rapid than one would imagine, with an average frequency of 45 bangs per minute and a reported range of 19 to 121 bangs per minute. The etiology of headbanging is not clearly identified. Although organic etiologies have been suspected on the basis of association with mental retardation, other researchers have supported psychopathologic etiologies. An alternative interpretation is that this is a learned behavior, reinforced by pleasurable sensations arising from the activity itself. There is a suggestion that the pleasurable sensations are mediated by the vestibular pathways as a form of self-stimulation.

Treatment approaches have included behavioral modification programs (which have been successful in many younger children). Psychiatric and neurologic evaluations may be indicated for older children when headbanging persists beyond 3 years of age. Benzodiazepines and tricyclic antidepressant medications have also been reported to be helpful in some cases.

Sleep and Seizures

One of the difficulties facing sleep clinicians, who frequently study sleep, is that many normal children do strange things in their sleep. Transitions out of stage 4 and events during partial arousals can be quite bizarre in nature. Although many of these are easily typified as partial arousals, one must also confront the statistic that seizures occur predominantly during sleep or on arousal from sleep in as many as 50 to 80% of epileptics (Shouse,

1989). The electroencephalographic synchronization occurring during non-REM sleep appears to be conducive to the spread of abnormal discharges. In addition, the transition into and out of sleep can activate seizures (this is one of the values of performing diagnostic EEGs in the sleep-deprived state). The relationship between sleep and seizures is complex and not well understood. For the purposes of this consideration, it is important to note that: (1) There are rare cases in which seizures occur only during sleep when a seizure disorder has not otherwise been considered. (2) An EEG overnight sleep study is not the equivalent of a clinical EEG evaluation. The limited number of EEG electrodes (usually only to 1 to 3 channels in sleep studies) and slow paper speed (to permit all-night recording) do not permit the specific EEG information obtained in a full 10/20 EEG for a neurologic evaluation. (3) Often it is necessary to obtain support from both a neurologist and sleep clinician working together to reach a diagnosis of unusual events occurring in sleep.

SLEEP CHANGES ASSOCIATED WITH PSYCHIATRIC DISORDERS

Disturbed sleep is a common symptom associated with many psychiatric disorders. In studies of adult psychiatric patients, these complaints are frequently accompanied by objective alterations in sleep. These measures of altered sleep have been used as psychobiologic markers, particularly with respect to adult affective disorders. EEG sleep studies of adult patients with major depressive disorder (MDD) have reported evidence of altered sleep in approximately 90% of the subjects (Reynold and Kupfer, 1987). The specific abnormalities described in adults during episodes of depression consist of: (1) difficulty initiating and maintaining sleep (problems falling asleep, increased nocturnal awakenings and early morning awakenings); (2) diminished delta sleep (stages 3 and 4 sleep); (3) earlier occurrence of the first REM sleep period of the night (re-

duced REM latency); and (4) an altered pattern of REM sleep, with longer and more intense early REM periods.

Child and Adolescent Depression

Sleep studies of child and adolescent affective disorders have not yielded the same consistent pattern of altered sleep (Dahl et al., 1990). Of the eight well-controlled drug-free studies in this age group, only three of the studies indicate reduced REM latency and a few have found some evidence of difficulty initiating and maintaining sleep. Most studies have failed to find any evidence of increased REM density, and none of the controlled studies has reported diminished delta sleep associated with depression in this age group. One possibility is that the large amounts of delta sleep and high sleep efficiency associated with younger subjects mask the sleep disturbances associated with depression. Researchers have also hypothesized that age and depression may interact in producing the sleep changes associated with depression.

In contrast to the paucity of objective evidence of sleep disturbances, subjective sleep complaints are very common in children and adolescents with MDD. These symptoms include difficulty falling asleep, middle-of-the-night awakenings, early morning awakening, and restless sleep. In addition, there are many children and adolescents who report hypersomnia in association with depressive episodes. In a recent review of the clinical picture of child and adolescent MDD (which included 187 subjects), 74% of the sample presented with significant complaints of disturbed sleep, while 25% had significant symptoms of hypersomnia (Ryan et al., 1987). Thirty-eight percent of this sample complained of severe insomnia, with many complaining they almost never sleep and always feel exhausted during the day. Again, it must be emphasized that in objective studies, including some drawn from this sample, there were no significant sleep disturbances in the children and adolescents complaining of insomnia. Although less frequent than insomnia, symptoms of hypersomnia are more common in child and adolescent depressed subjects than in adult depressed subjects. Some of these adolescents report significant daytime sleepiness despite 10 to 12 hours of sleep at night. One study of depressed adolescents and young adults found that depressed subjects were able to extend their sleep beyond baseline almost twice as frequently as the normal controls.

There are at least two interpretations to these objective/subjective discrepancies in child and adolescent depression. One interpretation is that major depressive disorder is associated with a change in the *perception* of sleep rather than physiologic changes in sleep as measured by EEG studies. The second interpretation is that our current methods of measuring sleep are not capable of reliably detecting the sleep disruptions associated with depression in these younger subjects due to maturational effects on sleep. In support of the second interpretation is evidence that although children with depression did not have significantly disturbed sleep compared with controls, when they were restudied in recovery they had small but significant improvement in sleep compared with their previous studies (Puig-Antich et al., 1983).

From a clinical perspective, when a child or adolescent presents with significant sleep complaints, the possibility of depression should be considered and the symptoms should be assessed in the context of other signs and symptoms of major depression. Likewise, a complete history of the child's or adolescent's sleep and schedule should be assessed for other causes of sleep disturbances, as described in the section entitled "Pediatric Sleep Disorders." There can also be considerable overlap between sleep schedule disturbances and major depression. Depressed adolescents can develop difficulties falling asleep, withdraw from school and social activities, take daytime naps, and develop very late-night and erratic schedules. In some cases it becomes necessary to address both the sleep schedule issues and symptoms of depression.

Another important consideration in the evaluation of sleep changes in affective disorders is the individual with a bipolar illness presenting with a dramatically decreased need for sleep. During manic episodes, these adolescents get by with very little sleep. One distinction between this situation and other causes of sleep loss in this age group is that the manic adolescents do not complain of daytime sleepiness during mania but present with decreased sleep requirements and feel energetic.

One additional clinical aspect of assessing sleep problems when an affective disorder is suspected is the need to consider the wide range of normal symptoms of sleep disturbances in this age group. Adolescents often have transient periods of fatigue, are undergoing many stresses and life changes, and often follow erratic schedules. The severity and chronicity of these problems in association with major depressive disorder are greater than in normal adolescents. It is also worth noting that adolescents can often be reluctant to voice these complaints to parents or clinicians. Clinicians assessing these problems must actively and specifically question adolescents about sleep symptoms and schedules and acquire a sense of the range of normal sleep patterns and complaints in this population.

Attention Deficit Disorder

Behaviors indicating inattentiveness, impulsivity, restlessness, hyperactivity, and disruptiveness in children are common sources of complaints by parents and teachers. In this clinical entity of attention-related problems, sleep complaints are also frequent. Parents of children with the diagnosis of attention deficit disorder (ADD) report significantly more difficulties in their children fall asleep, waking in the night, waking early, and having restless sleep (Kaplan, 1987). Despite convincing evidence of subjective sleep disturbances, objective sleep studies have not revealed significant sleep disruption in children with ADD.

As with affective disorders in this age group, subjective/objective discrepancies in sleep are a source of speculation and disagreement. One important consideration is the possibility that only a small subgroup of children within the overall diagnosis of attention deficit disorder have sleep disturbances of clinical significance. We have seen children with ADD who show increased behavioral symptoms after sleep loss. As mentioned in "Pediatric Sleep Disorders," there is evidence that inadequate sleep can cause behavioral symptoms in children that overlap with those of ADD. Specifically, inattention, irritability, distractibility, and impulsivity can be the result of sleep loss. We recently reported the case of a 10-year-old girl with a clear diagnosis of ADD and long-standing sleep difficulties (delayed sleep phase insomnia) with significant improvement of ADD and learning disability symptoms (as determined by blind raters in a controlled setting) following treatment of her sleep problem (Dahl et al., 1991).

Our approach to these problems is to recommend a careful assessment and treatment of sleep problems in children with ADD symptoms. When sleep disturbances are identified, treatment should address both behavioral and physiologic components of the sleep problems. One difficulty from a clinical perspective is the problem of defining adequate sleep. Because of the wide range of individual variations in sleep requirements, the definitions of sleep needs have traditionally been reported as the amount of sleep necessary for "optimal daytime functioning." In dealing with a population of children with ADD, attempts at defining optimal daytime functioning can be difficult. If inadequate sleep or sleep disturbances are suspected, one prudent approach is to attempt to increase or improve sleep and evaluate for signs of *improved* daytime functioning.

Another important consideration in the relationship of sleep and ADD is the sleep effects of the stimulants used to treat attention deficit disorder. Some children receive late doses of stimulants or long-acting preparations that can prolong sleep latency. We also have seen children whose families report significant *improvement* in their child's sleep when the child is placed on stimulants. Some children have further improvement in sleep when they are placed on later doses and long-acting preparations. This paradoxic improvement in sleep onset may result from better organized behavior around bedtime and compliance with going to bed. Objective sleep studies of children on stimulant medication have revealed small delays (15 to 20 minutes) in sleep onset during medicated condition compared with nonmedicated condition.

The control of arousal and attention, the regulation of sleep, and the psychobiology of attention deficit disorder are areas that are not well-understood but are likely to have some overlap. It appears that there is a need for more well-controlled studies addressing the relationship between ADD symptomatology and sleep regulation in children.

Tourette's Syndrome

Sleep disturbances are commonly reported in association with Tourette's syndrome and tic disorders and occur more frequently in family members of Tourette's syndrome patients. Although many neurologic textbooks report that all movement disorders cease during sleep, studies of younger Tourette's patients consistently indicate that tics occur throughout all sleep stages. In addition to both motor and vocal tics, these patients also show increased partial arousals out of deep sleep. These sudden and intense partial arousals can manifest as night terrors, sleepwalking, enuresis, or Tourette-like behaviors such as coprolalia or bird calls. Both tics and partial arousals from sleep appear to decrease with treatment of Tourette's syndrome. We recently treated a boy with Tourette's syndrome who had frequent partial arousals and tics during sleep but who demonstrated significant improvement following a change in his medication to include a dose near bedtime. His parents reported not only an improvement in sleep-related symptoms but also improvement in symptoms of daytime irritability and tiredness, which may have been caused by the chronic sleep disturbances.

Summary

Symptoms of sleep disturbances are common in child psychopathology. Differentiating the range of normal minor sleep complaints in children and adolescents and the more significant complaints associated with pathology must be based on clinical judgment and experience. Objective physiologic studies for the most part have not produced specific evidence of sleep disruptions that is of clinical benefit at this time. The reasons for this may be due to technical limitations of measuring sleep or may be due to maturational factors that protect the sleep of children and mask any disturbances. Because both the fields of sleep disorders and biologic approaches to child psychopathology are relatively new areas, further research resulting in a better understanding of the interaction of the regulation of sleep and the regulation of affect, arousal, and behavior remains promising.

USE OF THE SLEEP LABORATORY/ POLYSOMNOGRAPHY

Sleep studies are time-consuming, labor-intensive, and expensive (typically costing $500 to $1500). Polysomnographic studies are most helpful when they are being done to answer a specific question such as whether narcolepsy, obstructive sleep apnea syndrome, or an unidentified cause of daytime sleepiness exists. Sleep studies cannot confirm the diagnosis of depression, shed little light on most cases of insomnia, and rarely contribute to clinical decisions in adolescents with delayed sleep phase syndrome. Further, the appropriateness of obtaining sleep studies is influenced by the strengths and weaknesses of the particular lab and polysomnographer available to the referring clinician.

It is important to understand that many different types of evaluations fall under the rubric of "sleep studies." All-night measures can include EEG, EOG (electrooculogram), EMG (electromyogram), respiratory measures of chest movement and abdominal movement, nasal/oral thermistors estimating airflow, pulse oximetry, capnographs (assessment of CO_2 content of expired air), and infrared video camera recording (with a split screen to produce simultaneous images of the patient and the EEG record). Further, labs may use only one EEG channel or multiple channels in a full 10/20 montage for the detection of neurologic abnormalities or seizures. Some sleep labs perform only a few of these measures, while other labs have the capabilities for all of these measures. Although general standards have been set by the American Sleep Disorders Association, not all labs follow these guidelines. (For a list of accredited labs, one can contact the American Sleep Disorders Association directly at 604 2nd Street, SW, Rochester, MN 55902; (507)287-6006). All accredited labs have at least one clinical polysomnographer (an MD or PhD who meets all qualifications of training and performance as specified by the American Sleep Disorders Association to diagnose and treat sleep disorders). However, it is important to note that the background of the lab director (neurology, pulmonology, psychiatry, pediatrics, or psychology) can significantly contribute to the strengths and weaknesses of that particular laboratory.

This wide spectrum of laboratories and clinicians performing "sleep studies" is particularly relevant to the special problems posed by sleep evaluations in children and adolescents. The size of the equipment, the lab and lab setting, facilities to accommodate a family member to sleep over with frightened children, and the skill of the staff in dealing with children while performing wire-ups and putting the child to bed can all influence test results. Specifically, many sleep labs in smaller centers perform primarily adult pulmonary (sleep apnea) studies and have very little experience diagnosing a wide variety of problems in children and adolescents.

The important message to the referring clinician is that sleep evaluations in children are not standardized laboratory tests. In the ideal setting, the sleep "laboratory" should provide a comprehensive consultation that may or may not involve EEG sleep studies. As with any consultation, the clinical abilities of the consultant and quality of communication between consultant and referring clinician are major determinants in the likelihood that laboratory values will have clinical relevance.

There are some clear indications for polysomnographic studies in children and adolescents, such as: (1) Significant unexplained daytime sleepiness despite what appears to be adequate nighttime sleep (with or without signs of narcolepsy). (2) Complicated or ambiguous cases of suspected sleep apnea (when the clinical evidence strongly supports a straightforward case of enlarged tonsils and adenoids and probably OSAS, sleep studies are often *not* necessary). (3) Sleep studies can be an essential component of the evaluation in some cases when children present with bizarre or atypical behaviors in the middle of the night that may represent a partial arousal (parasomnia) but could be seizure related.

In the wide range of common cases involving straightforward parasomnias, probable sleep/wake schedule disorders, and insomnias, formal sleep studies are usually unnecessary. In many of these cases, however, consultation with a sleep clinician experienced with children and adolescents can be extremely valuable in assisting with evaluation and treatment as well as delineating which patients may warrant further studies.

ACKNOWLEDGMENTS

The author wishes to acknowledge the mentorship and inspiration of Joaquim Puig-Antich, MD; it is to his memory that this chapter is dedicated. Dan Buysee, MD, and Neal Ryan, MD, made helpful suggestions, and Deborah Small assisted in the preparation of this manuscript.

REFERENCES

Dahl RE, Puig-Antich J, Ryan ND, Nelson B. EEG sleep in adolescent depression. J Affective Disord 1990;19:63–75.

Dahl RE, Pelham WE, Wierson, M. The role of sleep disturbances in attention deficit disorder symptoms: a case study. J Pediatr Psychol 1991;16(2):229–239.

Ferber R. Circadian and schedule disturbances. In Guilleminault C, ed. Sleep and its disorders in children. New York: Raven Press, 1987A.

Ferber R. Sleeplessness, night awakening, and night crying in the infant and toddler. Pediatr Rev 1987B;9:69–82.

Ferber R. Solve your child's sleep problems. New York: Simon & Schuster, 1985.

Guilleminault C, Winkle R, Korobin R, Simmons B. Children and nocturnal snoring: evaluation of the effects of sleep related respiratory resting load and daytime functioning. Eur J Pediatr 1982;139:165–171.

Kaplan BI, et al. Sleep disturbance in preschool age hyperactive and non-hyperactive children. Pediatrics 1987; 6:839–844.

Klackenberg G. Incidence of parasomnias in children in a general population. In: Guilleminault C, ed. Sleep and its disorders in children. New York: Raven Press, 1987:99–113.

Kleine W. Periodische schlafsucht. Monatsschr Psychiatr Neurol 1925;57:285–298.

Kotogal S, Hartse KM, Walsh JK. Characteristics of narcolepsy in preteenaged children. Pediatrics 1990;85:205–209.

Levin M. Narcolepsy and other varieties of morbid somnolence. Arch Neurol Psychiatry 1929;22:1172–1200.

Moore-Ede MC, Czeisler CA, Richardson GS. Circadian timekeeping in health and disease. N Engl J Med 1983;309:469–476.

Puig-Antich J, Goetz R, Hanlon C, Tabrizi MA, Daview M, Weitzman ED. Sleep architecture and REM sleep measures in prepubertal major depressives. Arch Gen Psychiatry 1983;40:187–192.

Reynold CF, Kupfer DJ. State-of-the-art review: Sleep research in affective illness state of the art circa 1987. Sleep 1987;10:199–215.

Ryan ND, Puig-Antich J, Ambrosini P. The clinical picture of depression in children and adolescents. Arch Gen Psychiatry 1987;44:854–861.

Shouse MN. Epilepsy and seizures during sleep. In: Principles and practices of sleep medicine. Kreiger MH, Roth T, Dement WC, eds. Philadelphia: WB Saunders, 1989.

Chapter 13

STATIC ENCEPHALOPATHY AND RELATED DISORDERS

John M. Pellock, MD, and Edwin C. Myer, MD

STATIC ENCEPHALOPATHY

Cerebral Palsy

Cerebral palsy (CP) is a term that refers to a group of disorders characterized by motor deficits with onset in early infancy. The motor deficits can be paralysis, abnormality in tone (hypotonia or hypertonia), or movement disorder, including ataxia, athetosis, or chorea. CP encompasses a group of static encephalopathies that begin early in life, even in the first few months or before, and have *no associated progressive disease*. However, CP is not a single disease and the term is offered only as a description, rather than as a diagnosis, to the parents of children with delayed development and motor deficits (Bax, 1990). CP implies that there is nonprogressive pathology of the brain secondary to maldevelopment, disease, or damage during gestation, birth, or in early life (Naeye et al., 1989; Nelson and Ellenberg, 1978; Stanley and Alberman, 1984).

The classification of CP by symptoms (Table 13.1) includes spastic, athetotic, ataxic, hypotonic, and mixed forms. CP may also be classified by the topographic representation of the body, i.e., hemiplegia, diplegia (lower extremities more affected than upper extremities), quadriplegia, or monoplegia. Its severity may be mild,

moderate, or severe. Associated dysfunctions include numerous neurologic symptoms such as mental retardation, epilepsy, sensory impairments (vision, hearing), and behavioral, learning, and emotional disabilities (Table 13.2). The etiologies of CP include hereditary conditions; congenital malformations; intrauterine or neonatal infections, such as toxoplasmosis, rubella, cytomegalovirus, herpes and syphilis; intrauterine hypoxia/ischemia; perinatal mechanical, anoxic, and traumatic injuries; infants' small size for gestional age; prematurity; respiratory distress; and perinatally acquired infections. In the postnatal period, trauma, infections, toxins, hypoxia, stroke, and neuronal dysfunction may also cause CP. Children exposed to AIDS at birth may appear at first to have a static encephalopathy resembling CP, but when their progressive deficits are noted, a true diagnosis is made. Hence, CP is a symptom complex secondary to a static, one-time injury to the nervous system (Stanley and Alberman, 1984).

The diagnosis of cerebral palsy is usually made when a child fails to meet motor developmental milestones. A detailed history and examination should exclude progressive or degenerative causes. For example, if a child has evidence of neurofibromatosis or tuberous sclerosis, diagnosing cerebral palsy would be inappropriate be-

Table 13.1.
Classification of Cerebral Palsy

Spastic
  Hemiplegic
  Diplegic
  Quadriplegic
Athetotic
Ataxic
Hypotonic
Mixed (i.e., spasticity and athetosis)

cause the former illnesses are progressive. Multiple metabolic abnormalities and degenerative diseases first present in the same manner as CP. The most important diagnostic consideration is that there is *no evidence of progressive disease*. There can be no loss of previously obtained milestones and no increase in abnormal neurologic signs. Also, a family history of CP should suggest the possibly of a disease of a chromosomal or inherited metabolic nature, which might imply treatment or family counseling as well as mandate a revision in the diagnosis and prognosis.

Besides a routine history and a physical, neurologic, and developmental examination, the CP patient's evaluation should include a search for an etiology. Appropriate tests include screening for metabolic disease, imaging studies such as CT (computed tomography) and MRI (magnetic resonance imaging), electrophysiologic testing, neuropsychologic and/or developmental testing (to exclude mental retardation), and evaluation of hearing, vision, and other sensory systems. Occupational and physical therapy evaluations to assess function are particularly valuable (Myer and Pellock, 1983; Menkes, 1985).

Many factors affect the prognosis of a child with CP. In general, the greater the amount of motor inability, the greater the risk of a child's not being stimulated. Also, any associated mental retardation, epilepsy, or sensory, behavioral, learning, or emotional disabilities further ostracize the child (Table 13.2). Frequently, a motor disability is so great that severe maladaption occurs although there is no mental retardation or primary behavioral abnormality. This response is particularly common in children with severe movement disorders such as athetosis. Recent evidence reveals a shortened lifespan when mental retardation is associated with severe motor deficits (Eyman et al., 1990).

Determination of chromosome number and architecture and testing for fragile X (which requires special processing in folate-deficient media) should be considered in "CP" children who are dysmorphic or have a positive family history.

Treatment of CP aims to prevent further motor deterioration from musculotendon joint contractures that result from abnormal postures and disuse. Standard techniques are physical therapy, occupational therapy, and speech therapy (Palmer et al., 1988). Medication used for the amelioration of spasticity and movement disorders are baclofen, diazepam, and dantrolene. Surgery to reduce joint contractures and spasticity is frequently used (Black, 1987). Casting and physical therapy are usually employed before and after surgery to maximize its benefit. However, these techniques can allow only a certain amount of improvement. Certain therapies, including vitamin therapy, special diets, and complex motor therapies, are usually no more helpful than standard medical care. Dorsal rhizotomy to reduce spasticity is at present under evaluation (Peacock and Staudt, 1990).

An important component of the total treatment of the child and family is counseling, psychologic therapy, and educational planning (Rapin, 1982). The goal of rehabilitation is maximization of potential and reintegration into society. However, ease of movement and hence social acceptance, education, and employability

Table 13.2.
Cerebral Palsy: Associated Abnormalities

Sensory
Epileptic
Intellectual
Perceptual
Behavioral
Learning
Emotional
Bone/Joint

depend upon the severity of the CP and the presence or absence of associated neurologic symptoms. Psychiatric consultation can help both the individual and family cope with the disability and lack of fulfillment, and it is especially helpful when maladaptive behavior complicates the picture. It is sometimes most difficult for those who are trapped within their disabled bodies yet who have good intellectual potential to accept their motor disabilities. Social isolation is a problem for both the families and the patients. Parents may overinvest time in the child, and other family pathology develops. As parents age, placement of the child may become necessary. Depression on the part of the patient or family may soon surface.

When counseling these patients, it is extremely important to remember that their motor (and mental) deficit should be *nonprogressive*. Any progressive loss of function, perhaps manifested by decreased ability to perform as they previously were able to do, suggests the presence of a progressive disease. New symptoms, especially headaches, vomiting, incontinence, visual or auditory change, increased behavioral abnormality, hyperactivity, "depression," or dementia, require reinvestigation by a neurologist. Hydrocephalus or spinal cord anomalies, which are discussed in the following sections, may be present for a number of years as a seemingly static condition, only then to surface with progressive loss of mentation and motor function with increased spasticity, particularly in the lower extremities. Some symptoms may represent secondary effects of medications, while others are manifestations of ongoing disease.

Hydrocephalus

Hydrocephalus, a specific cause of macrocephaly (enlarged head), is usually associated with enlarged cerebral ventricles and raised cerebrospinal fluid (CSF) pressure. It can be the cause of deficient CSF reabsorption. Hydrocephalus is the physiologic result of an imbalance of CSF formation and absorption with a great enough dif-ference between the two to produce a net accumulation of fluid and increased intracranial pressure. It is usually caused by deficient CSF reabsorption. However, not every case of ventriculomegaly has associated increased pressure. Enlarged ventricles may occur because of cerebral atrophy without increased pressure, a condition referred to as *hydrocephalus ex vacuo*. The enlarged head or macrocephalic state should not be automatically diagnosed as representing hydrocephalus. Similarly, following shunting procedure for treatment, some patients with hydrocephalus may no longer have enlarged heads.

Increased skull size, or macrocephaly, commonly occurs in the young child as a consequence of increased brain size, intracranial mass, hydrocephalus, or raised intracranial pressure. All sutures remain open until 6 months of age, when fibrous closure occurs. However, complete ossification of the basal skull bones is accomplished only by 8 years of age, and by age 12 years, sutures are rarely separated by increased intracranial pressure (Stanley and Alberman, 1984). Figure 2.4 demonstrates the normal growth rate of the occipital-frontal head circumference through childhood and adolescence (see Chapter 2).

The differential diagnoses of macrocephaly include extracranial, cranial, and intracranial abnormalities (Myer and Pellock, 1983; Menkes, 1985). In the infant, skin contusions, subgaleal hemorrhage (hemorrhage into the subaponeurotic compartment), cephalohematoma (subperiosteal hemorrhage) are possible. Bony enlargement may occur through various metabolic diseases of bone, craniosynostosis (premature closure of cephalic bones), and hematologic disorders of young childhood in which bone marrow becomes active in response to anemia. In the case of craniosynostosis, the actual head circumference may be normal although the appearance is one of macrocephaly. Intracranial causes of macrocephaly include intracranial hemorrhage that may be subdural, subarachnoid, or intraparenchymal. In subarachnoid or intraventricular hemorrhage, head enlargement may be secondary to obstruction of CSF flow or re-absorption of CSF at the subarachnoid granulations. Hence, following child abuse and intracranial hemorrhage of various types, macrocephaly or hydrocephalus may develop, with signs and symptoms of increased intracranial pressure. Parenchymal causes include cerebral edema from various sources, including trauma, encephalitis, toxic substances such as lead, anoxia or hypoxia, Reye's syndrome, or pseudotumor cerebri. Intracerebral mass lesions may cause direct enlargement of the cerebral substance or, more commonly, partly obstruct CSF outflow by means of a combination of lesion size, surrounding edema, and obstructive hydrocephalus. Rarely, degenerative diseases with the accumulation of storage substances or other metabolic defects such as Tay-Sachs disease, Krabbe's disease, or mucopolysaccharidosis lead to macrocephaly. Lastly, congenital defects of brain structure may lead to macrocephaly through the production of cavities associated with aberrant neuronal migration, cerebral gigantism, or achondroplasia. Neurofibromatosis may also be associated with macrocephaly, both on a primary megalencephalic basis and because some with this disorder later develop aqueductal stenosis. Familial macrocoephaly may also present in entirely normal individuals and is verified by measuring the head circumference of the child's parents.

The understanding of hydrocephalus can be fully explained and appreciated only following a review of CSF production and absorption (Milhorat, 1978). CSF is produced by the choroid plexus. Although present in other areas, it is primarily localized in the lateral cerebral ventricles. These two lateral ventricles meet in the midline at the foramen of Monro, wherein the third ventricle begins and extends to the aqueduct of Sylvius. This narrow passageway leads to the fourth ventricle. From the fourth ventricle, CSF escapes through the foramina of Luschka and Magendie, as shown in Figure 13.1. CSF

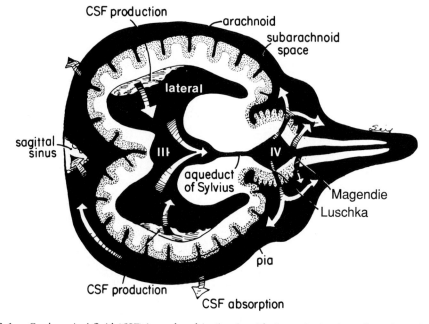

Figure 13.1. Cerebrospinal fluid (*CSF*) is produced in the choroid plexus; it circulates throughout the ventricles and exists within the foramina of Luschka and Magendie. The most common sites of obstruction to CSF flow are the bottlenecks at the aqueduct of Sylvius as well as the foramina.

then flows up over the convexities of the cerebral hemisphere, where it is absorbed mainly through the arachnoid villi. There is also a small amount of absorption across the wall of the ventricles, but obstruction of one of the outflow channels usually leads to hydrocephalus. The causes of hydrocephalus are generally divided into communicating and noncommunicating types. Noncommunicating types presume an obstruction to CSF flow, whereas communicating hydrocephalus presumes dysfunction in distal reabsorption. The condition of overproduction of CSF associated with choroid plexus papilloma usually presents in infancy. Causes of communicating and noncommunicating hydrocephalus are listed in Table 13.3.

The symptoms associated with hydrocephalus depend upon the stage of the process and whether there is an acute or more chronic increase in intracranial pressure. In the first few years of life, when sutures and fontanelles are open, in-

creased intracranial pressure is manifested by growing head circumference. This occurs in the young infant before papilledema is seen. In babies, the triad of macrocephaly, bulging fontanelle, and so-called sunsetting sign (eyes deviating downward, partly setting over the lower lid), caused by brainstem dysfunction disallowing upgaze, are classic symptoms. Nonspecific irritability and vomiting frequently accompany these symptoms. Because sutures do not fully close until early adolescence, head growth is still possible but less likely in later childhood. Sutural splitting associated with headaches and vomiting suggests increased intracranial pressure from any cause, as do all symptoms of hydrocephalus. In the acute process the bulging fontanelle, papilledema, increased blood pressure, slow pulse rate, and cranial nerve dysfunction (particularly that of nerves III and VI, including anisocoria and sluggish or nonreactive pupils) are common. Vomiting, headaches, and mentation changes are frequent. When increased intracranial pressure is slowly progressive or when shunts for treatment function intermittently, single or combined findings may be a slight increase in spasticity, particularly in the lower extremities, increased incontinence and enuresis, increased nonspecific headaches, or decline in school performance secondary to neuropsychologic dysfunction. Head tilt associated with other symptoms of raised intracranial pressure suggests the presence of posterior fossa hemiation. Hence, the slower the onset of increased intracranial pressure, the more difficult it may be to make the correct diagnosis, but the association and progression of symptoms are extremely important.

The treatment of hydrocephalus is to decrease CSF pressure by removing cerebrospinal fluid. This is typically done by shunting CSF either from the lateral ventricle through a subcutaneous system into the peritoneal cavity or into the jugular system and draining into the right atrium. CSF has also been shunted into many sterile body cavities (Milhorat, 1978; Jones et al., 1988).

Table 13.3.
Causes of Communicating and
Noncommunicating Hydrocephalus

Causes of hydrocephalus:
  Increased CSF production
  Decreased CSF absorption
Causes of noncommunicating hydrocephalus:
  Foramen of Monro obstruction
  Third ventricle obstruction
  Aqueductal stenosis
    Congenital
    Infection
    External compression
  IV ventricle: posterior fossa tumor
  Obstruction to Luschka and Magendie
      foramina
  Infection
Causes of communicating hydrocephalus:
  Congenital abnormalities
    Arnold-Chiari malformation
  Infections
    Pus and adhesions, especially base of brain
    Meningitis
  Subarachnoid hemorrhage
  Tumor
  Sinus thrombosis or obstruction of venous
      return

Unfortunately, this artificial means of controlling increased intracranial pressure is imperfect—leading to shunts that malfunction and/or become infected. Medications such as acetazolamide and isosorbide have been used, but they are an insufficient treatment of true, lasting hydrocephalus. These medications may also be associated with dehydration and acidosis (Milhorat, 1978).

As noted above, with the exception of the removal of the choroid plexus papilloma, the treatment of hydrocephalus is usually through shunting techniques, the single most important advance in the treatment of hydrocephalus. Unfortunately, the introduction of catheters and valves into the body cavity has disadvantages, in that: (1) a single shunting operation is rarely curative and repetitive revisions are required; (2) shunting operations and revisions are associated with numerous complications; and (3) shunt complications occur frequently in children and adults and have significant morbidity and mortality (Milhorat, 1978; Mickell and Ward, 1984). Indeed, the ultimate prognosis of the patient with hydrocephalus depends upon how infrequently they were subjected to bouts of increased intracranial pressure. An extracranial valve with a low-, medium-, or high-pressure system allows CSF to pass through the valve at a specific rate so that the ventricle is not overshunted. Overshunting can atually result in rapid collapse of the ventricular system, and possible subdural hematoma or symptoms of overshunting are difficult to differentiate from shunt failure (Epstein et al., 1988). Following shunting procedure, any breakdown or erythema of skin over the shunt tract may indicate malfunction or infection, and the presence of subcutaneous fluid surrounding the tubing requires urgent consultation.

As noted, acute shunt failure constitutes a true neurosurgical emergency, and it may be characterized clinically by a sudden onset of headache, vomiting, and lethargy (Mickell and Ward, 1984). The less dramatic presentation of irritability, vomiting, and lethargy over several days, particularly when associated with a presumptive infectious disease, is less easy to diagnose but still may represent shunt failure. In those with peritoneal shunt, abdominal pain or signs of intestinal obstruction may be secondary to shunt malfunction. Any increase in motor symptoms or complaints of headache, vomiting, and visual disturbance should prompt an urgent referral. Hence, although symptoms may be somewhat diffuse, they must be realized and proper referral made because of the potential emergency.

A psychiatrist may be consulted by a number of these patients for various reasons. One important reason might be a decline in school or work performance because of neuropsychologic dysfunction. This complaint should be considered secondary to shunt malfunction until another cause is proved. Drop in IQ or subtle neuropsychologic changes may occur with children failing in school or just not performing up to their potential. Several studies reveal this to be a recurrent theme of intermittent shunt failure, to the point at which some clinics are using repeat neuropsychologic testing along with head CT as a follow-up tool to predict or help aid in the diagnosis of slowing evolving shunt failure. Other symptoms such as ataxia, decreased motor performance, "depression", enuresis, increased spasticity, increased lethargy or alteration in sleep cycle, and suggestion of dementia must be considered symptoms of possible shunt failure.

Anomalies Associated with Hydrocephalus

Besides aqueductal stenosis, the most common lesions associated with congenital hydrocephalus are the Arnold-Chiari malformation and the Dandy-Walker or posterior fossa cyst-type malformation (Milhorat, 1978).

Chiari malformations are of three types, but all represent a type of dysraphism (see below) in which the cerebellum is elongated and protrudes through the foramen magnum into the cervical spinal cord. In the most common variety, type 2 form of Chiari malformation, which typically accompanies meningomyelocele, various anomalies of cerebellum and lower brainstem are associated with noncommunicating (obstructive) hydrocephalus. The foramina of Lushka and Magendie and the basal cisterns are occluded. This malformation may exist alone or in combination with aqueductal stenosis. Older children and adolescent patients may first present with hydrocephalus with a slowly progressive history suggesting increased intracranial pressure. Because of the herniation of cerebellar tissue and constriction of the spinal cord and medulla, apnea may be a presenting sign. Symptoms of torticollis, opisthotonus, cervical cord compression (motor and long tract signs), headache, vertigo, laryngeal paralysis, and progressive cerebellar signs of incoordination all may signal this abnormality as children grow (Dysta and Menezes, 1988; Dauser et al., 1988).

Other malformations involving the base of the skull and cervical spine—hydromyelia, syringomyelia, syringobulbia, and diastematomyelia—add a number of possible sensory and motor disorders to the symptom list. A syrinx represents an intrinsic cavitation of the spinal cord or brainstem. Diastematomyelia is characterized by a cartilaginous spicule that divides the cord in the midline. Both become symptomatic only when these structures impinge on spinal cord long tracts or neuronal aggregates. Hence, symptoms usually occur in later childhood, adolescence, or adulthood. Symptoms of dissociated anesthesia with involvement of pain and temperature along with sparing of position sense and touch are characteristic (Rowland, 1989). There may also be a cloak-like distribution of sensory symptoms. Atrophy and weakness, painless ulcerations, coldness, cyanosis, hyperhidrosis, and painless arthropathy (Charcot joint) are all reported. As the syrinx extends upward into the midline, lower cranial nerve symptoms, such as hoarseness, and a variety of motor long

tract symptoms develop (Milhorat, 1978; Rowland, 1989; Scatliff et al., 1989).

The Dandy-Walker type anomaly is characterized by fourth ventricular or posterior fossa cyst agenesis of the cerebellar vermis and obstructive hydrocephalus. The cyst-like lesions separate the cerebellar hemispheres posteriorly (Bordarier and Aicardi, 1990). Associated anomalies include agenesis of the corpus callosum, aqueductal stenosis, occipital encephalocele, polymicrogyria, syringomyelia, heterotopias, facial angiomas, cleft palate, and cardiac and renal anomalies (Menkes, 1985; Bordarier and Aicardi, 1990). This syndrome may present with symptoms of increased intracranial pressure but a bulging occiput, nystagmus, ataxia, and cranial nerve deficit are typical. Treatment of this disorder may require shunting of the cyst or fourth ventricle along with shunting of supratentorial ventricular dilation.

The variety of signs and symptoms noted in Arnold-Chiari and Dandy-Walker syndromes are not specific. Rather, they should expand the psychiatrist's scope of important associated clinical complaints. Also, onset need not occur in infancy; a series of chronic complaints may even be misdiagnosed in the older child or adolescent. The psychiatrist aware of these associated conditions should refer the patient for neurologic reevaluation.

Myelomeningocele

In the developing nervous system, neural tube defects may result in dysfunction of ectodermal and mesodermal development involving one or both of these elements. The final result is either spina bifida occulta when only vertebral arches fail to fuse, or spina bifida cystica or spinal dysraphism when more underlying elements are involved. These include a dermal sinus with or without a tag of skin or tuft of hair and a possible connection with underlying subarachnoid space. Protrusion of the meninges through the vertebral cleft is known as a meningocele or encephalocele, depending on the anatomic position. If the spinal cord or nerve roots protrude through the defect, this is a myelomeningocele (Fig. 13.2).

Pathogenesis. Various theories as to the anatomic causes have been proposed. The popular ones are failure of the closure of the neural tube during embryogenesis or faulty fluid dynamics at the fourth ventricle (Osaka et al., 1987).

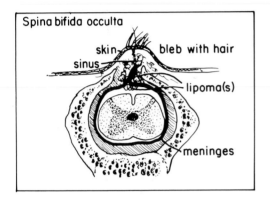

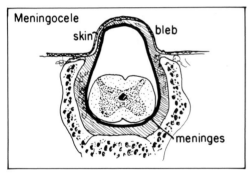

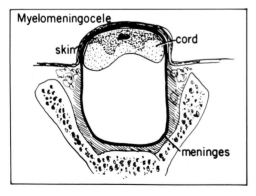

Figure 13.2. Illustrations of three common spinal neural tube defects of increasing severity.

These events occur during the 4th week of gestation.

Causes of these events have been suggested. A polygenic and environmental background may play a part, especially since there is a 4% risk of recurrence after the first involved pregnancy and a 10% risk if two previous infants have been affected. Various teratogens have been implicated, including valproic acid, radiation, and folic acid and vitamin D deficiencies. High levels of alpha-fetoprotein in the maternal blood and amniotic fluid samples frequently suggest the diagnosis, which can be confirmed in utero by ultrasonography.

The various types of spinal dysraphism have different clinical presentations that occur more frequently in some areas. *Spina bifida occulta,* which occurs in 5% of the population, is frequently asymptomatic (Anderson, 1975). *Occult spinal dysraphism,* frequently associated with a lipoma, or diastematomyelia or a tethered cord may be initially asymptomatic, but bowel and bladder symptoms may soon develop in the growing infant and child. Various symptoms may include repeated bladder and kidney infections, enuresis, decreased anal sphincter tone, pes cavus, and decreased ankle reflexes. The diagnosis is confirmed by MRI. Dermal sinus defects may result in recurrent meningitis. Treatment for spinal dysraphism is early surgery. Delay in surgery may result in irreversible loss of bladder and bowel control (Editorial, 1986). This may be due to the associated tethered cord's resulting in defects in the conus medullaris or cauda equina (S3–S5 nerve roots) as the vertebral growth outstrips the cord growth (Hood and Robinson, 1978).

Meningocele is not usually associated with neurologic deficits, but careful evaluation to rule out bladder, bowel, and gait disturbances is necessary. Elective surgery for meningocele is recommended.

Myelomeningocele (MMC) involves all layers of the spinal cord, nerve roots, vertebrae, and skin.

The incidence is 0.2–0.3%. It is associated with hydrocephalus 80% of the time. In the absence of treatment, 50% of infants will die from either hydrocephalus, meningitis, or renal failure, singularly or in combination.

Lumbosacral myelomeningocele is the most common form, occurring in 80% of cases, suggesting that this is associated with closure dysfunction of the posterior neuropore. The diagnosis is made by seeing a protuberant, fluctuant bleb surrounded by skin. Depending on the precise spinal cord level, varying symptoms are present. At the S1-S2 level, the patient is able to walk. In lesions above L2, walking does not occur and the patient is wheelchair-bound.

The paresis and sensory deficit depend on the level; however, all patients have sphincter dysfunction affecting bowel and bladder. Associated defects include hydrocephalus in 73% of cases of lumbosacral MMC. In thoracolumbar lesions, the involvement is much more severe, with potential kyphoscoliosis, and 90% have associated hydrocephalus.

If hydrocephalus is not present at birth, more than 80% will exhibit this within 6 weeks. Other associated anomalies of the spinal cord include diplomyelia, diastometomyelia, and syringomyelia. Central anomalies include Arnold-Chiari malformations of varying severity, microgyria, and interthalamic disconnections. Central nervous system (CNS) infections associated with the original dysfunction and subsequent treatment (shunts) may affect cortical function.

Management of MMC involves a multidisciplinary team (Colgan, 1981). The team consists of a neurosurgeon, neurologist, urologist, orthopedist, pediatrician, psychologist, psychiatrist, physio- and occupational therapist, educational consultant, special teacher, and social worker. The pediatrician should organize and lead this team.

At birth, the primary lesion requires surgical covering. The potential hydrocephalus requires appropriate shunting or following with ultra-sonography or CT scanning (McLaughlin et al., 1985).

Bladder and renal care are major problems and need constant attention to prevent chronic renal failure (Brem et al., 1987). Flaccid, distensible bladders are at low risk for renal complications. However, small, trabeculated bladder is a risk factor for loss of kidney function. Intermittent catheterization resulting in satisfactory dryness can be most helpful (Uehling, 1985) and can prevent renal problems.

Bowel incontinence requires appropriate management, and attempts at preservation of internal sphincter tone can be helpful. Subsequent fecal incontinence occurs in 90% of cases and may cause major social problems (Chapman et al., 1979), since the malodorous child tends to be ostracized by his or her peers. Suppositories, stool softeners, scheduled toileting, and manual removal are necessary. Biofeedback training has been of questionable use (Loening-Baucke et al., 1988).

Orthopedic intervention has helped subluxation of hips and feet deformities, and it prevents contracture. Therapists help develop alternate skills and appropriate mechanical aids to normalize life as much as possible.

Arnold-Chiari malformations may result in central ventilatory dysfunction, including stridor, respiratory distress, aspiration, and central apnea. Treatment may require intubation and tracheostomy, and supplemental oxygenation. Because of deficiency of arousal responses to hypoxia and hypercapnia constant monitoring may be necessary (Hays et al., 1989).

As growth and development proceed, the patient requires psychologic and educational evaluations for appropriate school placement. Dietary regimens to avoid gaining weight, which decreases potential mobility, is necessary, especially in the pubertal child. Both the patient and, especially, the parent or caretaker require counseling and emotional support. The child and adolescent may require psychiatric intervention, therapy, and counseling. Skills to cope mentally and avoid frequent depression are necessary. Of affected adults, especially those with lower lesions, 75% are sexually active (Cass et al., 1986). Twenty-eight percent of adolescents with myelomeningocele are sexually active. Three-fourths of the boys believe they are able to father children. Marriage is desired, although relationships are difficult to sustain. From various studies, it appears that sexual education is lacking (Cramer et al., 1990).

A constant problem is potential shunt failure. This can manifest acutely as headaches, fever, and vomiting. It must always be considered in spite of other repeated infections, especially renal. Chronic shunt failure may be difficult to diagnose. It may present as deterioration in school function, depression, or behavior change, and may simulate emotional problems. Repeated psychologic evaluations can be useful, since decreasing IQ suggests cortical dysfunction, possibly due to chronic increased pressure.

Seizure activity is a further problem, and partial complex seizures and antiepileptic drug effects may further complicate the total picture (Noetzel, 1989). Careful assessment of drug side effects must be considered when obtaining seizure control.

DISCUSSION

Treatment of myelomeningocele can be a medical, ethical, and moral dilemma. However, some neurosurgeons believe that procedures can be delayed for a short period until parents, the majority of whom wish to be involved in decisions about the care of their infant, are appropriately informed. In making the decision, accurate and up-to-date medical information is necessary (Charney, 1990). Emotional support of spouses and family is necessary. The physician must be well-informed and competent at conveying medical information to the parents. Early appropriate information and resources are essential (Evans et al., 1985).

As these children grow, in addition to multiple discipline problems, medical management, economic, and emotional costs arise not only in the patients but in families. Parents living with an impaired child need support. Siblings, especially, may feel deprived in many ways. Educational roadblocks and the fear of recurring illness must be overcome (Query et al., 1990). The worse the medical outcome, the poorer the family's life. In general, however, families and siblings with appropriate resource help appear to adjust well socially and psychologically (Kazak and Clark, 1986).

One must remember that teenage problems require attention. Many of the adolescents, although mobile in wheelchairs, are still in diapers and need continual catheterization. Many of these adolescents reveal cognitive disabilities as increased demands are made by higher education. They tend to have poor contact with classmates and usually feel isolated (Borjeson and Lagergren, 1990). This isolation may also affect families. Most adolescents are concerned about sex and the possibility of having children. Genetic risks are of major concern. All of these aspects should be addressed aggressively, especially in the teenager, and active therapy should be initiated (Greene et al., 1985). Suicidal thoughts occur in 25% of girls, and depression occurs frequently.

Various physical coping methods, such as dressing and undressing, must be taught. Handicapped children's teams (group therapy) may help prepare the developing youth for adult life, independence from parents, and breaking the social isolation. Gainful employment should be the aim of each patient. Adequate resources from many disciplines and special groups must be available for this ever-increasing population. Active support groups are present in MMC referral centers.

Family stresses are often aggravated, especially if present before the birth of the affected infant. On the other hand, family cohesion can occur.

Hence children with MMC have significantly

lower self-concepts, which may influence siblings and parents. Larger families appear to cope better.

Support for families—siblings and parents as well as MMC patients—is important. Both psychiatrist and psychologist should play an active role in helping parents, siblings, and the patient to cope (Lavigne, 1988). Depression is an important complication and should be constantly monitored. Psychiatric intervention for depression is imperative.

CONCLUSION

In the past, selective management of myelomeningocele was postulated (Jacobson, 1989). Today, aggressive total management of all MMC is advocated, with 80 to 90% survival and an average IQ of 88. The complexity of the problem necessitates multiple-discipline involvement. At all stages of development, psychiatric and psychologic involvement are necessary, not only for the patient but for the entire family. Continual, recurrent problems can devastate a family emotionally and financially.

REFERENCES

Anderson FM. Occult spinal dysraphism: a series of 73 cases. Pediatrics, 1975;55:826.

Bax M. Motor delay and cerebral palsy. Devel Med Child Neurol 1990;32:283–284.

Black EE. Orthopaedic management in cerebral palsy. London: Mac Keith Press, 1987.

Bordarier C, Aicardi J. Dandy-Walker syndrome and agenesis of the cerebellar vermis: diagnostic problems and genetic counselling. Devel Med Child Neurol 1990;32:285–294.

Borjeson MC, Lagergren J. Life conditioning of adolescents with myelomeningocele. Devel Med Child Neurol 1990;32:698–706.

Brem AS, Martin D, Callaghan J, Maynard J. Long-term renal risk factors in children with meningomyelocele. J Pediatr 1987;110:51–55.

Cass RA, Bloom BA, Luxenberg M. Sexual function in adults with myelomeningocele. J Urol 1986;136:425–426.

Chapman W, Hill M, Shurtleff DB. Prevention of the outhouse syndrome: management of colon, anorectal and genito urinary tract function in the myelodysplastic child. Oakbrook, IL: Eterna Press, 1979.

Charney EB. Parental attitudes towards management of newborns with myelomeningocele. Devel Med Child Neurol 1990;32:14–19.

Colgan MT. The child with spina bifida: role of the pediatrician. Am J Dis Child 1981;135:854.

Cramer BA, Enrile B, McCoy KS. Knowledge, attitudes and behaviors related to sexuality in adolescents with chronic disability. Devel Med Child Neurol 1990;32:602–610.

Dauser RC, DiPietro MA, Venes JL. Symptomatic Chiara I malformation in childhood. A report of 7 cases. Pediatr Neurosci 1988;14:71–76.

Dysta GN, Menezes AH. Presentation and management of pediatric Chiari malformation in children without myelodysplasia. Neurosurgery 1988;23:589–597.

Editorial. Tethered cord. Lancet 1986;2:549–550.

Epstein F, Lapras C, Wisoff JH. "Slit-ventricle syndrome": etiology and treatment. Pediatr Neurosci 1988;14:5–10.

Evans RC, Tew B, Thomas MD, Ford J. Selective management of neural tube malformations. Arch Dis Child 1985;60:415.

Eyman RK, Grossman HJ, Chaney RH, Call TL. The life expectancy of profoundly handicapped people with mental retardation. N Engl J Med 1990;323:584–589.

Greene SA, Frank M, Zachman M, Prader A. Growth and sexual development in children with myelomeningocele. Eur J Pediatr 1985;144:146–148.

Hays RM, Jordan RA, McLaughlin JF, et al. Central ventilatory dysfunction in myelodysplasia: an independent determination of survival. Devel Med Child Neurol 1989;31:366–370.

Hood VD, Robinson HP. Diagnosis of closed neural tube defects by ultrasound in second trimester of pregnancy. Br Med J 1978;417:931.

Jacobson RI. Congenital structural defects. In: Swaiman KF, ed. Pediatric neurology. St. Louis: C.V. Mosby, 1989:319–326.

Jones RFC, Currie BG, Kwok BCT. Ventriculopleural shunts for hydrocephalus: a useful alternative. Neurosurgery 1988:23:753–755.

Kazak AE, Clark MW. Stress in families in children with myelomeningocele. Devel Med Child Neurol 1986;28:220–228.

Lavigne JV, Nolan D, McClone DG. Temperament, psychological coping and psychological adjustment in young children with myelomeningocele. J Pediatr Psychol 1988;13:363–378.

Loening-Baucke V, Desch L, Wolraich M. Biofeedback training for patients with myelomeningocele and fecal incontinence. Devel Med Child Neurol 1988;30:781–790.

McLaughlin JF, Shurtleff DB, Lamers JY, et al. Influence of prognosis on decisions regarding the care of newborns with myelodysplasia. N Engl J Med 1985;312:1589.

Menkes JH. Textbook of child neurology. 3rd ed. Philadelphia: Lea & Febiger, 1985.

Mickell JJ, Ward JD. Evaluation and treatment of intracranial hypertension. In: Pellock JM, Myer ED, eds. Neurologic emergencies in infancy and childhood. Philadelphia: Harper & Row, 1984:71–106.

Milihorat TH. Pediatric neurosurgery. Philadelphia: FA Davis, 1978.

Myer EC, Pellock JM. Disorders of the nervous system. In: Maurer HM, ed. Pediatrics. New York: Churchill Livingstone, 1983:531.

Naeye RL, Peters EC, Bartholomew M, Landis RJ. Origins of cerebral palsy. Am J Dis Child 1989;;143:1154–1161.

Nelson KB, Ellenberg JH. Epidemiology of cerebral palsy. Adv Neurol 1978;19:421–435.

Noetzel MJ. Myelomeningocele: current concepts of management. Clin Perinatol 1989;16:311–329.

Osaka K, Matsumoto S, Tanimura T. Myeloschisis in early human embryos. Child's Brain 1987;4:347.

Palmer FB, Shapiro BK, Wachtel RC, et al. The effects of physical therapy on cerebral palsy: a controlled trial in infants with spastic diplegia. N Engl J Med 1988:318:803–808.

Peacock WJ, Staudt LA. Spasticity in cerebral palsy and the selective posterior rhizotomy procedure. J Child Neurol 1990;5:179–185.

Query JM, Ruchet CC, Christoferson LA. Living with chronic illness: a retrospective study of patients shunted for hydrocephalus and their families. Devel Med Child Neurol 1990;32:119–128.

Rapin I. Children with brain dysfunction: neurology, cognition, language and behavior. New York: Raven Press, 1982.

Rowland LP. Merritt's textbook of neurology. 8th ed. Philadelphia: Lea & Febiger, 1989.

Scatcliff JH, Kendall BE, Kingsley DFE, et al. Closed spinal dysraphism: analysis of clinical, radiological and surgical findings in 104 consecutive patients. Am J Neuroradiol 1989;10:269–278.

Stanley F, Alberman E: The epidemiology of cerebral palsies. London: Spastics International Medical Publications, 1984.

Uehling DT, Smith J, Meyer J, Bruskewitz R. Impact of intermittent catheterization program on children with myelomeningocele. Pediatrics 1985;76:892–895.

Chapter 14

PSYCHIATRIC SYMPTOMS IN THE PROGRESSIVE METABOLIC, DEGENERATIVE, AND INFECTIOUS DISORDERS OF THE NERVOUS SYSTEM

Abe M. Chutorian, MD, and Steven G. Pavlakis, MD

INTRODUCTION

Progressive metabolic, degenerative, and infectious disorders of the nervous system, commonly grouped as the "neurodegenerative disorders", can begin with alterations of behavior and thinking that cannot initially be distinguished from psychologic disorders. These diseases typically produce progressive, generalized cerebral dysfunction (encephalopathy) characterized by dementia that might be accompanied by thought disorders, changes in personality, and hallucinations. However, some of the disorders may cause episodic mental changes. On the other hand, psychiatric disturbances without other neurologic manifestations over months to years are unlikely to be the result of a neurodegenerative disorder.

The differential diagnosis of neurodegenerative disorders according to their initial clinical manifestations is a standard approach. The diagnosis of these disorders in a child should be raised by the following presentations:

1. Cognitive defects without apparent cause.
2. Deterioration of academic achievement.
3. Lack of seizure control and developmental regression despite skillful anticonvulsant treatment.
4. The appearance, or worsening, of cognitive, motor, visual, or auditory function.
5. Genetic history of similar problem.

On the other hand, subtle static disturbances of cognitive function, such as dyslexia, attention deficit disorder, and learning disability, are rarely due to established metabolic disturbances. Children with these disorders often also have a similarly affected relative. Patients with atypical features of static conditions, such as attention deficit disorder with hyperactivity (ADDH), should be evaluated by a neurologist. For example, children with ADDH and staring spells may have absence epilepsy in addition to distractibility.

For the psychiatrist, the most meaningful classification of neurodegenerative diseases is based upon clinical features. Primary classification based on neuropathologic, biochemical, or genetic data is less helpful, and cross-classification with clinical features is required. Conditions that affect brain function during infancy

Table 14.1.
Classification and Clinical Features of Progressive Metabolic, Degenerative, and Infectious Disorders of the Nervous System

Poliodystrophy[a]	Dementia, seizures
Leukodystrophy[a]	Progressive spasticity, paresis, or ataxia, optic atrophy and other special sensory deficits
Chronic viral encephalopathies	Seizures, dementia, immunodeficiency
Nonstorage metabolic encephalopathies	
Amino acidopathies	Episodic or progressive mental status, neurologic, and systemic changes
Organic acidurias	
Porphyrias	
System degenerations	
Basal ganglia	Postural and movement abnormalities
Spinal cord	Progressive paresis and/or spasticity
Cerebellum	Progressive ataxia

[a] Many conditions have systemic involvement (storage) that causes visceromegaly and/or malfunction.

(e.g., Tay-Sachs disease) or cause predominantly spinal cord or peripheral nerve dysfunction (e.g., Friedreich's ataxia) are not discussed because psychologic disturbances are not a primary clinical manifestation.

The following classification (Table 14.1) begins with the distinction between degeneration of cerebral cortical gray matter (poliodystrophy), which usually causes seizures and dementia early in the course and degeneration of cerebral cortical white matter (leukodystrophy), which usually cause blindness, spasticity, and other motor disturbances.

POLIODYSTROPHIES (GRAY MATTER DISEASES)

Lipidoses

The lipidoses result from excessive storage of lipids in the nervous system and, to a varying degree, the visceral organs because of a specific lysosomal enzyme deficiency (Table 14.2). Since the lipid storage affects mostly the cerebral cortex, these illnesses are characterized by dementia and seizures. Lysosomal enzyme determination in white cells and skin fibroblast culture can confirm the diagnosis of specific disorders.

The gangliosidoses, one of the major varieties of lipidoses, show storage of ganglioside because of hexosaminidase or B-galactosidase deficiency. Both Tay-Sach's and Sandhoff's disease, well-known examples that occur in infants, are characterized by motor and intellectual deterioration, seizures, macrocephaly, and macular abnormalities (including the retinal cherry-red spot). Varieties that occur in children are characterized by more subtle changes, slower deterioration of intellect, and ataxia.

The Tay-Sach's disease gene has a frequency of 1/27 among Jewish people and 1/380 among non-Jewish people. Adult carriers of Tay-Sach's gene and affected fetuses can be detected by de-

Table 14.2.
Poliodystrophies (Gray Matter Disease)

Metabolic storage diseases
Lipidoses
Neuronal ceroid lipofuscinoses
Mucopolysaccharidoses
Mucolipidoses
Glycogen storage disorders
Alpers syndrome
Mitochondrial disorders
Rett's syndrome
Epileptic encephalopathies
Infantile myoclonic
Lennox-Gastaut syndrome

termining the concentration of leukocyte or amniotic fluid hexosaminidase.

Niemann-Pick disease (sphingomyelinase deficiency) is classified into infantile and juvenile varieties. There are some relatively unique clinical features that aid in their identification apart from the usual mental, motor, macular, and visceral manifestations. Changes in behavior and intellect are the features that bring affected children to the attention of the psychiatrist.

In Gaucher's disease, glucocerebrosidase is severely deficient in infants who manifest the disease and is mildly decreased in adults. The juvenile variety is characterized by progressive spasticity and seizures, but the adult form chiefly has hepatic failure and anemia (i.e., nonneurologic problems).

Fabry's disease, which results from trihexosidase deficiency, causes a syndrome of dermal angiokerotosis, renal disease, hypertension, and attacks of painful, burning neuropathy.

The late-onset neuronal ceroid lipofuscinoses may present with behavior change and dementia before overt neurologic disturbances, such as seizures, abnormal movements (e.g., dystonia), and motor deterioration. The basic metabolic defect has not been determined, but abnormal quantities of ceroid lipofuscin accumulate in brain, muscle, and somatic tissues. The diagnosis depends on clinical suspicion and electron microscopic demonstration of inclusions in lymphocytes, skin, or muscle. Infantile and late infantile forms are characterized by retinal degeneration and seizures, while juvenile (Spielmeyer-Vogt disease) and adult (Kufs' disease) forms show retinal degeneration, followed by mild ataxia, dystonia and dementia.

Other disorders of lipid metabolism are associated with a variety of systemic and peripheral nervous system conditions that are important to general medicine and neurology but do not cause patients to have mental or behavioral changes of the type likely to prompt psychiatric consultation. These disorders include Refsum's disease, abetalipoproteinemia, vitamin E deficiency, Tan-

gier's disease, and disorders of carnitine metabolism. Although in carnitine deficiency, for example, acute encephalopathy (with stupor or coma) may occur, this group of disorders is not associated with chronic mental or behavioral changes of the type likely to prompt psychiatric consultation.

Mucopolysaccharidoses and Mucolipidoses

Mucopolysaccharidoses and mucolipidoses are characterized by dysmorphic features including certain skeletal changes called "gargoylism," corneal clouding and other ocular abnormalities, and visceromegaly. In most forms of these disorders there is progressive intellectual decline. When lipid storage occurs concomitantly, the disorder is known as a mucolipidosis. The dysmorphic features of gargoylism are short stature, macrocephaly, coarse facial features, short spadelike hands and feet, and protuberant abdomen. Sanfilippo's syndrome is characterized by dementia and behavioral problems in childhood, with fewer dysmorphic features.

The child's dysmorphic appearance should lead to urine screening for the mucopolysaccharidoses (excretion of dextran and herparan sulfate). The enzymatic defects include iuronidase, sulfatase, galactosidase, glucouronidase (mucopolysaccharidoses), mannosidase, fucosidase (glycoprotein disorders), and neuraminidase (mucolipidoses) deficiencies. Biopsy of a variety of tissues, and, above all, specific enzyme determination, will pinpoint the subclass of disorder involved.

Alpers Syndrome

Alpers syndrome is a progressive poliodystrophy characterized by seizures and dementia. It is inherited principally in an autosomal-recessive form. Progressive cortical atrophy, demonstrated on computed tomography (CT) or magnetic resonance imaging (MRI) by widening of the central sulci, cisterns, and fissures, results from

marked loss of neurons. Seizures are often refractory to treatment. Symptoms begin in early
childhood or in the teen years and progress to a
vegetative state and death. The exact cause is
unknown, and specific laboratory identification
is not possible.

Mitochondrial Encephalomyopathies

Mitochondrial encephalomyopathies may present with peripheral and/or central nervous system impairments. In these disorders, which have
different rates of progression and principal clinical manifestations, derangements of energy metabolism generally result in failure to thrive,
short stature, seizures, ophthalmoplegia, and dementia. These disorders can be inherited mater-
nally. Acute hemiplegia and migrainous syndromes occur in a form known as MELAS:
Mitochondrial Encephalopathy with Lactic Aci-
doses and Stroke-like episodes. Since lactic acidosis is common, serum lactate determination is
the most useful screening test. Cardiac and renal
disease may occur. One of the first patients who
presented with MELAS had visual hallucinations; later he developed seizures and a stroke-
like episode. Myopathy, whether clinically evident or silent can be demonstrated by the histologic presence of "ragged red fibers" on
trichrome stain of a muscle biopsy. Other mitochondrial syndromes include Kearns-Sayre
syndrome (ophthalmoplegia, retinal degeneration, dementia, and heart-block) and MERRF
syndrome: Myoclonic Epilepsy with ataxia and
Ragged Red Fibers. Since growth failure is a
common feature, short children with undiagnosed central and/or peripheral nervous system disorders should be screened by serum
lactate determination and, if suspicion is appropriate, undergo muscle biopsy.

Rett's Syndrome

Rett's syndrome is limited to girls. It is first
apparent at age 1 to 2 years and is slowly progressive. Its principal features are developmental
arrest with deceleration of head growth (second-

ary microcephaly), evolving autistic features and
dementia, and a striking loss of purposeful hand
function with unique hand-wringing. There is
also the development of gradual scoliosis spasticity, and seizures. Cases are usually sporadic.
Since no laboratory test for the disorder is available, the diagnosis of Rett's syndrome is entirely
clinical.

Epileptic Encephalopathies

This term refers to any situation in which developmental arrest and/or regression are presumed to result from severe epilepsy, regardless
of its etiology, that is refractory to treatment.
Syndromes complicated by epileptic encephalopathy include infantile spasms with hypsarhythmic electroencephalogram (EEG) (West's
syndrome) and generalized mixed seizures in
early childhood, including myoclonic, absence,
atonic, and major seizures (Lennox-Gastaut syndrome).

LEUKODYSTROPHIES
(WHITE MATTER DISEASES)

Unlike the poliodystrophies, which are characterized principally by seizures and dementia, the
leukodystrophies (Table 14.3), which cause
white matter abnormalities (dysmyelination), are
characterized by progressively more severe spasticity, ataxia, optic atrophy, and intellectual
decline. Relatively common illnesses in this
category are transmitted genetically and include
metachromatic leukodystrophy. Krabbe's disease, and adrenoleukodystrophy. Children and adolescents are also subject to acquired disorders
of cerebral myelin (demyelination). These in-

Table 14.3.
Leukodystrophies (White Matter Disease)

Metachromatic leukodystrophy
Krabbe's disease
Adrenoleukodystrophy
Pelizaeus-Merzbacher disease
Canavan's disease
Alexander's disease

clude multiple sclerosis, progressive multifocal leukoencephalopathy (PML), and subacute sclerosing panencephalitis (SSPE). Cerebral myelination is abnormal and can be detected by CT and even better delineated by MRI in both genetic and acquired conditions.

Metachromatic Leukodystrophy

Metachromatic leukodystrophy (MLD) usually becomes apparent in late infancy, but juvenile and later onset also occur. In MLD, a deficiency of the enzyme arylsulfatase A results in storage of sulfatide, which is metachromatically stained in tissue by cresyl violet stain applied either to peripheral or central myelin.

Juvenile MLD is characterized by ataxia and evolving spasticity, along with hyporeflexia due to peripheral nerve involvement. Dementia gradually occurs with advancing age. Juvenile-onset MLD can present atypically with dementia and schizophrenic symptoms. Cerebrospinal fluid (CSF) protein is characteristically elevated, nerve conduction velocity is slowed, and arylsulfatase-A is depleted in serum and fibroblasts. Sural nerve biopsy aids in diagnosis.

Krabbe's Disease

Krabbe's disease also called "globoid cell leukodystrophy" due to the histologic appearance of affected tissues, occurs as a rapidly progressive quadriparesis in infancy, but rare juvenile cases are characterized by dementia and progressive spasticity. As in MLD, CSF protein is elevated and nerve conduction velocity is slowed. Crystalline needle-like inclusions are seen on sural nerve biopsy. Enzymatic assay of fibroblasts demonstrates the deficiency of beta-galactosylcerebrosidase.

Adrenoleukodystrophy

Adrenoleukodystrophy, which is an X-linked genetic illness, is characterized by boys' and young men's developing visual loss, progressive spas-

ticity, and dementia. Seizures occur but usually are not prominent. Behavioral difficulty with emotional lability is very common at the onset. An early school-aged boy who presents with progressive behavior and learning problems should be suspected of harboring this disorder.

Abnormal myelination, most notable in the occipital regions, may be striking on CT or MRI. Peripheral nervous system involvement occurs, but it is prominent only in a variant in adolescents and young women. Adrenal insufficiency may be clinically silent or severe, particularly late in the illness, and cause increased dermal or gingival pigmentation, postural hypotension, a hypoglycemic glucose tolerance test, and lack of response to ACTH stimulation. The diagnosis may be confirmed by demonstrating an increase of very long chain fatty acids in the plasma. Characteristic lipid inclusions are found by histologic examination of testicular, adrenal, or nervous system tissue.

Pelizaeus-Merzbacher Disease

Although the congenital form, with infantile involvement and demise in early childhood, does not merit discussion here, older children with the disease typically have coarse nystagmus, roving eye movements, progressive spasticity, and dementia. Psychiatric manifestations likely occur in the context of an obvious neurologic syndrome. Dysmyelination can be demonstrated by slowed nerve conduction velocity. Brain biopsy is required for definitive diagnosis.

Canavan's Disease

Dysmyelination with spongy degeneration results in severe neurologic impairment in this rare, autosomal-recessive disorder presenting in infancy. The defect in Canavan's disease is lack of aspartoacyclase enzyme. It is diagnosed by an excessive N-acetylaspartic acid in urine and other body fluids. Macrocephaly may be striking. This condition is unlikely to mimic psychiatric disease.

Alexander's Disease

Although it has a later onset and a more gradual progression than Canavan's disease, Alexander's disease also causes macrocephaly and symptoms that are unlikely to mimic psychiatric disease. This illness is due to accumulation of eosinophilic material in astrocytic footplates throughout the brain. As in the other dysmyelination disorders, CT or MRI are helpful in the diagnosis, but definitive diagnosis requires brain biopsy.

"SLOW" VIRAL INFECTIONS OF THE CNS

On rare occasion, seizures and/or progressive dementia result from vital infection of the brain. Infectious disorders and their principal manifestations in children can induce neurodegenerative disease (Table 14.4).

Acquired immunodeficiency syndrome (AIDS) is playing an increasing role in chronic cerebral infection in children. An opportunistic infection can occur (e.g., toxoplasmosis), but the AIDS virus is neurotropic and results in a slowly progressive dementia with spasticity (see Chapter 17).

Progressive multifocal leukoencephalopathy (PML) is a subacute disorder found in children with compromised immune systems that is unlikely to be confused with degenerative disease. Although patients can present with altered behavior, the multifocal physical manifestations and evolving stupor help to differentiate PML from the chronic encephalopathies. Children with PML usually are already known to have AIDS, immunosuppressive drug treatment, radiation, or lymphomatous disease. On MRI, multifocal demyelination is evident.

Subacute sclerosing panencephalitis (SSPE) (and similarly progressive subacute rubella encephalitis) are more apt to appear as degenerative than infectious disorders. In these illnesses, following a latent period of 5 to 10 years after an acute measles (rubeola) or rubella infection, children develop behavioral change, impaired school performance, and, finally, myoclonic seizures and dementia. The disease may cause stupor, coma, and death within months or may progress over several years. The diagnosis depends upon

Table 14.4.
Chronic Viral Infections

Acquired immunodeficiency syndrome (AIDS)	Gradual dementia
	Progressive spasticity
	Secondary microcephaly
	Acquired immunodeficiency
Progressive multifocal leukoencephalopathy (PML)	Seizures, especially myoclonic
	Dementia
	Stupor
	Immunodeficiency
Subacute sclerosing panencephalitis (SSPE)	Seizures, especially myoclonic
	Dementia
	Rubeola CSF antibodies
Progressive rubella panencephalitis	Seizures
	Dementia
	Rubella CSF antibodies
Chronic enteroviral encephalitis	Seizures
	Dementia
	IgG deficiency
Jakob-Creutzfeldt disease	Myoclonus
	Dementia
	Ataxia
	Rigidity

demonstration of CSF antibodies and associated CSF immunochemical changes.

Chronic enteroviral encephalitis, which causes seizures and dementia, occurs in children with agammaglobulinemia who have multiple infections. The CSF pleocytosis and CSF virus persist in the immunocompromised child.

Jakob-Creutzfeldt disease, which is usually a disease of older adults, causes progressively more severe myoclonus, dementia, rigidity and spasticity. It has developed in children who have received infected protein or transplanted tissue (e.g., infected human growth hormone, infected corneal transplant).

METABOLIC ENCEPHALOPATHIES

Most children with inborn errors of metabolism present during infancy with seizure, metabolic encephalopathy, stupor and coma, or failure to thrive (Table 14.5); the reader is referred for discussion of these disorders to a comprehensive textbook. However, some of these disorders or their milder forms can present in school-aged children.

Aminoacidopathies

In the aminoacidopathies, protein ingestion leads to accumulation of either amino acids or intermediary metabolites that precipitate neurologic illness. Although most of these disorders cause illness during infancy and therefore are not described, some exist in a compensated state

Table 14.5.
Inborn Errors of Metabolism
Causing Encephalopathy

Aminoacidopathies
Organic acidurias
Urea cycle disorders (hyperammonemias)
Carbohydrate disorders
Disorders of purine and pyrimidine metabolism
Porphyrias

with chronic neurologic illness or they involve periodic or progressive seizures and dementia. For example, phenylketonuria is encountered in retarded children with seizure disorder. These children and others with aminoacidopathy become ill during infancy, but later-onset cases have been reported.

In general, children with unexplained retardation, seizures, or ataxia, with or without failure to thrive, should be tested for aminoaciduria. Aminoacidopathies are particularly responsive to treatment either by dietary manipulation or vitamin supplements. Genetic counseling is also mandatory.

Maple syrup urine disease may occur in a neonatal form, but a later-onset variant results in episodic ataxia or stupor.

Homocystinuria, resulting from cystathionine synthetase deficiency and accumulation of homocystine, leads to mild retardation and a tendency to suffer strokes. Marfanoid features are characteristic.

Hartnup disease, a defect in intestinal transport of certain amino acids, causes episodic ataxia, behavior disorder, and a pellagra-like rash. Urinary neutral amino acids are excreted.

Organic Acidurias

Organic acidemias result from defects in intermediary metabolism. These disorders are diagnosed by the specific metabolite accumulated; however, in general, they can be divided into disorders characterized by accumulation of ketones or glycine, or by the occurrence of lactic (and pyruvic) acidemia or glutarylacidemia. Lactic acidosis often occurs.

The severe disorders occur in infancy and are often fatal. Lesser severity is associated with chronic, intermittent, or progressive disease. Failure to thrive is common. Vomiting and cerebral dysfunction may occur. Exacerbation and remission of neurologic manifestations are common. Urinary organic acid analysis confirms the diagnosis, which may be partly responsive to treatment.

Urea Cycle Disorders

Hyperammonemia is the hallmark of this group of disorders. The most commonly occurring variety is ornithine transcarbamylase (OTC) deficiency, which is transmitted by X-linked inheritance. It is usually lethal to males but has variable expression in females. There is a spectrum of severity of the enzyme deficit in the urea cycle disorders. Survivors of neonatal encephalopathy typically have developmental delay. The episodic nature of these disorders should arouse suspicion in patients with milder, later-onset intermittent encephalopathies. The intermittent symptoms, which are correlated with high blood ammonia levels, are apt to occur during infection and consist of vomiting and drowsiness progressing to stupor. Dietary protein restriction may be effective treatment, especially for ornithine transcarbamylase deficiency. Benzoate, phenylacetate, and, in the acute situation, exchange transfusion are helpful.

Carbohydrate Disorders

These disorders, which include abnormalities of galactose, fructose, and glucose metabolism, lead to hypoglycemia. Defects in gluconeogenesis or glycolysis can produce severe progressive encephalopathy. However, further discussion is deferred since their manifestations are acute as well as chronic and therefore unlikely to present to the pediatric psychiatrist.

Purine and Pyrimidine Disorders

Phosphoribosyl transferase deficiency, better known as Lesch-Nyhan syndrome, is characterized by self-mutilation and other bizarre behaviors, mental deficiency, choreoathetosis, and spasticity in boys. It is an X-linked disorder. Uric acidemia in conjunction with the clinical syndrome is diagnostic.

The Porphyrias

Of the various porphyrias, acute intermittent porphyria (AIP) causes episodic abdominal pain with psychiatric disorder that may be precipitated by barbiturates and other drugs. AIP may also cause a severe polyneuropathy. Inheritance is dominant, and prepubertal occurrence is rare, but affected teenagers are reported. Uroporphyrinogen synthetase is deficient. Other porphyrias are associated with photosensitivity.

MOVEMENT DISORDERS OF KNOWN OR PRESUMPTIVE METABOLIC/ DEGENERATIVE TYPE

A variety of cerebral disorders due to involvement of the basal ganglia are characterized by abnormalities of muscle tone and posture. Other portions of the nervous system and even somatic viscera are involved in some of these disorders (see Chapter 7).

CHRONIC AND RECURRENT ATAXIA OF METABOLIC ORIGIN

Strictly speaking, ataxia can be caused by degeneration of any system of the CNS that functions in relay with the systems modulating coordination, such as the pontocerebellar, frontopontocerebellar, and spinocerebellar systems (Table 14.6). Moreover, ataxia in its purest sense means unsteady movement that can be caused by proprioceptive sensory impairment or, as in polyneuropathy, even peripheral weakness. In some disorders, such as maple syrup urine

Table 14.6.
Recurrent or Chronic Ataxia of Metabolic Degenerative Origin

Friedreich's ataxia
Other spinocerebellar degenerations
Myoclonic encephalopathies
  Ataxia/opsoclonus
  With organic acidemia
  With mitochondrial disease
  With aminoacidemia
  Lafora body disease
Subacute necrotizing encephalomyelitis
  (Leigh's disease)

disease, Hartnup disease, and multiple carboxylase deficiency, episodic ataxia is encountered.

Friedreich's Ataxia

Friedreich's ataxia is the classic inherited disorder of the spinocerebellar and peripheral nervous system. The affected child has progressive ataxia affecting the trunk, limbs, and oromotor function, together with progressive dysfunction of the long spinal cord tracts. Friedreich's ataxia causes proprioceptive sensory deficit and extensor plantar reflexes, but not encephalopathy.

Varieties of spinal, cerebellar, and peripheral nerve impairments may be encountered. Although clinical expression varies, cerebral function is usually spared.

Ataxia-Telangiectasia

Ataxia-telangiectasia is a neurocutaneous disorder in which ataxia develops early but mental deficiency is uncommon. Telangiectasia of the conjunctiva, earlobes, and malar areas occurs between 3 and 5 years of age in a child with ataxia. Other clinical manifestations include oculomotor apraxia, choreoathetosis, and dystonia. Serum alpha-fetoprotein is elevated, IgA may be absent, and cellular immunity is deficient. The immunodeficiency often causes recurrent infection, particularly sinopulmonary infection, and neoplasia, particularly lymphatic neoplasms. Faulty DNA repair is associated with the basic defect, which is of autosomal-recessive inheritance.

PEROXISOMAL AND OTHER ORGANELLE DISORDERS

Neurodegenerative disorders can also be separated by the affected organelle. Diseases of the peroxisome (Table 14.7), lysosome (Table 14.8), and mitochondria (Table 14.9) result in neurologic disease. In order to determine a diagnosis,

Table 14.7
The Peroxisomal Disorders[a]

Disease	Function Affected	Neurologic Findings
Refsum's disease	Phytanic acid oxidation	Neuropathy, pigmentary degeneration, deafness, ichthyosis
Acatalsemia	Reduction of hydrogen peroxide	None
Hyperoxaluria type I	Conversion of glyoxalate to glycine	None
X-linked Adrenoleukodystrophy	Beta-oxidation of fatty acids	Progressive dementia, impaired cortical vision and hearing, paralysis
Adrenomyeloneuropathy	Beta-oxidation of fatty acids	Spastic paraparesis, ataxia, dementia, polyneuropathy
Pseudoneonatal ALD	Beta-oxidation of fatty acids	Severe retardation and seizures
Pseudo-Zellweger's	Beta-oxidation of fatty acids	Profound retardation and seizures
Bifunctional enzyme deficiency	Beta-oxidation of fatty acids	Profound retardation and seizures
Rhizomelic chondrodysplasia punctata	Plasmalogen syntheses and phytanic acid oxidation	Severe retardation
Zellweger's syndrome	All functions deficient	Profound retardation with no psychomotor development; seizures
Neonatal ALD	All functions deficient	Profound retardation with little psychomotor development; seizures
Infantile Refsum's	All functions deficient	Severe retardation, blindness and deafness
Pipecolic acidemia	All functions deficient	Severe retardation, blindness
Benign variant	All functions deficient	Ataxia and peripheral neuropathy (normal cognition)

[a] These disorders are diagnosed by clinical features and plasma very long chain fatty acid determination.

Table 14.8.
The Lysosomal Disorders[a]

Disease	Function Affected	Neurologic Findings
Mucopolysaccharidoses	Lysosomal enzyme deficiency in degradation of dermatin, heparin, or keratin sulfate	Hydrocephalus, cervical myelopthy, dementia, multisystem involvement coarse features
Mucolipidoses II, III	Abnormal glycoprotein N-acetyl-galactoaminylphosphotransferase	Mental retardation, coarse features, seizures
Disorders of glycoprotein degradation	Fucosidase, neuraminidase, and aspartylglycosaminidase deficiency	Mental retardation, coarse features, seizures
Disorders of acid lipase	Acid lipase deficiency	Occasional retardation
Farber's	Ceramidase deficiency	Occasional retardation
Niemann-Pick	Sphingomyelinase deficiency	Mental retardation, hepatosplenomegaly
Gaucher's	Glucocerebrosidase deficiency	Mental retardation, spasticity, hepatosplenomegaly
Krabbe's	Galactocerebrosidase deficiency	Dementia, spasticity seizures, hepatosplenomegaly
Metachromatic leukodystrophy	Arylsulfatase deficiency	Dementia, blindness, neuropathy
Fabry's	Alpha-galactosidase deficiency	Skin lesion, painful neuropathy, strokes
GM1 and GM2 gangliosidoses	Beta-galactosidase and hexosaminidase deficiency	Dementia, seizures, large phenotypic variability

[a] These disorders are diagnosed by clinical features and biochemical markers. Enzymatic determinations are obtained on cultured white cells or fibroblasts.

cross-classification using clinical characteristics, involved organelles, biochemical derangements, and genetic markers, when available, is necessary.

METABOLIC/DEGENERATIVE DISORDERS AMENABLE TO TREATMENT

Some disorders amenable to therapy have been described above, according to their associ-

ated biochemical abnormalities, (Tables 14.10–14.12). In some cases, the disorders are due to coenzyme deficiency responsive to vitamin therapy, while in others, dietary or biochemical manipulation is possible.

SUMMARY

Although neurodegenerative disorders rarely present to the psychiatrist without obvious neurologic findings, an understanding by the psy-

Table 14.9
The Mitochondrial Disorders[a]

Disease	Function Affected	Neurologic Findings
MERRF	Electron transport (ET) defect	Myoclonus, epilepsy, ataxia
MELAS	Electron transport defect	Encephalopathy, seizures, stroke-like episodes
Kearns-Sayre syndrome (KSS)	?	Ophthalmoplegia, ataxia, retinal degeneration
Leber optic atrophy	?	Progressive optic atrophy
Infantile bilateral striatal necrosis	?	Encephalopathy and movement disorder

[a] Other biochemical mitochondrial defects of transport, substrate utilization, Krebs cycle, oxidation-phosphorylation coupling, and the electron transport chain are described. The clinical characteristics are protean.
    Diagnosis of these disorders is based on clinical characteristics, genetic markers (MELAS, MERRF, KSS, Leber optic atrophy), and biochemical derangements (enzyme assay in muscle, white cells, or skin culture). Abnormal muscle biopsy and lactic acidosis occur in MERRF, MELAS, and KSS.

Table 14.10.
Vitamin Deficiency

Disease	Biochemical Feature	Therapy	Clinical Feature
Combined systemic disease	Vitamin B_{12} deficiency	Vitamin B_{12}	Anemia Motor/sensory neuropathy, ataxia
Methylmalonic aciduria	Specific organic aciduria	Vitamin B_{12}	Failure to thrive, stupor-acidosis
Multiple carboxylase deficiency	Biotinidase deficiency	Biotin	Alopecia Ataxia Stupor, acidosis
Hartnup disease	Niacin deficiency	Niacin	Ataxia Aminoaciduria, rash
Pellagra	Niacin deficiency	Niacin	Rash, neuropathy, encephalopathy
Spinocerebellar	Vitamin E deficiency	Vitamin E	Steatorrhea Motor/sensory degeneration Neuropathy
Bassen-Kornsweig disease	Vitamin A and E deficiency	Vitamin A and E	Enteropathy, neuropathy Retinal degeneration, ataxia Acanthocytosis
Pyruvate-dehydrogenase deficiency	Thiamine deficiency	Thiamine	Leigh's syndrome

chiatrist of these disorders allows for prompt diagnosis, an appreciation of the condition, and, for several diseases, treatment. The clinical characteristics of neurodegenerative diseases are protean, yet discernible.

Gray matter diseases often start with behavioral alterations and school failure. Juvenile forms of gangliosidoses and Niemann-Pick disease present with dementia; neuronal ceroid lipofuscinosis can present in the adolescent with striking behavioral changes. Likewise, the mucopolysaccharidoses typically start at age 2 to 3 years with language regression and behavioral outbursts. Mitochondrial encephalopathies can

Table 14.11.
Organic Acidurias and Amino Acidurias

Disease	Biochemical Feature	Therapy	Clinical Features
Phenylketonuria	Phenylketonuria	Dietary	Mental deficiency Seizures, eczema
Maple syrup urine disease	Organic aciduria	Dietary	Acidosis, chronic or recurrent encephalopathy
Methylmalonic aciduria	Specific organic aciduria	Dietary: low protein	Acidosis, carnitine encephalopathy, chronic or recurrent
Proprionic acidemia	Specific organic aciduria	Dietary: low protein	Acidosis, carnitine encephalopathy, chronic or recurrent
Hyperglycinemia	Nonketotic hyperglycinemia	Diazepam folate	Intractible epilepsy Mental deficiency
Hyperammonemia	Arginosuccinic aciduria	Arginine	Lethargy, thin hair
Hyperphenylalaninemia	Dihydropteridine reductase deficiency	Neurotransmitter precursors	Seizures, mental deficiency

Table 14.12.
Miscellaneous Disorders

Disease	Biochemical Feature	Therapy	Neurologic Features
Glycogen storage disease	Hypoglycemia	Elevate glucose	Seizures Mental deficiency
Refsum's disease	Phytanic acidemia	Diet	Neuropathy, retinopathy ichthyosis
Labyrism	Oxalylaminoalaninemia	Diet	Spastic paraparesis
Wilson's disease	Copper deposition Low ceruloplasmin	Chelation	Dementia, extrapyramidal signs
Carbamyl-phosphate synthetase deficiency	Hyperammonemia	Benzoate low protein diet	Recurrent stupor and vomiting
Ornithine transcarbamylase deficiency	Hyperammonemia	Benzoate low protein diet	Recurrent stupor and vomiting
Galactosemia	Galactosuria	Diet	Hepatosplenomegaly Mental deficiency, cataract
Cretinism	Low serum T4	Thyroxine	Mental deficiency Slow metabolism Growth deceleration
Porphyria	Porphobilinogenemia and porphyrinemia	Prophylaxis Avoidance of painful crises Precipitating factors	Neuropathy, encephalopathy

present with psychosis. Rett's syndrome, probably the most common cause of autism in females, presents in girls aged 1 to 2 years with progressive microcephaly and autistic features.

The white matter diseases, as a rule, are associated less often with dementia and behavioral changes. However, this rule is often broken. For example, juvenile metachromatic leukodystrophy can start in the adolescent with alteration of behavior—either passivity or aggression—followed by school failure. Krabbe's disease usually occurs in infancy, but toddlers with developmental regression as the first symptom have been reported. X-linked adrenoleukodystrophy, the prototypical peroxisomal disorder, can present in preschool boys with visual failure, personality changes, and school problems.

Chronic viral infections, such as HIV encephalitis and SSPE, produce a progressive encephalopathy that may begin as a personality change and insidious school failure.

Prenatal diagnosis is potentially available for the numerous disorders with known genetic or enzymatic defects. Linkage analysis allows for prenatal diagnosis, and molecular markers are becoming available. Also, highly technical treatments, such as gene manipulation and bone marrow transplantation, as in metachromatic leukodystrophy, are undergoing trials.

Once a diagnosis is confirmed, the psychiatrist's role does not end. The psychiarist can provide individual and family support, with behavior modification playing a role in patient management. Major tranquilizers, stimulant medication, and antidepressants may improve behavior and mood. Finally, the psychiatrist can act as a liaison with community resources, providing maximum support to both the individual and the family.

SUGGESTED READINGS

Adrenoleukodystrophy
Kitchin W, Cohen-Cole SA, Mickel SF. Adrenoleukodystrophy: frequency of presentation as a psychiatric disorder. Bio Psychiatry 1987;22:1375–1387.

Menza MA, Blake J, Goldberg L. Affective symptoms and adrenoleukodystrophy: a report of two cases. Psychosomatics 1988;29:442–445.

Moser HW, Naidu S, Kumar AJ, et al. The adrenoleukodystrophies. Crit Rev Neurobiol 1987;3:29–99.

Panegyres PK, Goldswain P. Kakulas BA. Adult-onset adrenoleukodystrophy manifesting as dementia. Am J Med 1989;87:481–483.

Sadeghi-Nejad A, Senior B. Adrenomyeloneuropathy presenting as Addison's disease in childhood. N Engl J Med 1990;322:13–16.

Metachromatic Leukodystrophy

Galbraith DA, Gordon BA, Feleki V, et al. Metachromatic leukodystrophy (MLD) in hospitalized adult schizophrenic patients resistant to drug treatment Can J Psychiatry 1989;34:299–302.

Krivit W, Shapiro E, Kennedy W, et al. Treatment of late infantile metachromatic leukodystrophy by bone marrow transplantation. N Eng J Med 1990;322:28–32.

Naylor MW, Alessi NE. Pseudoarylsulfatase A deficiency in a psychiatrically disturbed adolescent. J Am Acad Child Adolesc Psychiatry 1989;28:444–449.

FitzGerald PM, Jankovic J, Glaze DG, et al. Extrapyramidal involvement in Rett's syndrome. Neurology 1990;40:293–295.

Mitochondrial Encephalopathies

Di Mauro S, Bonilla E, Zeviani M, Nakagawa M, de Vivo DC. Mitochondrial myopathies. Ann Neurol 1985;17:521–538.

Pavlakis SG, Rowland LP, DeVivo DC, et al. Mitochondrial myopathies and encephalopathies. In: Plum F, ed. Advances in contemporary neurology 1989;29:95–133.

Neuronal Ceroid-Lipofuscinoses

Kohlschutter A, Laabs R, Albani M. Juvenile neuronal ceroid lipofuscinosis (JNCL): quantitative description of its clinical variability. Acta Paediatr Scand 1988;77:867–872.

Santavuori P. Neuronal ceroid-lipofuscinoses in childhood. Brain Devel 1988;10:80–83.

Progressive Multifocal Leukoencephalopathy (PML)

Greenlee JE. Progressive multifocal leukoencephalopathy. Curr Clin Top Infect Dis 1989;10:140–156.

Hseuh C, Reyes CV. Progressive multifocal leukoencephalopathy. Am Fam Physician 1988;37:129–132.

Richardson EP. Our evolving understanding of progressive multifocal leukoencephalopathy. Ann NY Acad Sci 1974;230:358–364.

Porphyria

Holman JR, Green JB. Acute intermittent porphyria: more than just abdominal pain. Postgrad Med 1989;86:295–299.

Straka JG, Rank JM, Bloomer JR. Porphyria and porphyrin metabolism. Annu Rev Med 1990;41:457–469.

Rett's Syndrome

Budden S. Meek M, Henighan C. Communication and oral-motor function in Rett syndrome. Devel Med Child Neurol 1990;32:51–55.

Echenne B, Bressot N. Cheminal R, et al. Rett syndrome. A report of fifteen cases. Ann Pediatr 1989;36:661–668.

McIntosh RP, Simatos D, Weston HJ, et al. Rett syndrome: case reports and review. NZ Med J 1990;103:122–125.

Olsson B, Rett A. A review of the Rett syndrome with a theory of autism. Brain Devel 1990;12:11–5.

Subacute Sclerosing Panencephalitis (SSPE)

Duncalf CM, Kent JN, Harbord M, et al. Subacute sclerosing panencephalitis presenting a schizophreniform psychosis. Br J Psychiatry 1989;155:557–559.

Dyken PR. Subacute sclerosing panencephalitis. Current status. Neurol Clin 1985;3:179–196.

Okuno Y, Nakao T, Ishida N, et al. Incidence of subacute sclerosing panencephalitis following measles and measles vaccination in Japan. Int J Epidemiol 1989;18:684.

Robertson WC, Clark DB, Markesbery WR. Review of 328 cases of subacute sclerosing panencephalitis: effects of amantadine on the natural course of the disease. Ann Neurol 1980;8:422–425.

Tay-Sachs

Adams C, Green S. Late-onset hexosaminidase A and B deficiency: family study and review. Devel Med Child Neurol 1986;28:236–243.

Evans PR. Tay-Sachs disease: a centenary. Arch Dis Child 1987;62:1056–1059.

Specola N, Vanier MT, Goutiéres F, et al. The juvenile and chronic forms of GM2 gangliosidosis: clinical and enzymatic heterogeneity. Neurology 1990;40:145–150.

Streifler J, Golomb M, Gadoth N. Psychiatric features of adult GM2 gangliosidosis. Br J Psychiatry 1989;155:410–413.

General References

Scriver CR, Beaudet AL, Sly WJ, Valle D. The metabolic basis of inherited disease. 6th ed. New York: McGraw Hill, 1987.

Swaiman KF, ed. The practice of pediatric neurology. 3rd ed. St. Louis: Mosby, 1989

Menkes JH. Textbook of child neurology. 4th ed. Philadelphia: Lea & Febiger, 1990.

Chapter 15

MENTAL RETARDATION

Hart Peterson, MD

Mental retardation is not a disease but a state of intellectual subnormality. It affects 2 to 3% of the population and is generally, but not always, due to a "static" encephalopathy; moreover, it is commonly associated with other significant psychiatric problems such as pervasive developmental disorder.

Intellectual impairment is most comonly classified by the severity of deficit. A commonly accepted definition requires an IQ of less than 70 on one of the Wechsler intelligence tests. Using this system, *mild* mental retardation encompasses an IQ of 55 to 69; *moderate* mental retardation, an IQ of 40 to 54; *severe* mental retardation, an IQ of 25 to 39; and *profound* mental retardation, an IQ below 25. The use of IQ scores imparts a false sense of precision to these categories.

The level of mental retardation can also be graded by the degree of functional or educational impairment. Children with an IQ between 55 and 70 are considered *educable*. These are children whom we attempt to teach academic subjects such as reading and mathematics, some of whom will be able to be independent, or largely so, in society. Children with an IQ between 40 and 55 are considered *trainable*. They are individuals who can handle many of their own needs but require supervision for some aspects of travel and money management and will remain partly dependent. Many of these individuals can be trained to do productive and rewarding work in a sheltered environment. Most can become independent in activities of daily living. *Severe* mental retardation, with an IQ of 25 to 39, implies some ability to communicate but lack of full independence in activities of daily living. *Profound* mental retardation implies a high state of dependency, generally with only rudimentary ability to communicate. This functional classification has the considerable advantage of conveying the amount of outside supervision required for an individual retarded person.

The prevalence of various degrees of mental retardation is not equally distributed. Approximately 75% of cases fall into the educable range. Culturally disadvantaged individuals and minorities are heavily overrepresented in this group. Discrete brain anomalies or diseases are underrepresented in the educable group.

Classification by etiology is traditional in medicine. Indeed, classification of mental retardation by etiology has many virtues. Unfortunately, since most mental retardation represents dysfunction stemming from previous events (static encephalopathy), medically treatable forms of mental retardation are rare. Phenylketonuria, galactosemia, and other metabolic diseases are potentially treatable with dietary therapy, and early-life hypothyroidism is an important treatable cause of mental retardation. Hydrocephalus, which can be surgically treated with a shunt, is an important treatable cause of mental retardation. Premature craniosynostosis of multiple sutures that is impairing brain growth can be surgically treated, and osteopetrosis can be treated with bone marrow transplant. Unfortunately, the list is short.

Etiologic classification is important for prognosis. Knowledge of a major chromosome trisomy such as trisomy 13 virtually assures a substantially shortened life span. The presence of a major brain anomaly such as holoprosencephaly predicts a severe or profound handicap. On the other hand, Turner's syndrome (XO) and the fragile-X chromosome syndrome usually have only a mild intellectual deficit. Knowledge of the specific diagnosis and its natural history allows the physician to anticipate complications such as scoliosis and brain tumors is neurofibromatosis or epilepsy and renal cysts in tuberous sclerosis (Table 15.1).

Many causes of mental retardation are inherited in a predictable pattern. Parents want to know if there is increased risk for a similar problem in future pregnancies. Tuberous sclerosis is inherited in an autosomal-dominant manner, so that each pregnancy of a gene-carrying couple carries a 50% risk of transmitting the gene. Certain forms of agenesis of the corpus callosum are inherited in an autosomal-recessive manner, with a 25% risk for subsequent pregnancies. X-linked hydrocephalus in boys is well-described, and Duchenne muscular dystrophy, which is X-linked, has an increased risk of mild mental retardation. Women who have borne children with meningomyelocele or anencephaly carry at least a 5% risk of repetition in subsequent pregnancies, and this is a disorder that can be screened for by testing for alpha-fetoprotein in the mother by amniocentesis. In cases in which biochemical or chromosomal disturbance can be identified, the possibility of amniocentesis and therapeutic abortion exists. Screening of women older than 35 for Down's syndrome by amniocentesis is recommended if therapeutic abortion of an affected fetus would be elected.

Table 15.1.
Classification of Important Causes of Mental Retardation by Time of Insult to the Developing Brain[a]

PRENATAL:	
Inherited:	
Mendelian	Tuberous sclerosis
	Neurofibromatosis
	Incontinentia pigmenti
	Menkes' kinky-hair disease
	Mucopolysaccharidoses
	Aminoacidurias
	Aminoacidurias with hyperammonemia
	Galactosemia
Chromosomal	Down's syndrome
	Fragile-X syndrome
	Kleinfelter's syndrome
	Cri-du-chat syndrome
	Trisomy 13
	Trisomy 18
Dysgenetic syndromes	Cornelia de Lange syndrome
	Callosal agenesis syndrome
	Prader-Willi syndrome
Toxic insults	Maternal cocaine use
	Fetal alcohol syndrome
	Fetal hydantoin syndrome
Maternal infection	Acquired immunodeficiency syndrome
	Cytomegalovirus infection
	Toxoplasmosis
	Syphilis
	Rubella
PERINATAL:	Prematurity and its consequences
	Hypoxic-ischemic encephalopathy
	Meningitis
	Bilirubin encephalopathy
POSTNATAL:	Meningitis
	Encephalitis
	Head injury (accidents, child abuse)
	Lead poisoning
	Psychosocial

[a] This list is illustrative and not complete.

Roughly 65% of mental retardation stems from prenatal events; 15%, from perinatal events; and 20% from postnatal events.

PRENATAL EVENTS

As previously noted, mendelian inheritance is responsible for numerous cases of mental retardation. Examples of dominant inheritance include tuberous sclerosis, neurofibromatosis (von Recklinghausen's disease), and myotonic muscular dystrophy, in which mental retardation is seen in approximately 50% of cases. Dominantly inherited diseases tend to be extremely variable in their expression, and, frequently, careful examination of the parents of a child with a dominantly inherited form will reveal an unexpected carrier. Recessive inheritance, in which both parents are asymptomatic carriers, is common. Examples include many metabolic diseases such as phenylketonuria and galactosemia, as well as dysgenetic diseases such as the Lawrence-Moon-Biedl syndrome, with obesity, retinitis pigmentosa, hypogenitalism, and polydactyly. Unfortunately, in only a few cases can the carrier state be suspected before the birth of an affected child. Consanguinity greatly increases the possibility of expression of a recessive gene pair. Sex-linked inheritance is uncommon but is best understood. Boys with Duchenne muscular dystrophy have a high incidence of mental retardation, which is usually mild; however, Menkes' kinky-hair disease is associated with severe retardation and early death. Incontinentia pigmenti is highly associated with mental retardation but is seen almost exclusively in girls. This sex predilection is thought to be due to lethality for male fetuses.

Chromosome abnormalities are important causes of mental retardation. Abnormalities include triplications of entire chromosomes, as in Down's syndrome (chromosome 21) or trisomy 13, 18, or 22. Chromosomes are numbered from largest (number 1) to smallest (number 22). In general, the larger the chromosome triplicated, the more severe the mental retardation. Triplications of sex chromosome and deletion of the Y chromosome (Turner's syndrome) generally have a less severe effect on the intelligence. Deletions, triplications, and translocations of part of a chromosome are increasingly recognized as cytogenetic technique improves, and most are associated with some degree of mental retardation.

A special case is the fragile-X chromosome, a syndrome that occurs mostly in males, who are not severely retarded. Some have autistic features. At maturity, they have long faces and ears and large testes. This syndrome is familial but minimally symptomatic in the carrier mother. Karyotyping must be done in a folate-deficient medium, so routine studies do not permit the diagnosis.

Who should undergo chromosome studies? It depends upon the use to which the information will be put. Retarded children of families that desire more children but fear a repetition of the retardation should certainly be studied if multiple congenital anomalies are associated with the retardation but do not fit a described syndrome. Similarly, if more than one boy is retarded in a family, or perhaps when autism is present, a fragile-X chromosome search should be performed. There is no need to study chromosomes in parents and siblings unless an abnormality is found in the index case.

Dysgenetic syndromes of uncertain heredity are important contributors to mental retardation. Examples include Cornelia de Lange syndrome, which has short stature, wide-set nipples, synophrys, and abnormalities of the digits. Another is Prader-Willi syndrome, with short stature, obesity, and hypogonadism, although some of these patients have shown abnormalities of chromosome 17. Holoprosencephaly and lissencephaly are associated with severe to profound mental retardation. Agenesis of the corpus callosum is usually, but not always, associated with mental retardation.

Prenatal infectious causes are uncommon but important, because some of them are preventable. It is likely that numerous infectious causes of mental retardation remain to be identified. Important ones include cytomegalovirus infection, herpes simplex, toxoplasmosis, rubella, hepatitis, and syphilis. Human immunodeficiency virus (HIV, or AIDS) infection may be the most important of the prenatal infections. It can devastate the nervous system before the child dies of associated infections and may be found in 52% of infants born to HIV-positive mothers.

Toxic and traumatic insults comprise a large and mostly preventable group of causes of mental retardation. These can be divided into early gestational and late gestational insults. Early in gestation, the fetus is sensitive to many medications, including alcohol (fetal alcohol syndrome), phenytoin (fetal hydantoin syndrome), and numerous other medications such as adrenal steroids, which are teratogens in animals and probably so in humans. Proving that a medication is a mild teratogen in humans is extremely difficult and requires a large controlled study. For example, it is now considered that most anticonvulsants are mild teratogens and double or triple the incidence of congenital defects in epileptic mothers, from 2 to 5% to approximately 6 to 10%.

"Crack," a purified form of cocaine, poses a high risk to the infants of mothers who use it late in pregnancy. Cerebral infarcts are common, as is prematurity and its complications. Some of these mothers are also heroin users, and the infants suffer heroin withdrawal. Although it is safe to say that cocaine use by the pregnant mother is a risk to the fetus, the precise contribution is difficult to assess because most of these mothers' pregnancies are high-risk for multiple reasons.

PERINATAL EVENTS

Prematurity is the most important perinatal association with mental retardation. Fifty percent of infants at 32 weeks' gestation requiring respirator support suffer intraventricular hemorrhage. Not all of these infants become retarded, but hydrocephalus and cerebral palsy, both strongly associated with mental retardation, are common consequences of intraventricular hemorrhage. Periventricular leukomalacia is a common consequence of prematurity and appears to be related to hypoxia. Hypoxic-ischemic encephalopathy is an important cause of cerebral palsy in both premature and full-term infants. These infants show low 5-minute Apgar scores and depression of consciousness, impaired reflex responsiveness, and seizures in the 48 hours following birth. It is probable that most infants with spastic or athetoid cerebral palsy secondary to hypoxic-ischemic encephalopathy are mentally retarded. It is unlikely that a hypoxic-ischemic insult insufficient to cause a motor syndrome (cerebral palsy) can result in mental retardation. Jaundice at levels below those thought capable of causing kernicterus (20 mg/dl in the full-term infant, 15 mg/dl in premature) is thought by some investigators to cause a mild intellectual deficit.

Neonatal meningitis and bacterial sepsis are important causes of mental retardation. The etiology is from beta-hemolytic streptococcus or coliform bacteria, and the mortality approaches 50%, with permanent neurologic impairment that includes mental retardation in 50% of survivors.

POSTNATAL EVENTS

Postnatal insults are the least numerous but the most preventable cause of mental retardation. As in the perinatal period, infections are important. Bacterial meningitis, most often due to *Haemophilus influenzae* and *Diplococcus pneumoniae*, often leads to mental retardation. Viral encephalitis is uncommon and except for that due to herpes simplex, largely untreatable. Brain abscess is rare except in individuals at special risk, such as those with cyanotic congenital heart disease. Reye's syndrome is an uncommon cause of mental retardation, since recovery is usually complete in nonfatal cases.

Trauma is an important postnatal cause of mental retardation. Physical trauma from motor vehicle accidents is probably the most important single preventable cause of mental retardation.

Falls and drowning are other traumatic causes. Therapeutic radiation of brain tumors in early childhood is strongly associated with some degree of mental deficiency.

Metabolic insults capable of causing mental retardation can be divided into *endogenous insults*, such as hypoglycemia and hypernatremic and hyponatremic dehydration, and *exogenous insults*. Lead encephalopathy is now rare, but mild intellectual deficits are regarded by many as a common consequence of levels of body lead insufficient to cause frank encephalopathy. Other heavy metals and carbon monoxide poisoning are also contributors to the exogenous metabolic insults.

DIFFERENTIAL DIAGNOSIS

Certain conditions must be differentiated from mental retardation because their management or prognosis is substantially different. Deafness or partial deafness is extremely important to identify in the child with lagging language. The presence of hearing does not rule out high-tone hearing loss, which can severely impair intelligibility of speech, and all children with isolated language delays should have their hearing tested. Degenerative diseases of the nervous system such as Tay-Sachs disease or metachromatic leukodystrophy have been traditionally classified separately, since they tend to progress to death. However, many causes of mental retardation are actually slowly progressive. Examples include mucopolysaccharidosis type I (Hurler's disease), galactosemia, and neuronal ceroid lipofuscinosis. Children with severe systemic diseases or severe environmental deprivation may have retarded development without true mental retardation.

The relationship of pervasive developmental disorder to mental retardation is complex. The original idea that most of these children had normal intelligence that was occluded is probably incorrect. Most of these children have a degree of mental retardation, but their primary problem is not an intellectual one and their management is different.

Attention deficit disorder, especially when not associated with hyperkinesis, commonly presents with school failure and must be differentiated from true mental retardation.

EXAMINATION

Many times, findings on examination help in delineating the cause of mental retardation. Head circumference, especially in young children, is of great importance. Microcephaly for age predicts mental retardation with great accuracy. Small body size does not change this, and dwarfs with normal intelligence generally have normal-sized heads. There is a crude relationship between the severity of mental retardation and the degree of microcephaly. Large heads are seen in a number of mental retardation syndromes, including the mucopolysaccharidoses and hydrocephalus. Hydrocephalus, of course, is treatable by shunting. Large heads may also be familial.

In Menkes' kinky-hair disease, hairs are shiny and under the microscope appear irregular and twisted. Many mental retardation syndromes have characteristic facies.

Many clues may be found in the eye examination, such as optic atrophy, retinitis pigmentosa, cherry-red macular spot, colobomata, chorioretinitis, and cataract. Hypertelorism is said to be common in mental retardation and is correlated with midline developmental defects.

Low-set or malformed ears suggest a developmental defect. Webbing of the neck suggests Turner's syndrome. Organomegaly suggests a storage disease.

Since skin and brain are both ectodermal derivatives, it is no surprise that examination of the skin is frequently very helpful is diagnosing mental retardation syndromes. Gomez's excellent book *Neurocutaneous Diseases* lists 44 such syndromes. Particularly notable are multiple café-au-lait spots in neurofibromatosis. Tuberous sclerosis is characterized by depigmented nevi, shagreen patches, angiofibromata in the butterfly distribution, and periungual fibromata. Sturge-Weber syndrome, although not always associated with mental retardation, characteristically displays a facial angioma on the side ipsilateral to the angioma of the pial layer of the meninges.

PSYCHOMETRICS

Measurement of intelligence is necessary at some time in all children suspected of mental retardation. Office tests serve as a screening device. The Peabody Picture Vocabulary Test can be administered by a paraprofessional and for the English-speaking child gives a fair estimation of intelligence. This author has used the Goodenough "Draw-a-Person" test with great success. Once the scoring system is learned, which takes about 2 hours, the test can be scored in less than 5 minutes. It virtually never overestimates the IQ and so is an excellent screening device.

Formal tests that require a psychologist or psychometrician include the Wechsler Intelligence Scale for Children (WISC-R), which yields a performance and verbal IQ. The Stanford-Binet Form L-M, which is often used by schools, is heavily weighted toward language. The Leiter International Scale is nonverbal and useful for the non-English-speaking child.

LABORATORY TESTS

When the cause of mental retardation is not clear from the history and examination, certain laboratory tests may be appropriate. The author screens fairly routinely for hypothyroidism with T-4 and thyroid stimulating hormone (TSH). Urine is screened for amino acids, organic acids, and mucopolysaccharides. Chromosomes are studied in individuals with multiple congenital anomalies and boys clinically suspected of the fragile-X syndrome.

Electrophysiologic tests have little utility in mental retardation. Electroencephalograms are commonly abnormal, but in the absence of seizures this information has little practical value. Quantitative electroencephalogram (EEG) electrical brain mapping, and evoked response testing are generally not indicated.

Neuroimaging techniques such as magnetic resonance imaging (nuclear magnetic resonance imaging, or MRI) and computed tomography (CT) of the brain can demonstrate the gross anatomy of the brain. This may reveal agenesis of the corpus callosum, porencephaly, or schizencephaly, none of which is treatable. One of these techniques is essential if hydrocephalus is suspected. Positron emission tomography (PET) is a research technique only.

ASSOCIATED CONDITIONS

Cerebral palsy syndromes are commonly associated with mental retardation. This association is especially true when the form of cerebral palsy is spastic quadriplegia or so-called atonic diplegia. Hemiplegic forms and paraplegic forms are usually not associated with retardation, and those with spastic diplegia and the athetoid forms fall somewhere in between.

Approximately 25% of mentally retarded individuals have epilepsy. Many of these are the more severely retarded, with discrete brain lesions. Included in this list are tuberous sclerosis, Sturge-Weber syndrome, lissencephaly, and subacute sclerosing panencephalitis. Management of seizures in retarded individuals is no different from that in the remainder of the population with epilepsy.

Symptoms of attention deficit disorder are common in the mental retarded. Management should be the same, with the use of a structured environment and adjunctive use of methylphenidate, pemoline, or dextroamphetamine. Phenobarbital commonly produces hyperactivity in retarded children.

Aggressive behavior outbursts, sometimes called episodic dyscontrol syndrome, is not uncommon in the retarded. Such outbursts tend to occur for a recognized reason but are excessive in duration and severity. Control can sometimes be achieved with the use of carbamazepine or propanolol.

MANAGEMENT

The lack of specific medical treatment for most cases of mental retardation certainly does not mean that nothing can be done. The first goal is to make a diagnosis and carry out any investigations necessary for this. Mature parental acceptance of the nature and extent of the handicap is the goal. Parents who do not suspect mental retardation may reject the diagnosis. When this occurs, it is wise to suggest a second opinion. Many parents believe that the diagnosis of mental retardation means that the child will never grow or learn and are reassured to know that learning will occur, albeit at a slower pace. If the parents appear to reject the possibility of mental retardation even prior to the diagnosis formation, it may be wise to express only concerns regarding development. A useful way of interpreting developmental level is to ask the mother how old her child seems to her.

Telling a family that their child is retarded is painful and should be done gently, sympathetically, and without any attempt to minimize the facts. Unsuspecting parents will be terrified about what they are to do in dealing with such a handicap. Emotional support and concrete information about what is to come next should be provided. Prognostication is often very difficult and should be presented as a spectrum of possibilities, except when it is clear that the outlook is dismal and that there is no real possibility of a somewhat favorable outcome, as might be the case in severe microcephaly, trisomy 13, or holoprosencephaly.

Prompt referral to a therapy or educational program is essential. Special education for the retarded is clearly beneficial. Infant stimulation or early intervention programs are probably of value, if only by providing structured stimulation. These programs also provide an alternative to the numerous "nontraditional" therapies, which spring up with promises of cures or dramatic improvement for bereaved parents. One of the physician's important roles is to provide advice regarding the value of alternative therapies.

The school or therapy program will assess the child's problems and potential and, with this in mind, establish appropriate short-term and long-term goals. For the severely retarded, these will center on activities of daily living. For the mildly retarded, they will probably be academic. This is termed an *individualized educational program,* or IEP. The parents will generally be asked to participate in and approve the IEP. It is desirable that a similar set of short- and long-term goals be established at home. Encouraging attractive and compliant behavior is very desirable. Society is much more tolerant of sweet-natured persons with mental retardation than aggressive, impulsive ones.

There is a widespread belief that retarded children have substantially shortened life expectancies. This reflects institutional neglect, especially in the preantibiotic era. In general, only the profoundly retarded or those with progressive disease have shortened life expectancies.

PLACEMENT

The placement of retarded children in large residential institutions is no longer considered appropriate. Nursing home-type settings are occasionally resorted to when medical needs justify it. The current model is for children to remain at home until adolescence and then to be placed in group homes with approximately 10 similarly handicapped persons. From this setting, the children go out to school or a day program and are supervised by a staff of caregivers and consultants, who also develop a set of short- and long-term goals that are implemented within the group home. Parents are encouraged to participate in the planning process.

There is no requirement that a retarded person leave home for an institution, but for most, a time comes when the human and financial cost of remaining at home becomes such that placement is appropriate. It is wise for parents to make application of residental placement well before it is required; this will force them to explore their options and begin to come to grips with what is usually a sad time for any family.

SEXUALITY

Anyone who works with retarded adolescents is immediately aware that their sex drives are frequently as well-developed as those of any other adolescent. Group home programs are frequently designed to help the children function within societal norms, for example, by discouraging individuals from disrobing or masturbating in public areas. In some group homes sexual intercourse may occur, and when it does, the issue of birth control must be addressed. This problem is particularly difficult, since many of the group homes are sponsored by religious groups with strong prohibitions regarding premarital sex and the use of contraceptives. Many mothers ask for sterilization of retarded daughters. Unfortunately, current attitudes regarding involuntary sterilization are such that few physicians will perform such operations.

LEGAL RIGHTS

In the United States, retarded children are citizens and have the rights of citizens. In general, they cannot be deprived of those rights unless they are incompetent to exercise them.

The most important legal issue is guardianship. Until the child reaches age 18 or 21, parents are generally considered to be the legal guardians of the child and are entrusted to make decisions such as giving permission for medical treatment such as surgery. In the absence of a legal guardian, decisions are made on a case-by-case basis by the courts. Although parents of retarded adults frequently function as guardians, it is highly desirable to seek formal guardianship from the courts, especially since most retarded people will outlive their parents.

Mentally retarded individuals can apply for Supplemental Security Income (SSI) from the Social Security Administration. A small monthly sum of $35 is an entitlement based upon handicap.

Many issues remain to be resolved. Does a mentally retarded person have the right to refuse medication? Under what circumstances is it permissible to use chemical restraints such as sedation or psychotropics? To what extent are behavior modification techniques with noxious stimuli permissible? Always recall that retarded people have not surrendered their basic rights.

SUGGESTED READINGS

Berg JM, ed. Perspectives and progress in mental retardation. Vols. I and II. Baltimore: University Park Press, 1984.

Bergsma D, ed. Birth defects compendium. 2nd ed. New York: Alan R. Liss, 1973.

Committee on Bioethics, American Academy of Pediatrics. Sterilization of women who are mentally handicapped. Pediatrics 1990;85:868–871.

Gomez MR, ed. Neurocutaneous diseases. Boston: Butterworths, 1987.

Hogue HE, Jones KL, Dixon SD, et al. Prenatal cocaine exposure and fetal vascular disruption. Pediatrics 1990;85:743–747.

Miller ME, Sulkes S. Fire-setting behavior in individuals with Klinefelter syndrome. Pediatrics 1988;82:115–117.

Rosen M, Clark GR, Kintz MS, eds. The history of mental retardation. Vols. I and II. Baltimore: University Park Press, 1976.

Simko A, Hornstein L, Soukup S, et al. Fragile X syndrome: recognition in young children. Pediatrics 1989;83:547–552.

Smith DW, ed. Recognizable patterns of human malformation, 3rd ed. Philadelphia: WB Saunders, 1982.

Chapter 16

THE PSYCHIATRIST IN THE EMERGENCY ROOM: NEUROLOGIC EMERGENCIES

Mary Elizabeth Lell, MD

The psychiatrist may be one of the first physicians to see a child or adolescent brought to the emergency room (ER) for an acute change in behavior or alteration of mental status. There the physician must determine whether acute changes in behavior, orientation, short-term memory, or thought patterns are a manifestation of systemic or central nervous system (CNS) illness requiring further medical rather than psychiatric intervention.

Delirium, in the Diagnostic and Statistical Manual (DSM II-R) classification, is listed under "Organic Mental syndromes." It is an acute, potentially reversible disorder of organic etiology that affects the individual's memory; orientation to time, place, and person; concentration; and attention to external stimuli. In addition, there may be an alteration in level of consciousness. Delirium may also induce changes in behavior, agitation or confusion, and perceptual disturbances that include misinterpretation of sensory stimuli, illusions, and hallucinations. These symptoms typically fluctuate.

When first encountered, delirium may be difficult to differentiate from a primary psychiatric illness. Patients with psychosis may also show behavioral changes, such as agitation or confusion; however, they are more likely to remain oriented and their memory impairment is less pronounced. Although their interpretation of events may be distorted, patients with psychosis are able to provide an adequate history and their short-term memory remains intact. If not distracted, they should be able to recall four unrelated objects in 5 minutes. The most striking feature in psychotic patients is their disorganization of thought processes and the impairment of reality testing. In the psychotic patient, hallucinations and delusions tend to be systematized, whereas in the delirious patient, they are random and disorganized.

Patients with an organic etiology for their altered mental state, in addition to showing fluctuation of symptoms, may show progressive deterioration of function and signs of systemic illness. Serial examinations may be necessary to detect these findings. In particular, a progression from confusion or agitation to obtundation and coma (with or without focal neurologic signs or seizures) may represent increasing intracranial pressure and constitutes a medical emergency. Other clues, such as fever, sympathetic or parasympathetic excitation, or evidence of trauma, also indicate acute neurologic illness.

Common neurologic emergencies that occur in children and alter the child's mental status include metabolic encephalopathies, encephalitis, head trauma, ingestions, and seizures.

METABOLIC ENCEPHALOPATHIES

Metabolic encephalopathies are acute changes in mental status that result from an alteration in normal cerebral blood flow (ischemia), oxygen (hypoxia), or nutrition (hypoglycemia). Metabolic encephalopathies may also result from altered function or failure of vital organs, inherited enzymatic defects, or endocrine dysfunction. Despite multiple potential etiologies, the clinical picture is usually similar. The child appears confused and disoriented, and recent memory may be impaired. Over hours, he or she may have either fluctuations in ability to respond appropriately or progressive deterioration.

A staging system on serial examinations is often used to assess a child's level of function. In stage I, a child is drowsy and confused but can follow simple verbal or gestured requests. In stage II, the child is increasingly agitated but may follow some instructions. In stage III, the child is not responsive to verbal requests and shows decorticate posturing with stimulation (flexion of the upper extremities and extension of the lower extremities). In stage IV, the child has decerebrate posturing (extension of the upper extremities with internal rotation and extension of the legs). In stage V, the child is unresponsive to stimuli and has flaccid muscles.

In determining the etiology, a careful history and documentation of associated systemic findings is helpful. With ischemic insults, there may be a history of trauma, hypotension, or blood loss. With hypoxic insults, hypoventilation, carbon monoxide exposure, or choking may be reported. Hypoglycemia can be readily detected with a Dextro-stick in the emergency room and then confirmed with a specimen sent to the laboratory. Liver failure is frequently seen in association with jaundice, pruritis, and, in advanced cases, an abnormal flapping movement of the hands (asterixis). Liver function studies will show an elevation of serum glutamic-pyruvic transaminase (SGPT) and bilirubin concentra-

tions. If an infectious hepatitis is suspected, hepatitis antigens should be sent. Renal dysfunction can be detected by elevated concentrations of creatinine and blood urea nitrogen.

The most common cause of endocrine dysfunction that presents with altered mental status is hyper- or hypothyroidism. With hyperthyroidism there is a history of agitation, tachycardia, occasional night sweats, nightmares, and difficulty sleeping. Hypothyroidism is more commonly associated with poor school performance, weight gain, and sensitivity to cold.

In addition to these causes of metabolic encephalopathy, which may occur in any age group, an important cause of metabolic encephalopathy encountered virtually exclusively in children is Reye's syndrome. This condition, first reported by an Australian pathologist in 1963, is characterized by fatty changes in the liver and cerebral edema in children, who present with vomiting and agitation and progress to coma and death. Reye's typically follows a flu-like illness or varicella, and the child appears to improve but then presents to the ER with agitation or confusion. There is often a history of repeated vomiting. Autonomic dysfunction, which usually occurs, causes temperature elevation, dilated pupils, and deep, rapid respirations. As noted above, staging the patient and following the mental status with serial examinations can be important because deterioration of mental status indicates increasing intracranial pressure. Intracranial pressure monitoring and maintenance of adequate airway are essential. The most common causes of morbidity and mortality in Reye's syndrome are uncontrolled intracranial pressure and hypoxia. Laboratory data helpful in making the diagnosis of Reye's syndrome, which reflect severe liver damage, include elevated SGPT, prolonged prothrombin time (PT), elevated blood ammonia level, and decreased blood sugar. Treatment is supportive: hyperventilation and mannitol to control increased intracranial pressure; assisted ventilation to maintain adequate oxygenation; and maintenance of normal electrolytes and blood sugar. Mortality is highest when the patient presents in stage IV or V. Patients who remain only agitated and confused (stages I or II) usually recover without significant sequelae.

Since Reye's syndrome may occasionally be mimicked by drug ingestion or viral encephalitis, urine toxicology tests should be sent and a lumbar puncture (LP) should be performed. The cerebrospinal fluid (CSF) would be expected to show normal values with Reye's syndrome, but with viral encephalitis an elevated cell count with a predominance of lymphocytes would be expected. In rare instances, a similar syndrome has been reported as a recurrent phenomenon in patients with carnitine deficiency. This enzymatic defect should be considered if there is a history of recurrent episodes or a family history of a similar disturbance. Another consideration is nonicteric hepatitis because, like Reye's syndrome, it shows persistent liver function test abnormalities, confusion, and, finally, obtundation from hepatic encephalopathy. However, in contrast to Reye's, hepatitis is not comonly associated with fulminant brain edema and a rapid rise in intracranial pressure.

In metabolic encephalopathy, imaging studies, such as magnetic resonance imaging (MRI) or computerized tomography (CT), will not demonstrate a focal lesion, but they may show signs of diffuse edema, such as would be expected in Reye's syndrome. An electroencephalogram (EEG), a sensitive test for metabolic encephalopathy, usually shows diffuse slowing. Triphasic waves may be seen with hepatic failure. In many cases, the degree of abnormality seen on EEG correlates with the level of coma. This correlation has been particularly helpful in following patients with Reye's syndrome (Garrettson, 1984; Mistre and Berman, 1984).

VIRAL ENCEPHALITIS

The term *encephalitis* describes infection of brain parenchyma with an organism that may be viral, bacterial, or parasitic. There may also be involvement of the meninges surrounding the brain (meningoencephalitis) that produces symptoms of stiff neck and photophobia. Often, children with fever present with confusion and delirium, but the patient with encephalitis commonly has other neurologic signs, such as focal weakness, seizures, and lethargy.

Some viruses, such as herpes simplex, show a predilection for the frontal and temporal lobes. The inflammatory response elicited by these viruses frequently causes partial complex seizures whose manifestations may be subtle. These may include brief periods of staring or deviation of the eyes, repeated semipurposeful movement, such as wringing of the hands, or focal seizure activity. The patient may also have distortions of perception, memory impairment, or hallucinations. The EEG may be helpful in documenting both slowing associated with encephalitis and focal paroxysmal activity, often with temporal lobe discharges. Anticonvulsant medication, such as carbamazepine or phenytoin, are indicated for seizure control. Most often, temperature elevation is accompanied by an elevated white count. The CSF may show an elevated white count with a predominance of lymphocytes, and in herpes simplex encephalitis, there may be an elevation of red blood cells seen in a nontraumatic tap. Protein and glucose are usually normal. Treatment for herpes simplex is acyclovir.

Although herpes infections usually occur sporadically and thus may occur at any time of the year, other viruses, such as arbovirus, show a seasonal incidence because they are spread by insects. In addition, in endemic areas, particularly Westchester County, eastern Long Island, and Connecticut, physicians must also consider Lyme disease. This illness is an infection by a spirochete, *Borrelia burgdorferi,* which is transmitted by *Ixodes* ticks. The initial sign, which may be overlooked, is erythema at the site of the tick bite that is followed by a larger, target-shaped lesion. Headache, fatigue, and mild alteration of mentation often occur. In the next stage, with dissemination of the organism to the CNS, neck stiffness, photophobia, and frank neurologic deficits, especially facial palsy, may develop. Other manifestations include arthritis and carditis. In rare cases, progressive confusion, inappropriate behavior and violent outbursts have been the only manifestations. Serum Lyme titers by the enzyme-linked immunosorbent assay (ELISA) technique may be helpful in making the diagnosis. The titer may be positive in the serum 6 to 8 weeks after the initial infection. In the later stages, with CNS symptoms, the CSF would be expected to show an elevation of lymphocytes and a mild elevation of protein concentration. *Borrelia* may be cultured from the CSF. Antibody titers in the CSF would be detectable and should be compared with serum titers. Treatment consists of oral antibiotics for the early, localized stage and intravenous antibiotics when CNS manifestations are present (Pachner et al., 1989; Steere, 1989; Zaki, 1989).

In patients who are immunocompromised from either steroids, chemotherapy, or human immunodeficiency virus (HIV) infection, numerous organisms, some usually not pathogenic, may be infective. These organisms include cytomegalovirus (CMV), *Toxoplasma, Cryptococcus,* and HIV itself. As with all patients with meningoencephalitis, initial treatment consists of maintenance of normal electrolytes and support of vital functions. Fluid restriction may be necessary if the patient shows evidence of inappropriate antidiuretic hormone secretion or hyponatremia. Increasing obtundation, as with metabolic encephalopathy, may be associated with increased intracranial pressure and should be treated similarly. CT with contrast or MRI may be helpful in showing or excluding a mass lesion, such as is seen with toxoplasmosis. These studies may show periventricular enhancement, indicative of epididymitis—inflammation of the ventricular lining—associated with CMV. *Cryptococcus* infection is treated by Amphotericin, CMV by gancyclovir, and *Toxoplasma* by pyrimethamine and sulfa.

HEAD TRAUMA AND POSTCONCUSSIVE SYNDROME

Head trauma in children is a frequent problem in an emergency room. Children may have had transient loss of consciousness and then amnesia for events preceding (retrograde amnesia) or following the trauma (antegrade amnesia). The child may be confused or drowsy and show problems with short-term memory. Vomiting and headache are common in a young child. Repeated observations of children's mental function as well as motor function and pupillary responses are important in assessing patients.

Epidural hemorrhages, which occur in the space between the dura and the skull, are frequently associated with fractures in the temporal parietal region and tears of the middle meningeal artery. They caused arterial bleeding, which produces a mass lesion that compresses the underlying brain. Subdural collections, which are in the space between the dura and the brain, result from tears in veins that bridge this space. With venous bleeding, symptoms usually take longer to develop. However, in either case, patients show a progression of symptoms, including increasing obtundation, ipsilateral pupillary dilation, and weakness contralateral to the hemorrhage.

CT scans are helpful in showing epidural and subdural hemorrhages as well as contusions of the brain parenchyma. Skull x-rays are helpful in showing a fracture. Fractures through sinuses may be associated with a risk of intracranial infection, such as meningitis or brain abscess. Since the front lobes are closest to the sinuses, they are most frequently the site of brain abscess. Symptoms may initially be headaches, lethargy, and behavioral changes, but there will be little motor involvement. CT with contrast can identify and localize an abscess. Treatment with antibiotics on the organism, and surgical drainage is often required.

In addition to the complications of head trauma, the physician must be alert to the possibility of alcohol or drug usage altering the mental state of adolescents involved in accidents or trauma. These children may be agitated or obtunded, which raises the possibility of hemorrhage or contusion. Screening of individuals in ERs who have been involved in violent crimes or fatal motor vehicles accidents has shown a significant number with positive urine tests for cocaine, alcohol, or both (Lindenbaum et al., 1989; Marzuk et al., 1990; Sloan et al., 1989).

The physician in the ER must consider abuse in cases of trauma to the head or elsewhere on the body that the parent or caretaker cannot adequately explain. If there is suspicion of abuse, x-rays of the long bones and skull should be performed to document prior episodes of trauma. In cases of abuse, x-rays may reveal healed fractures or callous formation. When abuse is suspected, it should be reported to child welfare agencies.

ACUTE CEREBROVASCULAR INSULTS (STROKES)

Childhood stroke is characterized by sudden hemiplegia, often accompanied by seizures or alteration in consciousness, in a previously healthy child (Solomon, 1990). Although no specific cause can be found in many cases, numerous conditions can predispose children to ischemic or hemorrhagic strokes. Some common ones are congenital cyanotic heart disease; hematologic disease, such as sickle cell anemia and coagulopathies; and vascular disorders, such as an aneurysm, arteriovenous malformation (AVM), and lupus erythematosus and other collagen-vascular diseases (i.e., diseases of the heart, blood, and blood vessels). Trauma to the neck, oropharynx, or head can lead to vascular occlusions. For example, a child running while sucking an ice cream stick who falls may injure the cervical portion of the internal carotid artery, resulting in an arterial thrombosis and hemiplegia. Metabolic disorders that may lead to strokes

include homocystinuria, diabetes mellitus, progeria, and mitochondrial encephalomyopathy (MELAS) (see Chapter 14). Particularly in adolescents, strokes are induced by drug abuse, especially from crack-cocaine, phenylpropanolamine ("black beauties"), phencyclidine (PCP or "angel dust"), lysergic acid (LSD), mescaline, heroin, and amphetamine.

Another cerebrovascular disorder affecting children and adolescents is Moya Moya disease, which is a condition defined by its angiographic appearance (see Chapter 10). Unlike in adults, in whom most vascular occlusions are in the extracranial circulation, in children with Moya-Moya the supraclinoid portion of the carotid artery is typically the site of occlusion. Collateral circulation that develops in the basal ganglia is called Moya Moya (Japanese for "a puff of smoke") because of its soft, telangiectatic angiographic appearance. Some cases of Moya Moya, which has a higher incidence in Japan than in the United States, have been familial.

The signs of stroke must be differentiated from those of other structural lesions, such as brain tumor, abscess, and subdural hematoma; infection, such as encephalitis; and physiologic disturbance, such as hemiplegic migraine and postictal (Todd's) hemiparesis. The diagnostic evaluation begins with a detailed history and comprehensive physical examination for underlying medical conditions predisposing to the stroke. The laboratory tests include complete blood count, platelet count, coagulation studies, erythrocyte sedimentation rate (ESR), antinuclear antibody (ANA), biochemical profile, fasting glucose, urine analysis, and urine cyanide nitroprusside for homocystinuria. When considering emboli or underlying cardiac disease, such as subacute bacterial endocarditis or rheumatic heart disease, an echocardiogram and Holter monitor may be needed in addition to the routine electrocardiogram and chest x-ray.

For evaluation of the brain, CT shows an infarcted area of the brain as a region of decreased density. Although CT abnormalities are usually not apparent until 12 hours after the onset of the stroke, the CT can show whether the infarct is ischemic or hemorrhagic and reveal subarachnoid, subdural, or parenchymal bleeding. It can also show a calcified AVM (see Chapter 10).

MRI is more sensitive than CT in early detection of infarctions and in the diagnosis of venous sinus and cerebral vein thromboses. MRI shows vascular malformations in the brain without injections of contrast. The cerebral angiogram is definitive in visualizing occlusions, small vessel disease, AVMs, aneurysms, and the characteristic pattern of Moya Moya. Collaterals of a Moya Moya pattern may be seen with proximal supraclinoid carotid occlusions in neurofibromatosis, certain collagen-vascular diseases, including Kawasaki disease, radiation therapy, and sickle cell disease. (If angiography is required in a child with sickle cell disease, sickle hemoglobin concentration must be reduced to 20% by transfusion.)

In treatment, supportive care is the key factor (Solomon, 1984). The physician must provide an adequate airway, avoid aspiration, and give adequate hydration, electrolytes, and nutrients. Anticonvulsants may be needed for seizures. If a specific etiology is found, appropriate therapy is given. For example, if there is an embolic phenomenon, anticoagulation is used, and if there is a coagulation defect, the deficit is corrected. Surgery is usually the treatment of choice for aneurysms and AVMs.

Prognosis in stroke depends on the etiology, location, and size of the infarct or hemorrhage, and the age of the child. Many children are left with epilepsy, learning disabilities, and language problems as well as physical deficits. Children who have had strokes often require individualized management by multiple disciplines, including special education; psychological counseling; speech, occupational and physical therapy; and social service (see Chapter 13).

INGESTIONS

Accidental ingestion of medications can occur in the toddler or young child if the bottle is left out or not securely fastened. Increased parental education and new, "childproof" closures have decreased accidental ingestions.

Ingestion in adolescents with depression or impulsive behavior, or, occasionally, ingestion from experimentation, are frequently seen in the ER. The drugs most commonly taken in overdose are the tricyclic antidepressants, phenothiazines, barbiturates, and benzodiazepines. The effects of tricyclic overdose are roughly dose-related. If the amount ingested can be determined, the physician can predict the symptoms and outcome. Doses of less than 20 mg per kilogram usually cause confusion and agitation that progress to increasing sedation. Higher doses may produce myoclonic jerks (sudden, isolated, asymmetric jerks of the extremities) that may be associated with hallucinations and seizures. Ingestions of more than 20 mg per kilogram induce cardiac disturbances, especially tachycardia, arrhythmias, and conduction block.

Since treatment includes identification of the substance, and since multiple drugs may have been used, toxic screening of the urine is usually essential. Removal of the substance from the stomach, if the ingestion has been recent, should be attempted. If the patient is awake, vomiting can be induced. If not, a gastric lavage with a cuffed endotracheal tube in place to prevent aspiration should be instituted. Physostigmine has been used to control myoclonic jerks and seizures. As in any unresponsive patient, maintenance of the airway, fluid and electrolyte balance, and blood pressure are essential.

Ingestion of phenothiazines causes sedation, but frequently it induces dystonic posturing—prolonged twisting movements, which may mimic seizure activity, including arching of the trunk and rolling back of the eyes (oculogyric crisis). The child may also have dysarthria. However, the child is aware of the environment if not overly sedated. Treatment for the dystonia is an antihistamine (Benadryl) or benztropine mesylate (Cogentin). Hypotension and problems with temperature regulation, both hypo- and hyperthermia, may be seen. Hypotension is most frequently orthostatic, and it responds to the child's being kept supine and maintenance of adequate fluid volume.

Barbiturates are often taken alone or in combination with alcohol and other drugs. Once again, drug screening of the urine is appropriate to determine whether multiple substances have been ingested. The most threatening problem with barbiturate overdose is respiratory depression. Another characteristic manifestation is that the pupils are small and, in high doses, often pin-point, with little or no reaction to light. Benzodiazepines may also cause sedation and, in higher doses, especially in association with barbiturates, respiratory depression. In general, the treatment of overdose is to increase renal clearance of the drug.

Drugs that are commonly associated with hallucinations and delirium include antihistamines, amphetamines, and atropine. Hallucinations may be described or the physician may only note agitated, fearful behavior. With ingestion of high doses of these medicines, agitation and self-injury may occur. Young children, who may have difficulty describing what is occurring, may have flushing, sweating, tachycardia, and mild hypertension—as a result of excess sympathetic stimulation (American Academy of Pediatrics, 1987). If no other symptoms are noted, no further treatment is necessary and the patient may be observed (Commission on Classification and Terminology, 1981). However, if arrhythmia, hyperpyrexia, and further elevation of blood pressure occur, patients require treatment (Garrettson, 1984).

Atropine-like drugs may induce tachycardia, pupillary dilation, flushing, and dry mouth in association with hallucinations and agitated behavior—the "Mad Hatter" syndrome. Physo-

stigmine may be used for seizures and hyperthermia, but otherwise, treatment is supportive (Garrettson, 1984; Kuhlberg, 1986).

Alterations in mental status may also occur as a result of drug interactions. For example, the patient who is treated regularly for seizure control with carbamazepine (Tegretol) may become lethargic if erythromycin is prescribed for strep throat, because it raises the carbamazepine (Tegretol) level into the toxic range. Barbiturates taken with valproic acid (Depakene) can also cause lethargy and toxicity.

In addition to problems with combinations of prescribed drugs, the physician must also be alert to abuse of street drugs, such as PCP, cocaine, and heroin, and also alcohol.

PCP, also known as "angel dust," may cause hallucinations. PCP can be taken orally, intranasally, or intravenously. Other drugs or contaminants may be mixed with it and its purity may vary, and hence the toxicity for a given dose is unpredictable. PCP is rapidly absorbed and lipid-soluble. Following its ingestion, patients have an altered perception of pain, a distorted sense of their own strength, and aggressive, violent behavior. Sometimes patients exhibit a muted response to the environment and appear catatonic. Muscle rigidity, nystagmus, and pupillary dilation may also be found. Systemic signs that differentiate it from a primary psychosis include elevation of the blood pressure and hyperthermia. Correction of blood pressure is important to prevent intracranial hemorrhage. Hyperthermia must be treated to prevent muscle breakdown and kidney failure from myoglobinuria. After the acute ingestion is treated, thought disorders similar to those seen in schizophrenia have persisted.

Cocaine usage in adolescents has increased with the availability of "crack." Use of crack, which may be detected in urine and serum, commonly causes agitation, anxiety, and paranoia, and, sometimes, seizures. It also causes tachycardia, chest pain, and hypertension—excessive sympathetic stimulation—similar to that resulting from amphetamines and PCP. Chronic cocaine users may attempt to counter these sympathetic effects with alcohol, which acts as a CNS depressant. Because of crack's rapidly addictive nature, users become preoccupied with obtaining the drug. Their school performance deteriorates and their attendance becomes erratic. An increased incidence of chronic abuse has been reported in adolescents with chronic medical illness, but it is uncertain whether the drug use represents a higher incidence of underlying emotional problems, including depression, an attempt to gain peer approval, or adolescent impulsiveness and experimentation. A prior use of marijuana or alcohol is frequently reported (Gawin and Elinwood, 1988; Kuhlberg, 1986; Lindenbaum et al., 1989; Marzuk et al., 1990; Ringwalt and Palmer, 1989; Shannon et al., 1989; Sloan et al., 1989).

Although heroin or methadone addiction is less common than cocaine or crack addiction, they are important forms of intoxication. Heroin, which may be self-administered intravenously or intranasally, has a rapid onset of action. It, too, may be adulterated with other substances that cause systemic and psychic manifestations. Methadone causes agitation and hallucinations, often accompanied by miotic pupils, respiratory depression, and stupor. Evidence of intravenous drug use, such as needle tracks, should be noted. Intravenous drug users are also at great risk for systemic infections, such as subacute bacterial endocarditis, hepatitis, and HIV infection (see Chapter 17). Naloxone reverses narcotic-induced respiratory depression, and a positive response confirms the diagnosis. However, a response may not be apparent if multiple drugs have been used or if there is associated trauma. Respirations should be assisted by mechanical ventilation. Following the acute overdose, the patient should also be observed for withdrawal.

Alcohol remains the most readily available mood-altering drug. Euphoria, its immediate effect, is followed by increasing CNS depression with impairment of cognitive function. Alcohol

may be taken alone or in association with other drugs. At blood levels of 50 to 150 mg/ml, depending on past exposure and individual tolerance, speech may be dysarthric; gait, unsteady or ataxic; and skilled activities, such as driving, impaired. Blood tests for alcohol level as well as "drug screens" should be sent. As previously noted, a significant number of patients brought to urban trauma centers following violent crimes or motor vehicle accidents have tests that disclosed alcohol use. Recognition of drug use may help the physician in recommending further counseling and drug rehabilitation programs (American Academy of Pediatrics, 1987; Kuhlberg, 1986; Linderbaum et al., 1989; Marzuk et al., 1990).

Below is a table summarizing those drugs that cause pupillary changes and hallucinations:

Dilated:	Constricted:	
Amphetamines	Barbiturates	Antihistamines
Atropine	Opiates	Amphetamines
Cocaine		Cocaine
PCP		Heroin
		PCP

SEIZURES

Seizures may be associated with alteration of mentation but little or no apparent motor activity. Changes in mentation with virtually no physical activity may occur when the abnormal focus of electrical activity causes stimulation of the limbic system with its projections to both frontal and temporal lobes. Seizures result in staring episodes and semipurposeful and repetitive movements, such as chewing and handwringing. Often there are changes in autonomic function, such as increased sweating and tachycardia.

Where autonomic dysfunction represents the primary manifestations and there is no associated loss of consciousness, the physician must also consider an acute anxiety reaction. Helpful in differentiating an acute anxiety attack from a seizure is the anxious patient's ability to recall it in detail. In contrast, the seizure patient will be amnesic. Partial complex seizures tend to occur in flurries and last only a few minutes. If they become secondarily generalized, seizure activity will be overt, with tonic-clonic movements of the extremities. These patients will have a postictal period of drowsiness or confusion. If repetitive generalized seizures are not interrupted, the patient is considered to be in convulsive status epilepticus that should be treated with intravenous benzodiazepine or phenytoin (Kotagal and Rothner, 1987; Penry, 1986).

On rare occasions, patients can present to the emergency room with confusion, staring, eye blinking, or lip smacking that result from absence status. These seizures can be diagnosed by EEG, which shows a generalized, rhythmic 3-cycle-per-second discharge, and they can be controlled by benzodiazepine.

Adolescents with seizures also often have pseudoseizures that may be difficult to differentiate from their true seizures. In general, pseudoseizures are not associated with abnormal findings, such as Babinski signs or changes in muscle tone, in the postictal state. Also, a person with pseudoseizures is unlikely to be incontinent. A pseudoseizure is likely to be triggered by the suggestion that a seizure will occur. Movements tend to be bizarre and frequently involve thrashing or arching of the trunk and pelvis. At times, continuous video-EEG monitoring is necessary to determine whether abnormal EEG discharges correlate with the movements or altered behavior.

Children with migraine occasionally present with periods of confusion that may last for several hours with no headache or other manifestation. Such episodes are more common in adolescents, who are frequently evaluated, quite appropriately, for drug ingestion or seizures. Frequently there is a family history of migraine. A CT or MRI will rule out a mass lesion or hemorrhage.

The EEG may show slowing but paroxysmal activity that would be consistent with a seizure disorder. A follow-up EEG is usually normal.

In summary, a child or adolescent with metabolic encephalopathy, encephalitis, head trauma, ingestion, seizures, or migraine may present to the ER with alteration of mental status. Although the clinical presentation may be similar, there are multiple potential etiologies. A careful history, serial examinations, and pertinent laboratory studies will help in making the diagnosis.

REFERENCES

American Academy of Pediatrics. Committee on Adolescence. Alcohol use and abuse. Pediatrics 1987;79:450–453.

Commission on Classification and Terminology of the International League Against Epilepsy. Proposal for revised clinical and electroencephalographic classification of epileptic seizures. Epilepsia 1981;22:489–501.

Garrettson LK. Poisoning. In: Pellock JM, Meyer EC, ed. Neurologic emergencies in infancy and childhood. Philadelphia: Harper & Row, 1984:145–153.

Gawin FH, Ellinwood EH. Cocaine and other stimulants. N Engl J Med 1988;318:1173–1182.

Kotagal K, Rothner AD. Complex partial seizures in children: diagnosis and management. Int Pediatr 1987;2:182–188.

Kuhlberg A. Substance abuse: clinical identification and management. In: Pediatric toxicology. Pediatr Clin North Am 1986;33:325–361.

Lindenbaum GA, Stanton SF, Daskal I, Kapusnick R. Patterns of alcohol and drug abuse in an urban trauma center: the increasing role of cocaine abuse. J Trauma 1989;29:1654–1658.

Marzuk PM, Tardiff K, Leon AC, et al. Prevalence of recent cocaine use among motor vehicle fatalities in New York City. JAMA 1990;263:250–256.

Mestre JR, Berman WF. Reye's syndrome. In: Neurologic emergencies in infancy and childhood. Philadelphia: Harper & Row, 1984:145–153.

Nathan P. Alcohol dependency prevention and early intervention. Public Health Rep 1988;103:683–689.

Pachner AR, Duray P, Steere AC, Central nervous system manifestations of Lyme disease. Arch Neurol 1989;46:790–795.

Penry JK, ed. Epilepsy: diagnosis, management, and quality of life (a booklet from symposium). New York: Raven Press, 1986.

Ringwalt CL, Palmer JH. Cocaine and crack users compared. Adolescence 1989;24:851–859.

Shannon M, Lacoutre PG, Roa J, Woolf A. Cocaine exposure among children seen at a pediatric hospital. Pediatrics 1989;83:337–342.

Sloan EP, Zalenski RJ, Smith RF, et al. Toxicology screening in urban trauma patients: drug prevalence and its relationship to trauma severity and management. J Trauma 1989;29:1647–1653.

Solomon GE. Cerebrovascular disease in infants and childhood. In: Gellis SS and Kagan BM. Current pediatric therapy. 13th Ed. Philadelphia: WB Saunders, 1990:59–61.

Solomon GE. Acute treatment of strokes in children. In: Pellock JM and Myer EC. Neurologic emergencies in infancy and childhood. Philadelphia: Harper & Row, 1984:201–224.

Steere AC, Lyme disease. N Engl J Med 1989;321:586–596.

Zaki MH. Selected tickborne infections: a review of Lyme disease, Rocky Mountain spotted fever, and babesiosis. NY State J Med 1989;89:320–335.

Chapter 17

HIV-I AND THE CENTRAL NERVOUS SYSTEM*

Anita L. Belman, MD, Pim Brouwers, PhD, and Howard Moss, PhD

INTRODUCTION

Human immunodeficiency virus type I (HIV-I), the etiologic agent of acquired immunodeficiency syndrome (AIDS), was isolated in 1983 (Coffin et al., 1986). HIV-I, an RNA retrovirus, belongs to the lentivirus subfamily of nononcogenic retroviruses. Lentiviruses, or "slow viruses," have long incubation periods, cause persistent infection and chronic disease, and are generally neurotropic (Johnson et al., 1988). Nervous system involvement characteristically has a slow and progressive course. HIV-I, due to its trophism for the immune system, the central nervous system (CNS), and possibly other organ systems, causes a wide spectrum of disease in children; the most severe form of the disease results in AIDS.

DEFINITION OF "PEDIATRIC AIDS"

For the purpose of epidemiologic surveillance, the Centers for Disease Control (CDC) initially defined AIDS in children younger than age 13 years with the same restrictive clinical case definition as for adults (i.e., documentation of an opportunistic infection or an AIDS-related malignancy was required). In addition, primary (congenital) or secondary immunodeficiency disorders and congenital infections had to be excluded (CDC, 1984). After HIV-I was identified and with the advent of serologic testing, only a minority of children with HIV-I related disease manifestations were found to fit the case definition criteria for AIDS. Two subsequent revisions in the CDC case definition broadened the criteria. In 1985, biopsy-proved lymphoid interstitial pneumonitis was included as an indicator condition of AIDS in children (CDC, 1985). A major revision in 1987 substantially expanded the criteria (CDC, 1987). This definition is based on laboratory evidence of HIV-I infection, immunologic function, and a spectrum of clinical manifestations (Tables 17.1 and 17.2).

As greater understanding of the clinical aspects of HIV-I infection in children emerges, it is most likely that the CDC classification will again be revised and new staging systems developed. Hence, when reviewing information about children with "AIDS," it is imperative to be aware of the definition being used and the changing classification criteria.

---

* Portions of this chapter were previously reported in Belman AL. AIDS and pediatric neurology. In: Bodensteiner J, ed. Pediatric neurology. Neurol Clin 1990;8:571–603.

Table 17.1.
**Summary of the Definition of HIV Infection
in Children**[a]

Infants and children less than 15 months of age
with perinatal infection:
1. Virus in blood or tissues
        or
2. HIV antibody
        and
        Evidence of both cellular and humoral
            immune deficiency
        and
3. Symptoms meeting CDC case definition for
        AIDS
            one or more categories in Class P-1

1. Virus in blood or tissues
        or
2. HIV antibody
        or
3. Symptoms meeting CDC case definition for
        AIDS

[a] Modified from MMWR 1987;36:225–230, 235.

EPIDEMIOLOGY, MODE OF TRANSMISSION, AND RISK FACTORS

More than 2000 cases of pediatric AIDS were reported to the CDC as of 1990. Of these cases, approximately 11% had received contaminated blood products, 6% were infected during treatment of hemophilia or coagulopathy disorders, and approximately 80% had perinatally-acquired infection. Surveillance studies show that the incidence of transfusion-acquired AIDS has declined since 1985 (the year blood donor screening began). Unfortunately, the numbers of infants with perinatally (vertically) transmitted HIV-I infection continue to rise parallel to the percentage increase of HIV-I infected women of childbearing age (Oxtoby, 1990).

The most common risk factors for maternal infection in the United States and Europe are drug-related: women who are or were intravenous drug users (IVDU), women who traded "sex for drugs," women with sexual partners who are or were IVDU. Epidemiologic studies also in-

dicate that the numbers of women with heterosexually transmitted HIV-I infection are increasing.

The geographic distribution of children with vertically transmitted HIV-I infection reflects the demographics of infected women. Although most children with AIDS are from New York, New Jersey, Florida, California, and Texas, pediatric AIDS is spreading. HIV-I seropositive women and their offspring are increasingly being identified from other areas in the United States, including rural communities.

The number of children with asymptomatic or "mildly" symptomatic infection is unknown, as surveillance systems are based on children identified by clinical manifestations. It is currently estimated that half of the children with mild symptoms and all asymptomatic infected children remain excluded from CDC surveillance data (Krasinski et al., 1989).

INCUBATION PERIOD

The incubation period of HIV-I in children with vertically transmitted infection is not certain. Initially, two populations were recognized (Auger et al., 1988), with the first group manifesting symptoms in infancy (short incubation period, with a median of 4.1 months) and the second group manifesting symptoms in childhood (median of 6.1 years). However, asymptomatic and mildly symptomatic older (pre- and young adolescent) children with vertically transmitted HIV-I infection are increasingly being identified (Aiuti et al., 1987; Kelly et al., 1987; Burger et al., 1990). Thus it appears that latency to onset of symptoms in some children may be considerably longer than previously appreciated. Therefore, it can be anticipated that an increasing number of asymptomatic school age children will develop signs of CNS involvement (changes in behavior, mood, affect, or cognition) prior to or concomitant with onset of systemic signs of HIV-I infection, and even prior to an "AIDS"-defining illness (see below).

Table 17.2.
Summary of the Classification of HIV Infection in Children Less than 13 Years of Age[a]

Class P-0	Indeterminate infection
Class P-1	Asymptomatic infection
Subclass A	Normal immune function
Subclass B	Abnormal immune function
Subclass C	Immune function not tested
Class P-2	Symptomatic infection
Subclass A	Nonspecific findings
Subclass B	Progressive neurologic symptoms
Subclass C	Lymphoid interstitial pneumonitis
Subclass D	Secondary infectious diseases
Category D-1	Specified secondary infectious diseases listed in the CDC surveillance definition of AIDS
Category D-2	Recurrent serious bacterial infections
Category D-3	Other specified secondary infectious diseases
Subclass E	Secondary cancers
Category E-1	Specified secondary cancers listed in the CDC surveillance definition for AIDS
Category E-2	Other cancers possibly secondary to HIV infection
Subclass F	Other diseases possibly due to HIV infection

[a] Modified from MMWR 1987;36:225–236.

SYSTEMIC SIGNS AND SYMPTOMS OF "PEDIATRIC AIDS"

The most common clinical features of symptomatic pediatric HIV-I infection/AIDS includes failure to thrive, lymphadenopathy, hepatosplenomegaly, chronic diarrhea, recalcitrant thrush, recurrent bacterial infections, including sepsis and meningitis, and interstitial pulmonary disease (Rubinstein et al., 1983; Rubinstein, 1986; Rubinstein et al., 1986; Scott et al., 1984; Oleske et al., 1983; Novick, 1990; Falloon et al., 1989).

Clinical manifestations in children reflect the early insult to the immune system, with consequent B and T cell dysfunction (Rubinstein et al., 1983; Rubinstein, 1986; Novick, 1990; Falloon et al., 1989). Bacterial infections, a manifestation of the underlying B-cell defect, often occur early and are an important cause of morbidity (Bernstein et al., 1985). In fact, most young children generally do not present with signs of cellular immunodeficiency and T-cell dysfunction, but instead have histories of recurrent infections, such as otitis media, pneumonia, urinary tract infections, and cellulitis. These children have abnormal primary and secondary responses to antigens. This occurs despite a profound, polyclonal hypergammaglobulinemia and elevated numbers of circulating B cells. In vitro studies demonstrate diminished lymphocyte proliferation to B-cell mitogens. Hypogammaglobulinemia, another manifestation of B-cell dysfunction, has also been noted (Rubinstein, 1986; Novick, 1990; Falloon et al., 1989). T-cell abnormalities do develop and include lymphopenia, low absolute numbers of CD4 cells, reversed T4/T8 ratio, poor in vitro lymphocyte proliferation to T-cell mitogens, and cutaneous anergy. Children, like adults, may develop infections with opportunistic pathogens associated with defects in cell-mediated immunity. *Pneumocystis carinii* pneumonia (PCP) is the most common. Disseminated candidiasis, *Mycobacterium avium-intracellulare* (MAI), disseminated or invasive cytomegalovirus (CMV) infections, and cryptospiridiosis are the next most frequent.

Lymphoid interstitial pneumonitis (LIP), a common feature of HIV-I infection in children, unlike adults, is characterized by progressive bilateral diffuse reticulonodular infiltrates. The age of onset is usually between 16 and 37 months. Survival for children with LIP appears to be better than for children who develop PCP in infancy (Krasinski et al., 1989; Blanche et al., 1989; Scott, 1989).

HIV-I AND THE CENTRAL NERVOUS SYSTEM

Central nervous system involvement associated with pediatric HIV-I infection can be divided into two main categories: (1) CNS disease related to "HIV-I itself"; and (2) CNS complications secondary to immunodeficiency; infections caused by organisms other than HIV-I neoplasms; or strokes. However, the CNS in children with HIV-I infection may also be affected by metabolic and endocrinologic derangements related to systemic HIV-I infection. It must also be kept in mind that the developing CNS in HIV-I infected infants, as in non-HIV-I infected infants, may be adversely affected by material conditions during pregnancy (Table 17.3) and complications in the perinatal period (Table 17.4).

In addition, the HIV-I infected child's development may be adversely affected by numerous and complex psychosocial stressors, such as unstable family units, changing caretakers, impoverished environments, and frequent hospitalizations.

Table 17.3.
Factors Related to Pregnancy

Maternal substance use:
    In utero exposure to cocaine, crack, heroin,
      alcohol, methadone, etc.
Poor or no maternal prenatal care
Inadequate maternal nutrition
Maternal illnesses:
    Maternal HIV-I disease
    Infections caused by pathogens other than HIV-I
    HIV-I-associated diseases

Table 17.4.
Perinatal Conditions

Low birth weight (small for date)
Prematurity
Perinatal asphyxia
Hypoxic-ischemic encephalopathy
Intracranial hemorrhage (subependymal, intraventricular, intraparenchymal)
Periventricular leukomalacia
Neonatal illnesses (respiratory distress, necrotizing enterocolitis, infections, etc.)

As new antiviral and immunomodulating agents are developed, and new treatment protocols for HIV-I and "AIDS-related diseases" are designed and instituted, it is also quite possible that the nervous system may be adversely affected by metabolic/toxic complications of these new therapies.

This chapter's focus is on CNS complications secondary to immunodeficiency; the clinical, neuroimaging, and pathologic features of HIV-I related CNS disease; and behavioral and psychosocial aspects associated with HIV-I infection in children.

CNS COMPLICATIONS ASSOCIATED WITH IMMUNE DEFICIENCY

Neurologic complications associated with immunodeficiency are well described in children with symptomatic HIV-I infection: a 10 to 20% incidence is estimated. Children often develop more than one of these complications, and coexisting HIV-I related CNS disease is common (Belman, 1988).

CNS Infections

As discussed above, children with AIDS often have serious bacterial infections, including sepsis and meningitis. *Streptococcus pneumoniae, Hemophilus influenzae,* and *Escherichia coli* are the most common pathogens (Bernstein et al., 1985). Neurologic sequelae (as in the non-HIV-I infected child) may include variable degrees of sensorineural hearing loss, cognitive deficits, and long tract signs.

Opportunistic infections of the CNS occur, but less frequently in HIV-I infected children than in adults (Belman et al., 1988; Epstein et al., 1988B). In adult patients, the most common CNS lesions are due to reactivation of previously acquired infection, including toxoplasmosis, CMV, and papovavirus infection, which is the etiologic agent of progressive multifocal leukoencephalopathy (PML). Hence, reactivation of latent infection would not be expected in infants and young children but could be expected in adolescents. Because more "older children" (see above) are being identified with HIV-I infection, and because more children are surviving longer as a result of early therapy, it seems likely that the risk for primary and reactivated CNS infections will increase.

CMV encephalitis, although well-documented in pediatric AIDS patients (Belman et al., 1988; Belman et al., 1985; Sharer et al., 1986), also does not appear to occur as frequently in children as in adults. *Candida albicans* has been the most common CNS fungal infection reported in children and may cause meningitis or microabscesses (Belman, 1990).

Neoplasm

Primary CNS lymphoma, an unusual neoplasm of childhood, is well-described as a CNS complication in children with HIV-I infection (Belman et al., 1988; Epstein et al., 1988A; Dickson et al., 1989; Dickson et al., 1990). Systemic lymphoma metastatic to the CNS has also been reported (Belman et al., 1988; Dickson et al., 1990). Presenting signs of lymphoma include the new onset of focal neurologic deficits, seizures, or a change in mental status (Belman, 1990; Epstein et al., 1988A). At times, neurologic deterioration may be rapidly progressive and fulminant. In general, these signs can be distinguished from the more insidious neurologic deterioration of HIV-I related encephalopathy (see below). Hence, the new onset of

seizures, focal motor deficits, or change in mental status warrants a neuroimaging study (Belman, 1990).

Computed tomography (CT) characteristics of lymphoma are variable and include (1) hyperdense or isodense mass lesion(s) that may or may not enhance after injection of contrast material; (2) diffusely infiltrating contrast-enhancing lesions; and (3) periventricular contrast-enhancing lesions. Multiple lesions are common (Belman, 1990).

Examination of the CSF may reveal mild-to-moderate pleocytosis, elevated protein content, and hypoglycorrhachia (Epstein et al., 1988A).

Cerebrovascular Complications

Cerebrovascular complications are increasingly being recognized as a secondary CNS complication in children with symptomatic HIV-I infection; both hemorrhagic and nonhemorrhagic strokes have been described (Belman et al., 1988; Belman, 1990; Dickson et al., 1990; Frank et al., 1989; Park et al., 1990). Intracerebral hemorrhage usually occurs in the setting of immune-mediated thrombocytopenia (Park et al., 1990). Clinical presentation is variable and reflects the severity and location of hemorrhage. Strokes may be catastrophic and fatal, but clinically silent events have also been reported (Belman, 1990; Park et al., 1990).

Nonhemorrhagic infarctions are most often associated with pathologic changes of cerebral blood vessels, meningeal infections, or cardiomyopathy (Dickson et al., 1989; Dickson et al., 1990; Frank et al., 1989; Park et al., 1990; Kure et al., 1989).

The new onset of focal neurologic deficits, most commonly hemiparesis, at times associated with seizures, is the most common presentation of stroke in children with HIV-I infection/AIDS (Park et al., 1990). Neuroradiologic findings may show bland or hemorrhagic infarction. Intracranial hemorrhage is readily identified on CT or magnetic resonance imaging (MRI) scan. Hence, neuroimaging studies should be obtained in the child who develops focal neurologic deficits, seizures, or rapidly progressing neurologic deterioration (Belman, 1990; Park et al., 1990).

HIV-I RELATED CNS DISEASE

CNS impairment has been a frequent finding in infants and young children with symptomatic disease (Belman et al., 1988; Belman et al., 1985; Epstein et al., 1985; Epstein et al., 1986; Blanche et al., 1990). As HIV-I infection advances to severe symptomatic stages, cognitive, behavioral, and motor impairment of varying severity, duration, and progression are common findings (Belman et al., 1988). However, the true incidence of HIV-I related CNS disease is not known and awaits completion of prospective studies in progress in the United States, Europe, and Africa.

HIV-I CNS Infection

Clinical, pathologic, and laboratory studies have been able to establish that the CNS is infected with HIV-I. Immunocytochemical studies have localized HIV-I antigen in brain monocytes, macrophages, and multinucleated giant cells. HIV-I nucleotide sequences have been demonstrated in the brain by in situ hybridization techniques. HIV-I has been recovered from cerebrospinal fluid. Intrathecal production of anti-HIV-I antibody has also been documented. In addition, it seems that CNS invasion by the retrovirus may occur early in the course of the disease (see Johnson et al., 1988, and Belman, 1990, for literature review).

These studies implicate HIV-I as the causative agent for "HIV-I related CNS disease," in adults (AIDS-dementia complex) (Navia et al., 1986; Price et al., 1988; McArthur, 1987) and "HIV-I/AIDS encephalopathy" in children. However, many questions remain concerning the natural history and the pathogenetic mechanism of HIV-I CNS disease. These include the timing and route of CNS invasion by the virus; the relationship between CNS viral invasion, latency, and subsequent clinical course; the explanation for the varying rate of progression of CNS disease and the varied encephalopathic courses described; and the different pathologic lesions noted in the brain and spinal cord (Belman, 1990).

Different pathogenetic mechanisms probably account for the different clinical expressions of CNS disease in children (Belman, 1990). Both direct and indirect effects of HIV-I have been proposed, as reviewed by Johnson et al. (1988). These include direct effects of infection of neural cells (cytopathic or function-altering); effects of macrophages/monocytes producing cytokines and chemotactic factors; possible toxic effects of monolymphokines, altering function of glia or function of neurons; effects of viral proteins, blocking neuroreceptors or blocking neurotrophic factors; effects on endothelial cells, altering the blood-brain barrier; transactivation of other infectious agents; and autoimmunity (Johnson et al., 1988). In addition, viral strain differences and host-related factors may play a significant role.

MANIFESTATIONS OF HIV-I CNS DISEASE

The most frequent neurologic manifestations of HIV-I involvement in infants and children include cognitive impairment, developmental delays, acquired microcephaly, and bilateral corticospinal tract (CST) signs (Belman et al., 1988; Belman et al., 1985; Epstein et al., 1986). Movement disorders and cerebellar signs occur less frequently (Belman et al., 1988). Seizures are uncommon and are most often symptomatic of secondary neurologic complications (see above) (Belman et al., 1988; Belman, 1990). Although some degree of cognitive, behavioral, and motor impairment appears to occur in all children with HIV-I related CNS disease, some patients may have a marked discrepancy between progression and severity of motor dysfunction compared with more stable, although impaired, cognitive and socially adaptive abilities (Belman, 1990).

NEUROLOGIC FEATURES, PROGRESSION, AND COURSES OF HIV-I RELATED DISEASE: "PROGRESSIVE ENCEPHALOMYELOPATHY"

The following section describes the neurologic, neuropsychologic, neuroimaging, and neuropathologic features of pediatric HIV-I related CNS disease (Belman, 1990).

In most children neurologic deterioration appears insidiously. In the young child, there may be deterioration of play and loss of previously acquired language and socially adaptive skills (Belman et al., 1988). Progressive motor dysfunction is common (Belman et al., 1988) and may manifest in the toddler or child by a change in gait or toe-walking (Belan, 1990). CST signs may be progressive and result in spastic paraparesis or quadriparesis with or without pseudobulbar signs. Disorder of movement such as rigidity, dystonic posturing, and/or extrapyramidal tremor occur, but less frequently. Some children develop cerebellar signs (Belman, 1990).

The child may develop a characteristic facial appearance (an alert, wide-eyed expression with a paucity of spontaneous facial movements, although there is no facial weakness, as evidenced by full movement when crying) (Belman, 1990). Eye movement abnormalities (restriction of upward gaze, reduced eye blink, abnormal pursuit, or ocular motor apraxia) may also develop (Belman, 1990). With progression of disease, most of the children eventually become apathic, lose interest in play and the environment, and have decreased gestures and vocalizations. If death from infection or neoplasm does not intervene, the child at end stage is mute, dull-eyed, and quadriparetic (Belman et al., 1988).

Neurologic deterioration in some patients occurs more rapidly (over a period of 1 to 2 months). In others, the course is episodic, with periods of deterioration interrupted by variable periods of relative neurologic stability (Belman et al., 1988; Epstein et al., 1988B; Belman et al., 1985).

However, in most children the rate of neurologic deterioration is slow and the course more indolent (Belman, 1990). Cognitive impairment becomes evident as the rate of developmental progress declines. Over time, although the child gains further cognitive and language skills, the rate of acquisition of new skills is extremely slow and deviates not only from the norm but also from the child's previous rate of early developmental progress. IQ scores, or the Mental Developmental Index (MDI) of the Bayley Scales of Infant Development [BSID] in the infant or young child, decline (Belman et al., 1988; Belman, 1990). The equivalent mental developmental age may remain essentially the same over a period of months or may advance, but very slowly (Belman et al., 1989; Belman et al., 1990). Attention deficits are also common. Manifestations of motor involvement usually develop, but again, progression and severity may vary. Poor brain growth resulting in acquired microcephaly can be documented by serial head circumference measurements. When plotted on standardized growth charts (Nellhaus, 1964), the measurements show downward deviation and crossing of percentiles (Belman et al., 1988; Belman et al., 1985).

SCHOOL-AGED CHILDREN

Early signs of CNS impairment in older children may manifest as a loss of interest in school performance (Belman et al., 1986). Other signs reported include attention deficits or worsening of attention deficit disorders (ADD), psychomotor slowing, social withdrawal, increased emotional lability, and, in some, worsening of ADD with conduct disorders (Belman, 1990; Belman et al., 1986; Loveland and Stehbens, 1990; Lifschitz et al., 1989).

Some investigators suggest that two domains of cognitive function seem to be most affected by CNS HIV-I infection. On the basis of IQ subset profiles and behavioral assessments, expressive language and difficulties with attention have been recognized (Brouwers et al., 1989). As the disease progresses, motor dysfunction and long tract signs may manifest. Movement disorders and/or signs of cerebellar involvement may also develop. With progressive disease, the child shows cognitive impairment and at end stage is apathetic and abulic (Belman, 1990).

"STATIC ENCEPHALOPATHY"

Abnormalities in development, including histories of delays in acquisition of language and of motor milestones, associated with intellectual impairment of varying severity were reported in children with AIDS/AIDS-related complex (ARC) in 1985 (Belman et al., 1985). At follow-up many of these children were found to function in the low-average to borderline range of intelligence, some in the mild, and a few in the moderate range of mental retardation (Belman et al., 1988; Ultmann et al., 1985; Ultmann et al., 1987). The majority also had varying degrees of motor impairment. Attention deficit disorders with or without hyperactivity were also very common findings. In one study (Belman et al., 1988), serial examinations during a 4-year period showed that, although present, cognitive and motor impairment remained stable—unlike the course described above. These children continued to acquire additional developmental skills, and IQ scores and motor deficits remained fairly stable. Head circumference measurements in many patients were below the 50th percentile (range, 2 to 25%); however, most followed the same percentile curve, reflecting continued brain growth.

Because of the (at least short-term) "stable" nature of neurologic deficits, this group of children was initially described as having a "static" course. Subsequent studies have described deficits in perceptual and visual integrative abilities and difficulties with visual organization (Diamond et al., 1987; Cohen et al., 1991). Other investigators, however, have noted language-related problems as the predominant deficiency

(Nozyce et al., 1989; Condini et al., 1989; Walters et al., 1989).

Notably, many of these children also had in utero exposure to drugs, and some were born prematurely. None was followed prospectively from birth. These and other confounding gestational, perinatal, medical, and psychosocial factors have made analysis difficult to date (Belman 1990; Ultmann et al., 1985; Ultmann et al., 1987; Diamond et al., 1990). In addition, terminology among investigators has not been uniform. Hence, children described as having "static" encephalopathy remain ill-defined; moreover, the relationship of "static encephalopathy" to HIV-I CNS disease remains uncertain. Howeover, abnormal MRI findings (see below) in some children coupled with evidence of intrathecal HIV-I antibody synthesis suggest that "static encephalopathy", in at least some patients, is related to HIV-I CNS infection (Belman et al., 1988; Belman, 1990). It is also possible that some of these patients may even have had an undocumented encephalopathic event related to HIV-I CNS infection in infancy or early childhood resulting in cognitive and motor impairment (Belman, 1990).

Of course, the encephalopathy may appear to be static in some of these patients because maturation is proceeding faster than deterioration. (The CNS in children is constantly maturing and developing, and children are attaining new abilities and mastering already-existing skills.) Another possibility is that CNS disease is quiescent. Prospective longitudinal studies, in progress, should help clarify some of these complex issues.

In any case, optimism remains guarded for children with "static encephalopathy." Many of these children will go on to develop "progressive encephalopathy," CNS complications of immunodeficiency, or, as HIV-I disease advances, both (Belman et al., 1988.)

NEUROIMAGING FINDINGS

CT examinations show cerebral atrophy of variable severity and abnormalities of white matter

(Belman et al., 1988; Epstein et al., 1988B; Belman et al., 1985; Epstein et al., 1985). Some patients have bilateral symmetrical calcification of the basal ganglia and, less frequently, calcification of the frontal white matter (Belman et al., 1988; Epstein et al., 1988B; Belman et al., 1985; Epstein et al., 1985; Epstein et al., 1986; Belman et al., 1986). Serial studies may show progressive atrophy and white matter changes (decreased density) (Belman et al., 1988; Belman, 1990). Some children have progressive calcification of the basal ganglia (Figure 17.1). Magnetic resonance imaging (MRI), which often shows abnormalities not visualized on CT, reveals atrophy and abnormal high signal intensity in the white matter on T-2 weighted images (Belman, 1990; Belman et al., 1986). Abnormal signal may be noted in the basal ganglia region.

In some children with developmental arrest, serial CT examinations may show no significant change even though poor serial head circumference measurements show a deceleration in head growth (a reflection of poor brain growth) (Belman, 1990; Wiley et al., 1990).

CT examinations in children with static encephalopathy are usually normal or show mild atrophy (Belman et al., 1988). However, in some children, MRI studies may show abnormal high signal in the white matter and/or basal ganglia (T2 weighted images) (Belman, 1990).

CEREBROSPINAL FLUID FINDINGS

Cerebrospinal fluid (CSF) profiles are generally normal, but mild pleocytosis and elevated protein content may be seen in some children during the late stages of progressive encephalopathy and seem to correlate with severe white matter abnormalities on CT (Belman et al., 1988). Other findings reported include intrathecal production of anti-HIV-I antibody, detectable levels of HIV-I p24, and, at times, macrophage-derived cytokines (Epstein et al., 1986; Blanche et al., 1990; Epstein et al., 1987; Gallo et al., 1990).

NEUROPATHOLOGIC FINDINGS

Postmortem examinations of the brain show variable degrees of cerebral atrophy, ventricular enlargement, widening of sulci, and attenuation of deep cerebral white matter (Belman et al.,

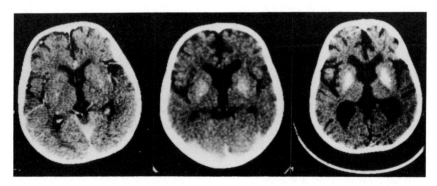

Figure 17.1. *Left,* Contrast-enhanced CT of a 15-month-old boy shows punctate area of increased density in the right posterior lateral lenticular region and contrast enhancement in the left basal ganglia region (medial to the enhancing middle cerebral arterial branches in the left sylvian fissure as well as sulcal and ventricular enlargement). *Middle,* Seven months later, punctate and diffuse areas/calcification are present bilaterally in the basal ganglia. There is also evidence of progressive cerebral atrophy. *Right,* Eight months later, CT without contrast shows that both basal ganglia calcification and cerebral atrophy have increased. (Used with permission from Belman AL, Lantos G, Horoupian D, et al. AIDS: calcification of the basal ganglia in infants and children. Neurology 1986;36:1192–1199.)

1988; Epstein et al., 1988B; Belman et al., 1985; Sharer et al., 1986; Dickson et al., 1989). The deep cerebral white matter may show diffuse and ill-defined or discrete and patchy staining pallor. Gliosis is a common finding (Belman et al., 1988; Epstein et al., 1988B; Belman et al., 1985; Sharer et al., 1986; Dickson et al., 1989).

HIV encephalopathy, also termed "subacute encephalitis," is defined as lesions containing multinucleated giant cells (Kozlowski et al., 1990). Often there is an inflammatory response of variable severity, characterized by perivascular mononuclear inflammatory cell infiltrates, microglial nodules, and multinucleated giant cells (Belman et al., 1988; Epstein et al., 1988B; Belman et al., 1985; Sharer et al., 1986; Dickson et al., 1989; Kozlowski et al., 1990). In situ hybridization and immunocytochemical studies have shown HIV-I antigen within multinucleated cells, monocytes and macrophages, and, more rarely, endothelial cells (Epstein et al., 1988B; Dickson et al., 1989; Wiley et al., 1990).

Calcific vasculopathy of the basal ganglia has been the most consistent pathologic finding in children with AIDS (Epstein et al., 1988B; Dickson et al., 1989; Kozlowski et al., 1990). Mineralization is most often found in the walls of small blood vessels, but in some cases calcific deposits have been seen in walls of vessels of all sizes (Epstein et al., 1988B; Dickson et al., 1989; Belman et al., 1986). Although calcification of the basal ganglia frequently coexists with "subacute AIDS encephalitis," this is not invariable, and patients may have basal ganglia calcification without inflammatory CNS disease or sign of acute infection (Belman et al., 1988; Belman et al., 1985).

In the spinal cord the most common histopathologic finding is corticospinal tract (CST) "degeneration", characterized by striking staining pallor of myelin that is restricted to the CST (Dickson et al., 1986; Weidenheim et al., 1990). This contrasts with the vacuolar myelopathy described in adult patients that predominantly affects the posterior columns (Petito et al., 1985).

BEHAVIORAL MANIFESTATIONS ASSOCIATED WITH HIV-I DISEASE AND PSYCHOSOCIAL ISSUES

The preceding descriptions of CNS HIV-I disease are from studies of children with symptoms of systemic HIV-I disease. On initial evaluations, the majority of children had evidence of CNS dysfunction, although of varying severity and duration. Therefore, the earliest manifestations of neurologic involvement, neuropsychologic profiles, and behavioral manifestations of HIV-I CNS disease have not yet been well-defined and are currently being investigated in prospective studies.

Behavioral manifestations of HIV-I infection in children are also currently being addressed but to date have not been studied sufficiently in large series to draw definite conclusions. Nevertheless, it has been the impression of clinicians that many young pre- and early school-aged children show levels of hyperactivity and attention difficulties that are disruptive and maladaptive. Many children have also been reported to exhibit learning and behavioral problems in school, and some have been held back one or two grades. This is even the case for some children with above-average to superior IQs. It is as yet unclear whether this is due to HIV-I CNS infection and/or confounding coexisting conditions related to both medical and psychosocial factors. Analysis becomes especially difficult when one considers the high prevalence or base rate of these disorders in the general population and especially in the children with in utero exposure to drugs and alcohol.

Although these behavioral manifestations may be the first or early signs of HIV-I encephalopathy, confounding gestational and psychosocial conditions must also be considered in the differential diagnosis. It is also possible that psychosocial stressors may even exacerbate manifestations of the underlying "organic basis" of these conditions. Clearly, these issues must be addressed in future studies.

In addition, the psychologic impact of HIV-I infection on the school-aged child and adolescent is often enormous. Salient efects may be direct, such as HIV-I associated CNS manifestations, or indirect, such as reactions to a myriad of illness-related stressful experiences.

DIRECT EFFECTS: HIV-I ASSOCIATED CNS MANIFESTATIONS IN COGNITIVE AND MOTOR ABILITIES

Most of the evidence for the direct effects of HIV-I on behavior comes from psychometric test results. As mentioned above, two domains of cognitive function seem to be most susceptible to the effects of CNS HIV-I infection: attention processes and expressive behavior. Attention difficulties have been recognized almost universally in pediatric (Brouwers et al., 1989) and adult patients with HIV-I disease, both on the basis of IQ subtest profiles and on behavioral assessment. In fact, it is one of the hallmark observations in adults with AIDS/dementia complex (Price et al., 1988). As mentioned above, in children with HIV-I disease, however, it is not clear whether attention problems are directly attributable to HIV-I or are related to other factors, or both.

Subclinical effects of HIV-I on the CNS have also been documented in a number of older children (Pizzo et al., 1988). Minimal deficiencies often noted by parents and caregivers are psychomotor slowing, increased fatigue, and, in some, mild-to-moderate signs of depression (Belman, 1990; Loveland and Stehbens, 1990; Pizzo et al., 1988).

With respect to the realm of expressive behavior, investigators have reported expressive language to be deficient despite relatively intact receptive verbal functioning, suggesting the specific vulnerability of this component of human functioning to HIV-I associated disease. Similarly, these patients frequently seem to have difficulty in expressing their emotions, both verbally and nonverbally (Moss et al., 1989).

Some young children with progressive encephalopathy as defined earlier in this chapter exhibit behavior found in childhood autistic syndromes, whereas signs and symptoms of depression occur in older children. It is possible that the same behavior at different ages is labeled differently because of conventional interpretations. Hence, autistic-like behaviors occasionally seen in young children may be similar to what has been called depression in older children. That is, children in both diagnostic groups may exhibit flattened affect, lack of social responsiveness, muteness, withdrawal, and minimal interest in the outside world.

INDIRECT EFFECTS: INFLUENCE OF FACTORS ASSOCIATED WITH HIV-I ON BEHAVIOR

Behavioral reactions to HIV-I infection can arise indirectly from the psychologic stress associated with having HIV-I disease. The stress associated with HIV-I infection can be classified into three primary categories based on the source of the stress: (1) *medical factors* (e.g., medical procedures and hospitalizations; recurring interfering medical symptoms; loss of abilities; pain and discomfort): (2) *psychologic stressors* (secrecy; fear of ostracism; death; guilt; uncertainties of future; inhibited sexual activity (adolescents); need to alter future perspectives); and (3) *social stressors* (ostracism by school, community and extended family; underachievement due to absenteeism). Some of these stressors are omnipresent, whereas others are transient or modulated by prevailing medical and psychosocial conditions and by the developmental status of the child.

HIV-I infected children can also be divided

into different subgroups based on background, personal characteristics, and disease parameters. Differences in environmental and predisposing medical conditions among patients may color the behavioral, neuropsychologic, and neurologic development and confound the evaluation of possible HIV-I associated deficits in these children. In addition, the age of the child may determine some of the behavioral consequences of HIV-I infection.

Relationship of Age to Patient Characteristics and Biomedical Background

It has not yet been possible to determine whether psychologic differences between age groups are due to timing of CNS invasion of the virus, developmental factors, or perhaps family structure and social class factors that also happen to co-vary with age for this population. There is a historic basis for the co-variance of these "social" factors with age in the pediatric AIDS population. Since the blood supply has been safe since the early spring of 1985, the youngest children born in the USA who acquired HIV-I through blood product or coagulation factor transfusion are now at least 5 years of age. Indeed, the majority of older children with symptomatic HIV-I disease entered into studies were infected through the transfer of blood products. Many of these patients were boys (hemophiliacs) who had received multiple transfusions of blood products.

In summary, most information on children older than 6 had transfusion-acquired HIV-I disease and were boys, while children younger than 6 had vertically acquired HIV-I. Differences in family structure and psychologic support between younger vertically infected children and older children infected through transfusion are discussed later.

Predisposing Conditions

Patients with transfusion acquired HIV-I may have been affected by potential adverse CNS se-

quelae from medical conditions that required transfusion in the first place. For example, CNS complications-associated prematurity (Spreen et al., 1984), cardiac surgery (Terplan, 1973), and some forms of childhood cancer (Poplack and Brouwers, 1985) have all been reported. Hence it may sometimes be difficult to distinguish between these effects and the more acute HIV-I CNS manifestations.

In patients with vertically transmitted infection, the adverse effect of in utero exposure to drugs must be considered for infants whose mothers have a history of IV drug use. Use of heroin (Naeye et al., 1973), cocaine (Chasnoff et al., 1989), and alcohol (Macgregor et al., 1987; Iosub et al., 1981; Day et al., 1989) have all been associated with adverse effects on the newborn. Differentiating between the contribution of HIV-I and of prenatal drug exposure to neurobehavioral dysfunctioning is complex.

Environment

Children infected through transfusion tend to come from intact, stable families with a higher level of economic and social support systems than that of vertically infected children. In addition, these families often have had to cope previously with chronic potentially life-threatening medical illness (hemophilia, cancer, major surgery, etc.), and may have grown somewhat accustomed to the stress and uncertainty associated with serious illness.

Vertically infected children will have parent(s) who are also infected with HIV-I. Because the parent's infection is often associated with specific high-risk behaviors, vertically infected children are more likely to be from unstable, nonsupportive family situations. Frequently, one encounters single parents, multiple substance abuse, low socioeconomic environment, prostitution, etc. In addition, the disease in the parent(s) may also have rendered them incapable of optimally caring for their children. In many cases, the child may have been placed in an institution or shifted among various foster homes.

The deleterious effect of the impoverished home environment and the other adverse conditions on psychosocial adjustment, mental growth, and development have been well-documented (Capron and Duyme, 1989).

Disease Status

Although behavioral abnormalities and encephalopathy have been reported as the first and sometimes only signs of HIV-I infection, neurologic and neuropsychologic defects seem to occur in the later stages of the disease, when the children have symptomatic HIV-I disease. Current information suggests that the likelihood of observing severe neurologic deficits as a first or only sign is higher in younger children and infants than in older children and adults. It has not yet been documented whether subtle deficits are present in older, asymptomatic pediatric patients, as has been observed in adult asymptomatic HIV-I positive patients (Grant et al., 1987).

ADAPTIVE BEHAVIORAL PATTERNS

During those periods when older HIV-I infected children are relatively symptom-free, they show few "outward signs" of adjustment difficulties, at least as they may relate to their illness. There is a tendency to be private and not want to talk about their illness, even with parents. Instead, they seem to prefer and are able to focus effectively on their typical everyday activities. Many of these children seem remarkably resilient, are active, exhibit appropriate positive and negative affect, are outgoing, and engage in usual social interactions with peers and adults. This is not to say that they may not be preoccupied and privately dealing with aspects of their illness and feel under great tension. However, as a group they seem to have things under control, want to continue with their lives, and are usually able to cope effectively. One 8-year-old boy recently stood up during a "show and tell" in his school and announced that there were rumors circulating for the past few years that someone in their school had AIDS and that he wanted to let everyone know that it was him. He felt under too much tension maintaining this secret and had a strong enough self-concept and sufficient confidence in his social status that he was able to risk divulging this guarded fact to his schoolmates.

THERAPY

Preliminary reports from phase I and II therapeutic trials of antiviral agents have been promising, with improvements in neurologic and intellectual function documented in small series of patients (Pizzo et al., 1988).

As noted above, deficits in expressive language despite intact receptive verbal functioning were noted in some children with HIV-I infection. Preliminary studies have suggested that treatment with zidovudine may lead to greater improvement in expressive as compared with receptive language abilities (Wolters et al., 1989).

Preliminary studies have also shown improvements in general adaptive behavior with zidovudine (AZT, formerly known as azidothymidine) therapy using a Q-sort rating scale technique (Moss et al., 1989). A moderate decrease in irritability was also observed for children without signs of HIV-I related CNS disease, but little or no change on this variable was noted for the group with CNS disease. Hyperactivity seemed unaffected by AZT treatment for either group. However, there are no data concerning attention or hyperactivity level of HIV-I infected children compared with a medically healthy cohort using the Q-sort technique.

In any case, preliminary data from these small cohorts of patients are promising. It also appears that the incidence of these symptom patterns may be lower with early anti-HIV-I interventions. However, large cohorts of patients in phase III therapeutic trials will be needed to confirm these findings.

Methylphenidate has been used for adult patients with HIV-I infection with depression, lack of energy, and/or psychomotor slowing. Preliminary reports (Holmes et al., 1989) have been encouraging, but the efficacy of this intervention has not yet been systematically studied in children with HIV-I infection.

EDUCATIONAL INTERVENTION

Educational interventions for HIV-I patients with neurodevelopmental deficits as well as HIV-I encephalopathy should take an individual approach. Specific deficits, as well as strengths and average abilities, should be assessed with a comprehensive neuropsychologic evaluation. In addition, patients should be taught how to increase concentration, sustain attention, and decrease distractibility. Adjustments, particularly in classroom settings, are frequently required.

CASE STUDIES

JD

A 10-year-old boy with hemophilia A developed insidious loss of interest in school performance over a 3-month period of time, although he was still capable of doing grade-appropriate work. He was in a class for the intellectually gifted and had been described as a highly motivated and excellent student. An "AIDS-defining" systemic illness was not diagnosed until several months after the change in behavior. CNS HIV-I related encephalopathy was relentlessly progressive, resulting in abulia, bilateral frontal release signs, and the ability to follow only one-step requests (Belman et al., 1986).

NM

At age 6 years, a girl with vertically transmitted HIV-I infection became shy, fearful, and withdrawn. Her teachers described a change in her interactions with the other children as well as adults. HIV-I infection had been diagnosed at age 3 years (HIV-I seropositivity; P-2C lymphoid interstitial pneumonitis). Serial neurologic examinations, psychometric evaluations, and neuroimaging studies performed between ages 3 and 5 years were normal.

CT scan at age 6 years showed mild atrophy. Manifestations of HIV-I CNS involvement were slowly progressive over the next 8 months. She became "clingy" and "weepy", and her behavior was immature. She gradually lost interest in the toys and books that she had previously enjoyed.

JS

JS was born to an IVDU mother. At age 2½ years he was placed in the home of a warm, supportive, and stable foster family. Although early developmental milestones were delayed, he made steady developmental progress. At age 3½ years, examination showed a playful, socially interactive child who was functioning at approximately a 24 to 30 month level. He continued to attain further developmental skills during the next year. His parents related that several months before the Christmas of his 5th year, they selected toys at an appropriate level for his mental age. However, by Christmas he showed little interest in these new toys. He was still alert, playful, and interactive but preferred toys designed not only for a much younger child but those he had "outgrown" months before.

REFERENCES

Aiuti F, Luzi G, Mezzaroma I, Scano G, Papetti C. Delayed appearance of HIV infection in children. Lancet 1987;2:858.

Auger I, Thomas P, De Gruttola V, et al. Incubation periods for paediatric AIDS patients. Nature 1988;336:575–577.

Belman AL. AIDS and pediatric neurology. Neurol Clin 1990;8:571–603.

Belman AL, Calvelli T, Nozyce M, et al. Neurologic and immunologic correlates in infants with vertically transmitted HIV infection. Neurology 1990;1(suppl):40:409.

Belman AL, Diamond G, Dickson D, et al. Pediatric AIDS: neurologic syndromes. Am J Dis Child 1988;142:29–35.

Belman AL, Diamond G, Park Y, et al. Perinatal HIV infection: a prospective longitudinal study of the initial CNS signs. Neurology 1989;39(suppl):278–279.

Belman AL, Lantos G, Horoupian D, et al. AIDS: calcification of the basal ganglia in infants and children. Neurology 1986;36:1192–1199.

Belman AL, Ultmann MH, Horoupian D, et al. Neurologic complications in infants and children with acquired immune deficiency syndrome. Ann Neurol 1985;18:560–566.

Bernstein LJ, Krieger BZ, Novick BE, Sicklick M, Rubinstein A. Bacterial infections—the acquired immunodeficiency syndrome in children. Pediatr Infect Dis 1985;4:472–475.

Blanche S, Rouzioux C, Moscato M-L, et al. A prospective study of infants born to mothers seropositive for human immunodeficiency virus type 1. N Engl J Med 1989;320:1643–1648.

Blanche S, Tardieu M, Duliege AM. Longitudinal study of 94 symptomatic infants with perinatally-acquired HIV infection. Am J Dis Child 1990;144:1210–1215.

Brouwers P, Moss H, Wolters P, Eddy J. Pizzo P. Neuropsychological profile of children with symptomatic HIV infection prior to anti-retroviral treatment. V International Conference on AIDS, Montreal, June 4–9, 1989.

Burger H, Belman AL, Grimson R, et al. Long HIV-I incubation periods and dynamics of transmission within a family. Lancet 1990;336:134–136.

Capron C, Duyme M. Assessment of effects of socioeconomic status on IQ in a full cross-fostering study. Nature 1989;340:552–554.

Centers for Disease Control. Update: acquired immunodeficiency syndrom (AIDS)—United States. MMWR 1984;21:688–691.

Centers for Disease Control. Revision of the case definition of acquired immunodeficiency syndrome for national reporting—United States. MMWR 1985;34:373–377.

Centers for Disease Control. Classification system for human immunodeficiency virus (HIV) infection in children under 13 years of age. MMWR 1987;103:665–670.

Chasnoff IJ, Griffith DR, MacGregor S, Dirkes K, Burns KA. Temporal patterns of cocaine use during pregnancy. JAMA 1989;261:1741–1744.

Coffin J, Haase A, Levy JA, et al. Human immunodeficiency viruses. Science 1986;232:697.

Cohen S, Mundy T, et al. Neuropsychological function in children HIV infected through neonatal blood transfusions. Pediatrics 1991;88:58–68.

Condini A, Cattalen C, Viaro F, et al. Psychic development of children born to HIV infected Italian mothers. T.B.P.178. V International Conference on AIDS, Montreal, June 4–9, 1989.

Day HNL, Jasperse D, Richardson G. Prenatal exposure to alcohol: effect on infant growth and morphologic characteristics. Pediatrics 1989;84:536–541.

Diamond GW, Belman AL, Park YD, et al. Characterization of cognitive functioning in a subgroup of children with congenital HIV infection. Arch Clin Neuropsychol 1987;2:1–16.

Diamond GW, Gurdin P, Wiznia A, Belman AL, Rubinstein A, Cohen HJ. Effects of congenital HIV-I infection on neurodevelopmental status of babies in foster care. Devel Med Child Neurol 1990;32:999–1005.

Dickson DW, Belman AL, Kim TS, Horoupian D, Rubinstein A. Spinal cord pathology in pediatric acquired immunodeficiency syndrome. Neurology 1986;39:227–235.

Dickson DW, Belman AL, Park YD, et al. Central nervous system pathology in pediatric AIDS: an autopsy study. APMIS 1989;8(suppl):50–57.

Dickson DW, Llena JF, Weidenheim KM, et al. Central nervous system pathology in children with AIDS and focal neurologic signs—stroke and lymphoma. In: Kozlowski PB, Snider DA, Vietze PM, Wisniewski HM, eds. Brain in pediatric AIDS. Basel: Karger, 1990;147–157.

Epstein LG, Dicarlo F, Joshi V, et al. Primary lymphoma of the central nervous system in children with acquired immunodeficiency syndrome. Pediatrics 1988A:82:355–363.

Epstein LG, Goudsmit J, Paul DA, et al. Expression of human immunodeficiency virus in cerebrospinal fluid of children with progressive encephalopathy. Ann Neurol 1987;21:397–401.

Epstein LG, Sharer LR, Goudsmit J. Neurological and neuropathological features of HIV in children. Ann Neurol 1988B;23(suppl):S19–S23.

Epstein LG, Sharer LR, Joshi VV, et al. Progressive encephalopathy in children with acquired immune deficiency syndrome. Ann Neurol 1985;17:488–496.

Epstein LG, Sharer LR, Oleske JM, et al. Neurologic manifestations of human immunodeficiency virus infection in children. Pediatrics 1986;78:678–687.

Falloon J, Eddy J, Weiner L, Pizzo PA. Human immunodeficiency virus infection in children. J Pediatr 1989;114:1–30.

Frank Y, Lim W, Kahn E, et al. Multiple ischemic infarcts in a child with AIDS, Varicella zoster infection and cerebral vasculitis. Pediatr Neurol 1989;5:64–67.

Gallo P, Laverda AM, DeRossi A, et al. Macrophage-derived cytokines in the cerebrospinal fluid of HIV-I infected patients. Acta Neurol (Napoli) 1990;12:62–65.

Grant I, Atkinson J, Hesseling, J, et al. Evidence for early central nervous system involvement in the acquired immunodeficiency syndrome (AIDS) and other human immunodeficiency virus (HIV) infections. Ann Intern Med 1987;107:828–836.

Holmes VF, Fernandez F, Leve JK. Psychostimulant response in AIDS related complex patients. J Clin Psychiatry 1989;50:5–8.

Iosub S, Fuchs M, Bingol N, Gromisch DS. Fetal alcohol syndrome revisited. Pediatrics 1981;68:475–479.

Johnson RT, McArthur JC, Narayan O. The neurobiology of human immunodeficiency virus infections. Fed Am Soc Exp Biol J 1988;2:2970–2981.

Kelly DA, Hallet RJ, Saed A, et al. Prolonged survival and late presentation of vertically transmitted HIV infection in childhood. Lancet 1987;1:806–807.

Kozlowski PB, Sher JH, Dickson DW, et al. Central nervous system in pediatric HIV infection. A multicenter study. In: Kozlowski PB, Snider DA, Vietz PM, Wisniewski HM, eds. Brain in Pediatric AIDS. Basel: Karger, 1990;132–146.

Krasinski K, Borkowsky W, Holzman R. Prognosis of human immunodeficiency virus in children & adolescents. Pediatr Infect Dis 1989;8:216–220.

Kure K, Park YD, Kim TS, et al. Immunohistochemical localization of an HIV epitope in cerebral aneurysmal arteriopathy in pediatric AIDS. Pediatr Pathol 1989;9:655–662.

Lifschitz M, Hanson C, Wilson G, Shearer WT. Behavioral changes in children with human immunodeficiency virus (HIV) infection. T.B.P.175. V International Conference on AIDS, Montreal, June 4–9, 1989.

Loveland KA, Stehbens JA. Early neurodevelopment signs of HIV infection in children and adolescents. In: Koslowski PB, Snider DA, Victze PM, eds. Brain in pediatric AIDS. Wisniewski: Karger, 1990:72–79.

Macgregor SN, Keith LG, Chasnoff IJ, et al., Rosner MA, Chisum GM, Shaw P. Adverse perinatal outcome. Am J Obstet Gynecol 1987;157:686–690.

McArthur JC. Neurologic manifestations of AIDS. Medicine 1987;66:407–437.

Moss H, Wolters P, Eddy J, Wiener L, Pizzo P, Brouwers P. The effects of encephalopathy and AZT treatment on the social and emotional behavior of pediatric AIDS patients. V International Conference on AIDS, Montreal, June 4–9, 1989.

Naeye RL, Blanc W, Leblanc W, Khatamee MA. Fetal complications of maternal heroin addiction: abnormal growth, infections and episodes of stress. J Pediatr 1973;83:1055–1061.

Navia BA, Jordan BD, Price RW. The AIDS dementia complex. I. Clinical features. Ann Neurol 1986;19:517–524.

Nellhaus G. Composite international and interracial graphs. Pediatrics 1964;41:106.

Novick BE. The spectrum of HIV infection in children. In: Transplacental disorders: perinatal detection, treatment and management (including pediatric AIDS). New York: Alan R. Liss, 1990:191–206.

Nozyce M, Diamond G, Belman A, et al. The course of neurodevelopmental functioning in the infants of IVDA and HIV-seropositive parents. M.B.O.41. V International Conference on AIDS, Montreal, June 4–9, 1989.

Oleske J, Minnefor A, Cooper R, et al. Immune deficiency syndrome in children. JAMA 1983;249:2345.

Oxtoby MJ. Perinatally acquired HIV-I infection. In: Pizzo PA, Wilfert CM, eds. Pediatric AIDS. The challenge of HIV infection in infants, children, and adolescents. Baltimore: Williams & Wilkins, 1990:3–21.

Park YD, Belman AL, Kim T-S, et al. Stroke in pediatric acquired immunodeficiency syndrome. Ann Neurol 1990;28:303–311.

Petito CK, Navia BA, Cho E-S, et al. Vacuolar myelopathy pathologically resembling subacute combined degeneration in patients with the acquired immunodeficiency syndrome. N Engl J Med 1985;312:874–879.

Pizzo PA, Eddy J, Balis FM, et al. Effective of continuous intravenous infusion of Zidovudine (AZT) in children with symptomatic HIV infection. N Engl J Med 1988;319:889–896.

Poplack DG, Brouwers P. Adverse sequelae of central nervous system therapy. Clin Oncol 1985;4:263–285.

Price RW, Brew B, Sidtis J, Rosenblum M, Scheck AC, Clearly P. The brain in AIDS: central nervous system HIV-I infection and AIDS dementia complex. Science 1988;239:586–592.

Rubinstein A. Pediatric AIDS. Curr Probl Pediatr 1986;16:399.

Rubinstein A, Morecki R, Silverman B, et al. Pulmonary disease in children with acquired immune deficiency syndrome and AIDS-related complex. J Pediatr 1986;108:298–503.

Rubinstein A, Sicklick M, Gupta A, et al. Acquired immunodeficiency with reversed T4/T8 ratios in infants born to promiscuous and drug-addicted mothers. JAMA 1983;249:2;350–2356.

Scott G. Survival in children with perinatally acquired human immunodeficiency virus type infection. N Engl J Med 1989;3211:1791–1796.

Scott GB, Buck BE, Leterman JG, et al. Acquired immunodeficiency syndrome in infants. N Engl J Med 1984;310:76–81.

Sharer LR, Epstein LG, Cho ES, et al. Pathologic features of AIDS encephalopathy in children. Hum Pathol 1986;17:271–284.

Spreen O, Tupper D, Risser A, Tuokko H, Edgell D. Prematurity and low birth weight. In: Spreen O, et al., eds. Human developmental neuropsychology. New York: Oxford University Press, 1984.

Terplan JL. Patterns of brain damage in infants and children with congenital heart disease: association with catherization and surgical procedures. Am J Dis Child 1973;125:175–185.

Ultmann MH, Belman AL, Ruff HA, Novick BE, Cone-Wesson B, Cohen HJ, Rubinstein A. Developmental abnormalities in infants and children with acquired immune deficiency syndrome (AIDS) and AIDS-related complex. Devel Med Child Neurol 1985;27:563–571.

Ultmann MH, Diamond G, Ruff, HA, Belman AL, et al. Developmental abnormalities in infants and children with acquired immune deficiency syndrome (AIDS): a follow-up study. Int J Neurosci 1987;32:661–667.

Weidenheim KM, Kure K, Belman AL, Dickson DW. Pathogenesis of corticospinal tract degeneration in pediatric AIDS encephalopathy? In: Kozlowski PB, Snider DA, Vietze PM, Wisniewsi HM, eds. Brain behavior and pediatric AIDS. Karger: Basel, 1990;170–182.

Wiley CA, Belman AL, Dickson D, Rubinstein A, Nelson JA. Human immunodeficiency virus within the brains of children with AIDS. Clin Neuropathol 1990;1:1–6.

Wolters PL, Moss H, Brouwers P, Edd J, Pizzo P. The adaptive behavior of children with symptomatic HIV infection and effects of AZT therapy. M.B.O.43. V International Conference on AIDS, Montreal, June 4–9, 1989.

INDEX

Page numbers in *italics* denote figures; those followed by "t" denote tables.